Therapeutic Strategies

EPILEPSY

Therapeutic Strategies

EPILEPSY

Edited by

Jacqueline A. French
Norman Delanty

CLINICAL PUBLISHING

OXFORD

Clinical Publishing
an imprint of Atlas Medical Publishing Ltd

Oxford Centre for Innovation
Mill Street, Oxford OX2 0JX, UK
Tel: +44 1865 811116
Fax: +44 1865 251550
Email: info@clinicalpublishing.co.uk
Web: www.clinicalpublishing.co.uk

Distributed in USA and Canada by:
Clinical Publishing
30 Amberwood Parkway
Ashland OH 44805, USA

Tel: 800-247-6553 (toll free within U.S. and Canada)
Fax: 419-281-6883
Email: order@bookmasters.com

Distributed in UK and Rest of World by:
Marston Book Services Ltd
PO Box 269
Abingdon
Oxon OX14 4YN, UK

Tel: +44 1235 465500
Fax: +44 1235 465555
Email: trade.orders@marston.co.uk

A catalogue record for this book is available from the British Library

ISBN-13   978 1 904392 80 4
ISBN e-book   978 1 84692 594 8

The publisher makes no representation, express or implied, that the dosages in this
book are correct. Readers must therefore always check the product information and
clinical procedures with the most up-to-date published product information and
data sheets provided by the manufacturers and the most recent codes of conduct
and safety regulations. The authors and the publisher do not accept any liability for
any errors in the text or for the misuse or misapplication of material in this work

Typeset by Prepress Projects Ltd, Perth, UK
Printed by TG Hostench SA, Barcelona, Spain

Cover image of subdural grid kindly donated by Dr Dileep Nair, Epilepsy Center,
Neurological Institute, The Cleveland Clinic, Cleveland, Ohio, USA

Contents

Editors   vii

Contributors   vii

Section I: Overview

1   Overview of therapeutics in epilepsy: anti-epileptic drugs   3
    J. A. French

2   Overview of therapeutics in epilepsy: epilepsy surgery   27
    D. M. Gazzola, C. Carlson, P. Ryvlin, V. M. Thadani,
    J. Taylor, S. Rheims

3   Neurostimulation for the treatment of epilepsy – vagus
    nerve stimulation   51
    E. Ben-Menachem

Section II: Childhood epilepsy

4   Treatment of severe epilepsies with onset under 2 years of age   63
    C. M. Eltze, J. H. Cross

5   Treatment of the child or adolescent with newly diagnosed epilepsy   85
    R. A. Shellhaas, D. J. Dlugos

6   Treatment of the child or adolescent with treatment-resistant epilepsy   103
    B. F. D. Bourgeois

Section III: Epilepsy in adulthood

7   Treatment of adults with newly diagnosed epilepsy   119
    J. P. Leach, R. Mohanraj

8   Treatment of adults with treatment-resistant epilepsy   135
    P. Kwan, H. Leung

9   Treatment of women with childbearing potential and beyond   153
      C. L. Harden

10   Treatment of the elderly with epilepsy   173
      J. I. Sirven

Section IV: Idiopathic epilepsy

11   The treatment of idiopathic generalized epilepsy   191
      M. Carreño

Section V: Complicating conditions

12   Treatment of the hospitalized patient with new-onset seizures   213
      K. J. Abou Khaled, L. J. Hirsch

13   Treatment of the epilepsy patient with concomitant medical conditions   229
      S. M. Murphy, N. Delanty

14   A rational approach to the treatment of status epilepticus   251
      P. Kinirons, C. P. Doherty

15   Treatment of common co-morbid psychiatric disorders in epilepsy:
      a review of practical strategies   281
      A. M. Kanner, M. Frey

16   The treatment of epilepsy in individuals with moderate
      to severe intellectual disability   305
      M. Scheepers, M. Kerr

Abbreviations   323
Index   327

Editors

Norman Delanty, FRCPI, ABPNT (Dip), Honorary Senior Lecturer Neurology (RCSI); Consultant Neurologist; Director of Epilepsy Services, Department of Neurology, Beaumont Hospital, Dublin, Ireland

Jacqueline A. French, MD, Professor of Neurology, NYU Comprehensive Epilepsy Center, New York, USA

Contributors

Karine J. Abou Khaled, MD, NYU Comprehensive Epilepsy Center, New York, USA. Currently at Hôtel-Dieu de France Hospital, Department of Neurology, Saint Joseph University, Beirut, Lebanon

Elinor Ben-Menachem, MD, PhD, Professor of Neurosciences, Institute of Clinical Neurosciences, Sahlgrenska Academy at Göteborg University, Göteborg, Sweden

Blaise F. D. Bourgeois, MD, Professor in Neurology, Harvard Medical School; Director, Division of Epilepsy and Clinical Neurophysiology, Children's Hospital Boston, Boston, Massachusetts, USA

Chad Carlson, MD, Assistant Professor, NYU Comprehensive Epilepsy Center, New York, USA

Mar Carreño, MD, PhD, Director, Epilepsy Unit, Hospital Clínic de Barcelona, Barcelona, Spain

J. Helen Cross, MB, ChB, PhD, FRCP, FRCPCH, University College London Institute of Child Health and Great Ormond Street Hospital for Children NHS Trust, London, UK

Dennis J. Dlugos, MD, MSCE, Associate Professor, Division of Neurology, The Children's Hospital of Philadelphia, University of Pennsylvania School of Medicine, Philadelphia, Pennsylvania, USA

Colin P. Doherty, MD, MRCPI, Consultant Neurologist, Department of Neurology, St James's Hospital, Dublin; Honorary Senior Lecturer, Royal College of Surgeons in Ireland

Christin M. Eltze, MSc, MD, MRCPH, University College London Institute of Child Health and Great Ormond Street Hospital for Children NHS Trust, London, UK

MARLIS FREY, MSN, Rush Epilepsy Center, Rush University Medical Center, Chicago, Illinois, USA

DEANA M. GAZZOLA, MD, Assistant Professor, NYU Comprehensive Epilepsy Center, Department of Neurology, NYU School of Medicine, New York, USA

CYNTHIA L. HARDEN, MD, Professor of Neurology, Epilepsy Division Chief, Department of Neurology, University of Miami, Miami, USA

LAWRENCE J. HIRSCH, MD, Associate Clinical Professor of Neurology, NYU Comprehensive Epilepsy Center; Department of Neurology, Columbia University, New York, USA

ANDRES M. KANNER, MD, Professor of Neurology, Department of Neurological Sciences, Rush Medical College and Rush Epilepsy Center, Rush University Medical Center, Chicago, Illinois, USA

MIKE KERR, MBChB, MRCPsych, MRCGP, MSc, MPhil, Professor of Learning Disability Psychiatry, Welsh Centre for Learning Disabilities, Cardiff, UK

PETER KINIRONS, MRCPI, PhD, Epilepsy and Neurophysiology Fellow, Massachusetts General Hospital, Boston, Massachusetts, USA

PATRICK KWAN, MD, PhD, Division of Neurology, Department of Medicine and Therapeutics, The Chinese University of Hong Kong, Prince of Wales Hospital, Hong Kong, People's Republic of China

JOHN PAUL LEACH, MD, FRCP, Consultant Neurologist and Neurophysiologist, Department of Neurology, Southern General Hospital; Epilepsy Unit, Western Infirmary, Glasgow, UK

HOWAN LEUNG, MD, Division of Neurology, Department of Medicine and Therapeutics, The Chinese University of Hong Kong, Prince of Wales Hospital, Hong Kong, People's Republic of China

RAJIV MOHANRAJ, PhD, MRCP, Consultant Neurologist, Hope Hospital, Manchester, UK

SINEAD M. MURPHY, MB, BCh, MRCPI, Specialist Registrar in Neurology, Department of Neurology, Beaumont Hospital, Dublin, Ireland

SYLVAIN RHEIMS, MD, Institut Des Epilepsies de l'Enfant et de l'adolescent, Hospices Civils de Lyon, Université Claude Bernard Lyon 1, Lyon, France

PHILIPPE RYVLIN, MD, PhD, Institut Des Epilepsies de l'Enfant et de l'adolescent, Hospices Civils de Lyon, Université Claude Bernard Lyon 1, Lyon, France

MARK SCHEEPERS, MBChB, MRCPsych, Consultant Psychiatrist, 2gether NHS Foundation Trust, Gloucestershire, UK

RENÉE A. SHELLHAAS, MD, Division of Pediatric Neurology, C. S. Mott Children's Hospital, University of Michigan, Ann Arbor, Michigan, USA

JOSEPH I. SIRVEN, MD, Professor, Department of Neurology, Mayo Clinic College of Medicine, Scottsdale, Arizona, USA

JOHN TAYLOR, DO, Section of Neurology, Dartmouth Hitchcock Medical Center/Dartmouth Medical School, Lebanon, New Hampshire, USA

VIJAY M. THADANI, MD, Section of Neurology, Dartmouth Hitchcock Medical Center/Dartmouth Medical School, Lebanon, New Hampshire, USA

Section I

Overview

1

Overview of therapeutics in epilepsy: anti-epileptic drugs

Jacqueline A. French

INTRODUCTION

Treating epilepsy has become a daunting task over the last 15 years, as the number of available anti-epileptic drugs (AEDs) has skyrocketed. With so many options, it is difficult for all but the specialist to know how to select and manage therapy for the many types and stages of epilepsy. Turning to guidelines may not provide substantial assistance. Most guidelines rely on randomized controlled trials to provide evidence of benefit. Unfortunately, there are many gaps in the evidence base, which leads to similar gaps in the guidelines. For example, recent guidelines written by the International League Against Epilepsy could only advise the use of phenytoin, carbamazepine and valproate as initial treatment for adults with partial seizures. Clearly, there are circumstances under which none of these would be an optimal choice.

This chapter will provide a pragmatic framework for AED therapy in adults with epilepsy. Paediatric epilepsy will be covered in Chapters 4–6. The chapter will begin with an overview of each commonly used AED, after which treatment strategies will be addressed.

AED CHARACTERISTICS

PHENYTOIN

Phenytoin has been used for over 50 years. Thus, the characteristics and side-effects have been well elucidated. Its primary use is for treatment of partial epilepsy, including simple and complex partial seizures, as well as generalized tonic–clonic seizures, whether of primary or partial onset [1]. Phenytoin can be initiated with a 'loading dose' of 13–20 mg/kg, or with a starting dose of 3–5 mg/kg/day. Phenytoin was one of the first AEDs that became associated with a 'therapeutic range' (10–20 mg/l in most laboratories), which represents serum concentrations most likely to produce a therapeutic effect without substantial dose-related side-effects. The phenytoin dose [2] should be selected using therapeutic monitoring rather than a predetermined dose, such as 300 mg/day. As the serum level increases, side-effects such as lethargy, ataxia, dysarthria, fatigue, diplopia, abnormal movements, mental confusion and cognitive changes may occur. This is particularly true at concentrations above 20 mg/l. However, the therapeutic range represents an average. A number of patients

Jacqueline A. French, MD, Professor of Neurology, NYU Comprehensive Epilepsy Center, New York, USA

may remain seizure-free at serum concentrations below the range, or may tolerate levels substantially above the range. However, it is very important to understand the properties of phenytoin metabolism. As serum concentrations rise, particularly to levels above 15 mg/l, the metabolism of phenytoin slows substantially (Figure 1.1). This is called 'zero order kinetics'. At levels below 15 mg/l, doubling the dose will lead to a doubling of serum concentration, and the half-life is 24 h. As metabolism slows at higher concentrations, even a 50-mg change in dose can double the serum concentration, and the half-life increases to 48–70 h. Since the half-life is so prolonged, a steady state after dose adjustments may not occur for weeks, with serum levels slowly rising over this time. This can easily lead to serious phenytoin toxicity. Hospitalization due to phenytoin toxicity under these circumstances is not uncommon [2]. *Dosage adjustments must be made with great care*, and levels should be repeated a month after any adjustment. In addition to dose-related toxicities, patients receiving phenytoin may experience side-effects that are relatively independent of dose. These include gingival hyperplasia, acne and hirsutism. Visits to the dentist every 6–12 months, accompanied by daily flossing, can help prevent gingival hypertrophy. There is now fairly substantial evidence that long-term phenytoin use can lead to reduced bone density and risk of fracture [3]. Obviously, this is a major issue for patients who fall with their seizures. All patients receiving phenytoin should receive supplemental calcium and vitamin D, and should be screened with bone densitometry. Allergic rash may occur. Although idiosyncratic side-effects are not common, they can occur, and patients should be advised of this possibility. These include Stevens–Johnson syndrome, aplastic anaemia, hepatic failure and a lupus-like syndrome. Monitoring of blood counts, liver function tests and electrolytes are warranted for the first 6–12 months of therapy. Drug interactions are relatively common, both with other epilepsy drugs and with drugs taken for other conditions. Interactions with other AEDs are listed in Tables 1.1 and 1.2. Phenytoin is less expensive than many alternatives, which is important for patients who are paying for their own medications. Because of phenytoin's relatively long half-life, it can be administered only once or twice a day.

CARBAMAZEPINE

Carbamazepine has long been considered a first-line agent for simple partial, complex partial and generalized tonic–clonic seizures [1]. Recently, many studies have compared the newer AEDs to carbamazepine as the 'gold standard' in patients with newly diagnosed epilepsy,

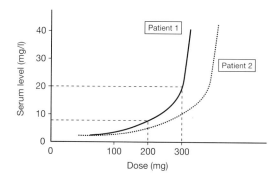

Figure 1.1 Graph showing relationship between phenytoin dose and serum concentration in two patients with slightly different metabolisms. In patient 1, dotted lines indicate that the serum level would be 8 mg/l if the patient was taking 200 mg/day, and 20 mg/l if the patient was taking 300 mg/day. At 350 mg/day, the serum concentration would be extremely high. This is because the patient has gone into 'zero order kinetics'.

Table 1.1 Pharmacokinetic impact of old anti-epileptic drugs (AEDs) on new AEDs. ↓, levels decrease (faster clearance); ↑, levels increase (slower clearance) [117]

	Gabapentin/pregabalin	Lamotrigine	Topiramate	Tiagabine	Levetiracetam	Zonisamide	Oxcarbazepine (MHD)
Phenytoin/carbamazepine/phenobarbital/primidone	None	↓	↓	↓	None	↓	↓
Valproate	None	↑	None	None	None	None	Slight ↓

MHD, monohydroxy- derivative.

Table 1.2 Pharmacokinetic impact of new anti-epileptic drugs (AEDs) on old AEDs. ↓, levels decrease (faster clearance); ↑, levels increase (slower clearance) [117]

	Phenytoin	Carbamazepine	Valproate	Phenobarbital	Primidone
Gabapentin/tiagabine/zonisamide/levetiracetam/pregabalin	None	None	None	None	None
Lamotrigine	None	None	↓ 25%	None	None
Topiramate	May ↑	None	None	None	None
Oxcarbazepine	May ↑	None	None	Slight ↑	None

and to date, none has been found to be more effective. However, lamotrigine, topiramate and oxcarbazepine all caused fewer dropouts due to side-effects than carbamazepine [4–9]. Of note, it is considered 'narrow spectrum', and may actually worsen generalized epilepsies, particularly those associated with absence or myoclonus [8]. Initiation must be done with titration, to avoid appearance of dose-related side-effects. Dose selection should be done using clinical response and serum levels. Typically, a level of 8–12 mg/l will provide the best response, and few patients will tolerate serum concentrations above 15 mg/l. Dose-related adverse effects include ataxia, drowsiness, vertigo, difficulty concentrating, diplopia and blurred vision. Using sustained-release formulations of carbamazepine will reduce some of these side-effects by reducing peak serum concentrations. The other advantage is the ability to use twice-a-day dosing, rather than the three- to four-times-a-day dosing that would otherwise be necessary due to the short half-life of carbamazepine. Gastrointestinal (GI) symptoms such as nausea, vomiting, diarrhoea and constipation may also be seen. The other side-effects of carbamazepine are not necessarily linked to dose. These include more common, but less serious, effects such as leucopenia, hyponatraemia and rash as well as life-threatening but extremely rare idiosyncratic reactions such as Stevens–Johnson syndrome, aplastic anaemia and hepatic failure. Mild leucopenia can be disregarded. Rarely, more profound leucopenia (with leucocyte counts $<2.5\times10^9$) may necessitate discontinuation of therapy [10]. Hyponatraemia does not necessitate discontinuation in all patients, as it can often be managed with water restriction. However, in some patients water restriction does not work, or too severely impacts lifestyle, and in these patients an alternative AED should be sought [11]. Because of the potential for all of the above issues, monitoring of liver function tests, white blood counts and electrolytes are necessary during the first 6–12 months of therapy, and yearly thereafter. The potential for carbamazepine to produce decreased bone density is under study. Of note, chronic carbamazepine use has been associated with some reduction in serum testosterone levels and increases in cholesterol levels [12, 13]. The clinical implications of these changes are under study. As with phenytoin, carbamazepine is associated with many drug interactions affecting AEDs and other drugs (see Tables 1.1 and 1.2). Because many drugs can inhibit or induce the metabolism of carbamazepine, and cause acute toxicity or reduced effect, it is a good idea to tell patients to inform their neurologist when starting any prescription drug. Carbamazepine, even in the extended-release formulations, is substantially less expensive than the newer anti-epileptic drugs.

PHENOBARBITAL

Phenobarbital is the 'grandfather of anti-epileptic drugs'. It has been available for over 100 years. It is effective for most seizure types and the fact that an intravenous (i.v.) formulation is available means it is often used for treatment of status epilepticus. In the modern era, it is rarely used as first-line therapy, as studies have demonstrated that it causes more dose-related side-effects, particularly sedation, than other options [14]. Also, once started it is very difficult to withdraw without causing seizure exacerbation. Abrupt withdrawal is not recommended, and even slow withdrawal can lead to problems. The initial dose is 30–50 mg, which is best administered at bedtime. Titration to optimal dose can be achieved over several weeks. Optimal effect is usually achieved at serum concentrations of 15–45 mg/l. Other dose-related side-effects include irritability, difficulty concentrating, memory loss, sedation, dysarthria and ataxia. Other reported adverse reactions include hyperactivity, mostly in children, and depression. As with phenytoin and carbamazepine, hypersensitivity syndrome, rash, hepatic failure and aplastic anaemia may occur. Since many patients who are currently on phenobarbital have been on it long term, an understanding of long-term side-effects is important. Some unique side-effects occur with long-term phenobarbital use, affecting the skin and connective tissue. These may include contractures, frozen shoulder and general pain [15]. Drug interactions may occur with phenobarbital (see Tables 1.1 and 1.2). It is the least expensive anti-epileptic drug, costing pennies a day, and its long half-life permits once-a-day dosing, which is important for potentially non-compliant patients.

PRIMIDONE

Primidone is no longer considered a first-line drug, and its use has diminished substantially. It is metabolized to a number of active metabolites, including phenobarbital and phenylethylmalonamide (PEMA), although the parent compound is also active. When obtaining serum levels, therapeutic effect will be associated with both the parent primidone levels and phenobarbital levels. In the presence of enzyme-inducing drugs, primidone levels will go down, and phenobarbital levels will rise. Primidone causes all the problems seen with phenobarbital use, described above.

VALPROATE

Valproate has been available since the 1970s, but remains the first-line drug for many epilepsy syndromes, including juvenile myoclonic epilepsy and syndromes associated with absence seizures. Valproate may be the only effective agent for some patients. A recent large randomized open-label trial demonstrated superior efficacy compared with lamotrigine, and superior tolerability compared with topiramate, in adults and children with idiopathic generalized or unclassified epilepsy [16]. Seizure control was maintained in the majority for 5 years.

In some countries, valproate is also used as first-line therapy for partial seizures. In a head-to-head study, valproate was as effective for generalized tonic–clonic convulsions as carbamazepine in patients with partial epilepsy, but was found to be less effective for complex partial seizures [17]. However, in other studies, the efficacy was equivalent in all seizure types, when valproate was compared with phenytoin, carbamazepine or oxcarbazepine [18–22]. Valproate is available in a variety of formulations, including sustained release, sprinkles and i.v.. With the availability of i.v., valproate has become more popular for treatment of status epilepticus [23]. Typical initiation in outpatients is at a dose of 10–15 mg/kg/day, with subsequent increases of 5–10 mg/kg/week as needed to control seizures [24]. Serum levels between 50 and 100 mg/l are typically therapeutic and well tolerated, but higher concentrations may be necessary in some patients.

Skin rashes are less common with valproate than with carbamazepine, phenytoin and lamotrigine, and therefore valproate is a reasonable choice for patients with a history of hypersensitivity [25]. The main side-effects are GI upset, nausea, vomiting, tremor, weight gain and hair loss [26]. Tremor and weight gain are dose related. GI upset can sometimes be avoided by using alternative formulations, such as sustained release or sprinkles. Elevated ammonia levels can be seen commonly, affecting 20–50% of patients [26]. In some patients this is well tolerated and not problematic, while in others elevated ammonia can be associated with encephalopathy, triphasic waves and even coma [27]. It is not recommended to monitor ammonia in asymptomatic patients. However, if patients demonstrate encephalopathy, particularly in the presence of asteryxis and/or delta slowing on the electroencephalogram (EEG), it is reasonable to check for hyperammonaemia. Carnitine supplementation has been recommended to improve valproate-induced hyperammonaemia [28, 29]. Idiosyncratic side-effects include rare fatal hepatotoxicity. The incidence is 1 in 20 000 in adults on monotherapy, but much more common in polytherapy, in children under 10 years old, and even more so in children under 2 years old [14]. Children who have seizures resulting from metabolic disorders may be at extremely high risk, and as a rule should not be treated with valproate. When children on polytherapy under the age of 2 are treated, the reported incidence is as high as 1 in 600–800 [26]. The greatest risk is in the first 6 months of use, and clinical as well as blood monitoring is indicated during this time. Pancreatitis may also occur, which may have a frequency of up to 1 in 3000. The risk of pancreatitis does not diminish over time. Aplastic anaemia is rare, but thrombocytopenia and altered bleeding time are common [30]. These are usually not clinically worrisome, and low platelet counts can usually be tolerated as they do not portend more significant blood dyscrasias. Some case reports note increased risk of bleeding during surgery in patients on valproate, whereas many others note no increase in bleeding [31]. Recently, a number of studies have reported adverse fetal outcomes in offspring of women receiving valproate [32–39]. Spina bifida is seen in up to 2% of children exposed to valproate before birth [26]. This makes valproate a poor choice for women contemplating pregnancy. In some studies, valproate has also been associated with development of polycystic ovarian syndrome. This appears to be more prevalent when valproate is initiated in women under 40 [40]. Reports of menstrual cycle irregularities are common.

One property of valproate that must be kept in mind is that it is a hepatic metabolic inhibitor. This has a number of consequences, including a number of interactions with other AEDs as well as drugs of different classes. In addition, intrinsic substances such as oestrogen may be inhibited. Valproate is highly protein bound. It may displace phenytoin from binding sites, causing emergence of phenytoin toxicity in the absence of an increased plasma level.

ETHOSUXIMIDE

Ethosuximide has a very narrow therapeutic indication, with use limited to patients with absence seizures [41]. In most cases, it should be used as the sole agent only in patients who experience this seizure type in isolation, a condition seen primarily in childhood [42]. Occasionally, in patients with primary generalized epilepsy with seizure types other than absence, addition of ethosuximide as an adjunctive medication may improve seizure control. Ethosuximide can be started at 500 mg/day, and titrated as tolerated, with weekly increments. Serum concentrations of 40–100 mg/l are usually optimal. The most common side-effects noted with ethosuximide use include nausea and abdominal discomfort, drowsiness, anorexia and headache [41]. In rare cases, behavioural changes may be seen, including psychosis. Blood dyscrasias have been reported. Drug–drug interactions are minimal.

BENZODIAZEPINES

Available benzodiazepines for chronic use include clonazepam, clorazepate and clobezam. Most benzodiazepines are not good choices for long-term therapy and should not be used as first-line agents. Patients may develop tolerance to the therapeutic effects of many of the benzodiazepines. Seizures may initially be decreased, but as tolerance develops over time, seizures may recur, necessitating dosage increases to regain control. Among the available benzodiazepines, clobezam has been touted as having less propensity for tolerance development. The most common dose-related side-effects of this drug class include drowsiness, ataxia and behavioural problems. Clonazepam is particularly useful for myoclonus. Clorazepate and clobezam may be used for both generalized and partial epilepsies. They tend to be used in patients with drug-resistant epilepsy. Starting dose for clonazepam is 0.5–1 mg twice daily, increasing as needed. Chlorazepate can be initiated at 7.5 mg twice daily or thrice daily. Clobezam can be started at 5 mg twice daily and increased by 5–10 mg every 1–2 weeks to achieve the best seizure control without development of excessive sleepiness. Abrupt withdrawal from chronic benzodiazepines may precipitate status epilepticus. Even slow withdrawal may exacerbate seizures. Acute benzodiazepines such as diazepam, lorazepam and midazolam may be used as intermittent 'rescue therapy' in patients who experience seizure clusters or status epilepticus.

SECOND-GENERATION AEDs

Drugs are listed in order of approval in the USA, from oldest to newest.

FELBAMATE

Felbamate is a broad-spectrum anti-epileptic drug. It is not considered to be a first-line drug because of its potential for serious idiosyncratic side-effects, including potentially fatal aplastic anaemia (incidence of 1 in 3000) and hepatic failure (incidence of 1 in 10 000) [43]. Recent analyses indicate that aplastic anaemia and liver failure occur almost exclusively within the first year of therapy. During this period, safety monitoring consisting of liver function tests and blood counts is recommended with a frequency of up to twice monthly, despite lack of evidence that early detection of changes will prevent serious health problems, even if the drug is discontinued. Yet, felbamate may still be an important drug in the armamentarium for refractory patients, because it may control seizures when other drugs fail, and tends to be alerting rather than sedating. It has been found to be particularly effective in patients with Lennox–Gastaut syndrome [44]. Felbamate should be started at 300–600 mg twice daily, and increased as necessary over several weeks, up to 3600 mg, or higher in some cases. Drug levels may be useful, and serum concentrations of 30–80 mg/l are recommended [45]. Three-times-a-day dosing may improve tolerability. Dose-related side-effects include insomnia, decreased appetite and weight loss, ataxia, GI upset and headache. Other serious idiosyncratic adverse events include rash and Stevens–Johnson syndrome. Felbamate has a complex metabolism and elimination, by both the hepatic and renal routes, and inhibits the metabolism of some drugs while inducing others (see Tables 1.1 and 1.2). Adjustments in these medications may be necessary.

LAMOTRIGINE

Lamotrigine is a broad-spectrum anti-epileptic drug that has been widely accepted as a first-line drug for both partial and generalized epilepsy syndromes. Clinical trials have supported its use in partial seizures, primary generalized tonic–clonic seizures, absence seizures and seizures associated with Lennox–Gastaut syndrome [46, 47]. There is some controversy regarding the use of lamotrigine in juvenile myoclonic epilepsy. It is commonly used, but may worsen myoclonus in some patients. Lamotrigine has been the subject of a number of head-to-head studies in newly diagnosed partial and generalized epilepsy. Lamotrigine was equally effective but better tolerated than phenytoin and carbamazepine in several somewhat under-powered studies [4, 48]. Several studies indicated that lamotrigine is better tolerated than carbamazepine in the elderly [49, 50]. A recent very large, randomized open-label study indicated that lamotrigine might be the drug of choice in patients with partial epilepsy, as it was equally effective but better tolerated, but in a companion study it was substantially less effective than valproate in patients with generalized or unclassified epilepsy [16, 51]. Some studies have advocated combining lamotrigine with valproate in refractory patients, to achieve maximum efficacy through a favourable pharmacodynamic interaction [52]. However, side-effects are also enhanced when the drugs are combined. Initiation of lamotrigine is somewhat more complex than for other drugs. Slow titration is mandatory to reduce occurrence of serious rash. In monotherapy, initiation with 25 mg/day for 2 weeks, then 50 mg/day for another 2 weeks, followed by increases of 25–50 mg/week is appropriate. If the patient is receiving valproate at the time of initiation, starting doses and doses during titration should be cut in half, whereas if they are receiving enzyme-inducing AEDs such as phenytoin, carbamazepine or phenobarbital, doses can be doubled [53]. Doses can then be increased as necessary. Typical doses for patients with newly diagnosed epilepsy are 100–200 mg/day. In refractory patients, doses may be as high as 500–1000 mg/day. There is a great deal of variability in serum concentrations that produce optimal effects. Some patients may do well at serum concentrations of 2 mg/l, while others may need levels of up to 20 mg/l. Common dose-related side-effects of lamotrigine include mild tremor, double vision, headache and insomnia. Rash, including Stevens–Johnson syndrome and toxic epidermal necrolysis, can occur. Risk is increased for children under 16, and is also more common with concomitant valproate use, and in patients who have experienced rash on other AEDs [54]. Rash almost always occurs within the first 8 weeks of therapy. Other hypersensitivity reactions, although much rarer, may be seen, including lymphadenopathy, fever, hepatic or renal failure, disseminated intravascular coagulation and arthritis [55]. Discontinuation of lamotrigine is recommended in the presence of rash or other indication of hypersensitivity, and it is very important to tell patients to call immediately with such symptoms. Rapid discontinuation can prevent a more severe, potentially life-threatening reaction. In the absence of any clinical symptoms of hypersensitivity, it is unclear that routine monitoring of liver function tests, blood counts or electrolytes is useful. Lamotrigine does not alter the metabolism of other drugs that are given concomitantly. However, other drugs may impact on the metabolism of lamotrigine (see Tables 1.1 and 1.2). One important and common drug interaction that bears noting is that with oral contraceptives, which double the clearance and halve the half-life of lamotrigine [56]. Women on lamotrigine should be told to notify their doctor of any changes in oral contraceptive pill use, something they might not otherwise think to do.

GABAPENTIN

Gabapentin is a narrow-spectrum drug. It is useful only in patients with partial epilepsy, that is those with simple or complex partial seizures, or partial-onset generalized tonic–clonic convulsions. Gabapentin is felt to be more useful in newly diagnosed patients with mild epilepsy and in the elderly, who benefit from the relatively mild side-effect profile and lack of drug interactions, but less useful in patients with refractory epilepsy. Although gabapentin can be initiated at a therapeutic dose of 1200–2400 mg/day, it appears to be better tolerated when titrated [57]. Typically, 300 mg two times a day is well tolerated as a starting dose, but lower starting doses are needed in some patients. Clinical trials have only tested efficacy to 2400 mg/day [46]. However, in clinical experience, higher doses can be useful. However, gabapentin displays dose-dependent, saturable absorption. At higher doses, less may be absorbed across the gut, leading to diminishing returns [58]. The amount of absorption varies from person to person. Determining if serum levels are rising after dose increments can help ascertain whether increasing doses are futile. Gabapentin is not bound to plasma proteins, is eliminated renally and does not interfere with the metabolism of other medications, including AEDs or psychotropic agents [56, 59]. This makes it an ideal drug for the elderly and patients with chronic illness, who are likely to be taking other drugs. Common dose-related side-effects include somnolence, dizziness, ataxia and fatigue. Weight gain is also seen, and appears to be dose related. Peripheral oedema may occur in some patients. Occurrence of myoclonus has been reported, as well as occasional behavioural disturbance in children [60, 61]. There are no reports of serious idiosyncratic side-effects. Therefore, routine monitoring of liver function tests, blood counts and electrolytes is probably not warranted.

TOPIRAMATE

Topiramate is another AED that is felt to be broad spectrum. It has been studied and found effective in patients with partial-onset or primary generalized tonic–clonic seizures, and in patients with seizures associated with Lennox–Gastaut syndrome [46]. Topiramate is felt to be first-line therapy in all these conditions. One head-to-head study in newly diagnosed patients found topiramate to be equal in efficacy with valproate in patients with mostly generalized seizures, and with carbamazepine in patients with mostly partial seizures, although the study was under-powered and has been criticized methodologically [7]. A recent open-label randomized study in newly diagnosed adults and children indicated that topiramate was as efficacious as any other drug for partial and generalized seizures, but was less well tolerated [16, 51]. However, the open-label nature of the study could have produced some bias. Topiramate should be started at a low dose and slowly titrated for best tolerabiiity, although there are no safety concerns related to starting more rapidly. It is best tolerated when initiated at 25 mg/day and increased by 25 mg/week. Typical doses necessary for newly diagnosed patients are in the range of 100–200 mg, while, as is the case for most drugs, refractory patients may require much higher doses. Up to 1000 mg has been tested in clinical trials, although few can tolerate such high doses. As with lamotrigine, serum levels needed to achieve control are variable, from 2 to 20 mg/l. Monitoring serum levels may be useful. Topiramate is well absorbed and has minimal protein binding [62]. Topiramate is partially metabolized by the liver and approximately 60% is excreted unchanged in the urine. Interactions between topiramate and other AEDs are listed in Tables 1.1 and 1.2. The more common dose-related adverse events include somnolence, paraesthesias (especially of fingertips), fatigue, taste perversion, weight loss and dizziness. One of the side-effects that is relatively specific to topiramate is psychomotor slowing, which particularly affects speech. Patients may complain of word-finding difficulty or slowing of speech. Academic performance can be affected. This side-effect is significant in some patients, while others may escape it entirely, even at high doses. Potential, more serious side-effects that occur infrequently include nephrolithiasis, open-angle glaucoma, causing transient and reversible visual loss, and hypohidrosis in children [63–65]. Rarely, the hypohidrosis has caused heat stroke with serious consequences. Children receiving topiramate have also rarely developed clinically significant metabolic acidosis. Milder forms are common. Topiramate has rarely been associated with hepatic failure, and this seems to happen more commonly when topiramate is combined with valproate [66]. Topiramate does not impact the metabolism of most concomitant drugs, but it does raise phenytoin levels when added to patients with baseline higher phenytoin levels (e.g. above 15 mg/l), which can potentially cause phenytoin toxicity. Therefore, phenytoin levels should be monitored. In addition, the classic hepatic enzyme-inducing AEDs, such as phenytoin and carbamazepine, will increase the metabolism of topiramate, and higher doses may be required [59].

OXCARBAZEPINE

Oxcarbazepine, an analogue of carbamazepine, is a narrow-spectrum drug that is considered to be a first-line therapy for the treatment of partial seizures [46, 47]. Although it is similar to carbamazepine, it is effective in some patients for whom carbamazepine has failed and is believed to have additional mechanisms of action. Oxcarbazepine is actually a prodrug for a mono-hydroxylated form, to which it is rapidly converted after oral administration. Several studies have been performed in patients with newly diagnosed epilepsy, comparing oxcarbazepine with older AEDs. In all of these studies, oxcarbazepine was equally efficacious. It was better tolerated than phenytoin and carbamazepine, and as well tolerated as valproate [6, 22, 67, 68]. Oxcarbazepine has been noted to exacerbate myoclonic seizures as well as absence [69].

Oxcarbazepine should be initiated with titration to avoid side-effects. However, in one inpatient study, 2400 mg/day was started, and caused few dropouts, thus rapid initiation in an emergency is possible [70]. In outpatients, initiation of 300 mg twice daily and titration of 600 mg/week is usually well tolerated [71]. Effective doses range from 900 to 2400 mg, but higher doses are not well tolerated in combination with other drugs, particularly those with similar side-effect profiles. If side-effects develop as the dose is being increased, spacing out dosing to three times daily, or even four times daily sometimes permits achievement of higher, more efficacious doses. Plasma concentrations of up to 45 mg/l have been well tolerated. Frequent dose-related adverse events include somnolence, dizziness, headache, ataxia, nausea and vomiting, diplopia, blurred vision, vertigo and tremor [72]. One problematic potential adverse event is hyponatraemia [72]. In a recent study, hyponatraemia was substantially more common for oxcarbazepine (29.9%) than carbamazepine (35.5%), and serum sodium levels of <128 mEq/l occurred in 12.4% [11]. Risk factors for hyponatraemia include older age and diuretic use. Hypersensitivity syndromes, including rash and Stevens–Johnson syndrome are rare consequences of oxcarbazepine use [73]. Oxcarbazepine does not have the strong enzyme-inducing properties of carbamazepine, and also does not induce its own metabolism. Oxcarbazepine also acts as an inhibitor of phenytoin metabolism, and its own metabolism is induced by the classic inducing anti-epileptic drugs such as phenytoin and carbamazepine (see Tables 1.1 and 1.2).

TIAGABINE

Tiagabine is a drug that is considered second-line therapy, and is effective for partial seizures only [46]. Like other drugs that work via γ-aminobutyric acid enhancement, tiagabine may exacerbate absence and myoclonic seizures [74]. Tiagabine was compared with carbamazepine in a study of newly diagnosed patients with partial seizures, and was found to be less efficacious. However, it was fairly effective as add-on therapy in patients with refractory epilepsy [46]. Nonetheless, its use has waned in recent years. Of note, some reports of seizures have surfaced when tiagabine has been used off-label for psychiatric indications [75]. Tiagabine is best tolerated when titrated. Initiation of 4 mg once or twice daily is recommended, with dose increments of 4 mg/week. A three–four-times-a-day regimen is recommended, due to the short half-life. Doses of up to 64 mg have been used in add-on trials. Patients receiving enzyme inducers will need higher doses than patients taking non-inducing AEDs. Serum levels have not been very clinically useful, due to the short half-life, which results in wide fluctuations in levels from peak to trough. Tiagabine is 96% protein bound, but no protein-binding interactions have been identified clinically. Common dose-related side-effects include tiredness, nervousness, dizziness, headache, tremor and abnormal thinking [76]. An unusual side-effect has been identified, consisting of a stuporous state accompanied by a slow wave or spike–wave pattern on EEG [77]. This resolves promptly with discontinuation of the drug. Another atypical side-effect is described as weakness or asthenia [46]. No metabolic, hepatic or blood-related adverse events have been identified. Therefore, monitoring of complete blood counts, electrolytes and liver function tests is not clinically warranted. Tiagabine does not impact on the metabolism of other drugs. Other AEDs can impact on the metabolism of tiagabine [56, 59] (see Tables 1.1 and 1.2).

LEVETIRACETAM

Levetiracetam is a broad-spectrum drug that has undergone extensive testing. Therefore, more syndromes have been explored than for some of the other newer AEDs. It is effective in partial seizures [46]. A study of patients with newly diagnosed partial or generalized tonic–clonic seizures showed no differences in efficacy or tolerability between levetiracetam and carbamazepine [5]. Levetiracetam is the only newer AED approved for use in juvenile myoclonic epilepsy [78]. It was also effective for idiopathic generalized tonic–clonic seizures in an add-on situation. Case series have indicated efficacy in other idiopathic epilepsy syndromes [79, 80].

One reason levetiracetam has become a very popular choice, for both initial and add-on therapy, is that it is easy to use. It can be started at a therapeutic dose, and data indicate that onset of action is within a day [81]. Patients can be started on either 500 mg once daily or 500 mg twice daily. The dose can then be increased gradually as necessary, with maximal dose typically being 3000 mg/day. If necessary, it can be started at a higher dose, although it is not clear if this is clinically necessary. In one study [82], levetiracetam was started at 4000 mg/day, and was well tolerated. Serum levels are typically within the range of 10–40 mg/l, but will vary substantially over the course of a day, because of the short half-life of the drug. Another advantage of levetiracetam is that it is associated with no drug interactions because it is predominantly renally excreted, and shows limited metabolism in humans. As with other renally excreted drugs, lower doses should be used in the elderly, because they have a reduced creatinine clearance [83].

Side-effects of levetiracetam include irritability, somnolence, dizziness, asthenia and headache. Other uncommon adverse events include behavioural problems, depression and psychosis [84]. Levetiracetam does not often cause rash, and is therefore a reasonable choice in patients with a history of hypersensitivity syndrome. To date, there has been no indication that levetiracetam can cause idiosyncratic safety problems such as aplastic anaemia or hepatic failure [83]. Therefore, routine monitoring of liver function tests, blood counts and electrolytes is not clinically warranted.

Levetiracetam was recently approved in an i.v. formulation. It is being used more frequently for inpatients with other medical conditions who require immediate AED therapy, and in status epilepticus, but no formal studies have been done.

ZONISAMIDE

Zonisamide is felt to be broad spectrum [85, 86]. Unfortunately, trials in generalized seizure syndromes have not been performed to confirm this clinical impression. The only randomized controlled trials were performed in adults with partial seizures [46]. Randomized trials in patients with newly diagnosed epilepsy have also not been done. Case series and open studies support a role for zonisamide in the treatment of syndromes associated with myoclonus, including juvenile myoclonic epilepsy and progressive myoclonic epilepsies [87, 86, 88]. Zonisamide is better tolerated when it is titrated at initiation. It can be started at 50 mg/day or 100 mg/day. The dose should then be titrated by 50 mg/week or 100 mg every other week [71]. Doses of 200–300 mg are common, and up to 500 mg can be necessary in difficult-to-treat patients. Serum concentrations of 20–40 mg/l are considered therapeutic. Since the half-life is long (up to 60 h), serum concentrations can be expected to be steady over the course of the day. Common dose-related adverse events include fatigue, weight loss, dizziness, somnolence, anorexia and abnormal thinking, and decreased sweating [89]. Zonisamide has also been associated with idiosyncratic side-effects. These include hypersensitivity syndromes such as rash and Stevens–Johnson syndrome and renal calculi [89]. Patients living in hot climates, who are on high doses and have a family history of renal calculi may be at higher risk. Patients receiving zonisamide should be advised to drink plenty of fluids. The recurrence rate, even if zonisamide is continued, is not 100% [90]. Hypohidrosis has also been seen, again more common in hot climates, and may infrequently lead to heat stroke in children [89]. Zonisamide is well absorbed and is not extensively bound to plasma proteins. Since enzyme-inducing drugs such as carbamazepine and phenytoin can significantly reduce the half-life of zonisamide, higher doses will be needed in patients taking them in combination [56]. Zonisamide metabolism can also be inhibited by a number of medications as well as by grapefruit juice. Zonisamide has essentially no impact on the pharmacokinetic parameters of other drugs [56, 59].

PREGABALIN

Pregabalin has a similar efficacy profile to gabapentin, that is to say its use is restricted to partial seizures [91]. No formal monotherapy studies have been completed, in either newly diagnosed or refractory patients. An advantage of pregabalin when compared to gabapentin, is that it is highly bioavailable, and does not require active dose-dependent transport in the GI tract [92]. Pregabalin is better tolerated when titrated. A recent study indicated that starting at the highest dose of 600 mg, while safe, led to 32% dropouts [93]. Pregabalin can be initiated at 50–75 mg twice daily, and titrated by 50–75 mg every week or two weeks. There are very few clinical data available regarding the safety and tolerability of doses above 600 mg/day. Twice-daily dosing is commonly used, despite the short half-life of the drug. A study comparing efficacy and tolerability of the same total daily dose, given as twice daily or thrice daily showed no statistically significant difference, but there was a trend to both better efficacy and tolerability when thrice daily was used [94]. Therefore, it is reasonable to start off with a twice-daily regimen, and switch to thrice daily only if side-effects are present and/or breakthrough seizures are occurring. Pregabalin levels have only recently become available, and their clinical utility is unknown. Common dose-related side-effects predominantly affecting the central nervous system include dizziness, somnolence and ataxia. Weight gain and peripheral oedema are also seen. Weight gain is also dose related [91]. To date, no idiosyncratic side-effects have been identified. Need for routine monitoring of liver functions, electrolytes and blood counts is therefore not established. Pregabalin is almost exclusively excreted unchanged in the urine, and does not undergo metabolic changes. To date, no drug–drug interactions have been uncovered, and none are expected.

VIGABATRIN (NOT APPROVED IN THE USA)

Vigabatrin, like felbamate, is an AED that has been associated with a significant adverse drug effect (irreversible visual field restriction) that limits its use to those patients who have severe epilepsy which has not responded to other AEDs [95]. In adults, vigabatrin appears to have a narrow spectrum of action, and its use is primarily restricted to those patients with refractory partial epilepsy [96]. It has been found inferior in efficacy to carbamazepine in trials of newly diagnosed patients [97]. It has also been known to worsen myoclonus [98]. In infants, however, vigabatrin was found to be highly effective in the devastating childhood epilepsy known as infantile spasms, or West syndrome [99]. In a randomized trial, there was a 78% reduction in seizures on vigabatrin, compared with 26% on placebo. Moreover, in the open-label phase, 38% of children were completely spasm free [100]. Vigabatrin is particularly effective in patients with spasms associated with tuberous sclerosis [101]. Vigabatrin can be initiated at 500–1000 mg, given once or twice a day. The dose can be increased in 500–1000 mg weekly increments, up to 3000 mg. Some patients worsen at higher doses. Vigabatrin has unique pharmacokinetic properties, in that its mechanism of action involves changes in brain chemistry that far outlast its presence in the bloodstream. Therefore, vigabatrin levels are not useful for therapeutic monitoring [102].

As noted, the main safety concern relates to irreversible peripheral visual field defects. This problem is estimated to occur in 30–50% of patients receiving the drug. Often, this will be picked up on screening visual field testing, but the patients will not spontaneously report any problems [103]. Since early development of this problem has not been seen in controlled studies, there may be a 3-month 'window of opportunity' to see if the drug works before there is a risk of the visual field defect [103]. However, once it occurs, it is not reversible.

Other side-effects of vigabatrin include drowsiness, depression, weight gain, dizziness and rare psychosis [104].

AED SELECTION

Selection of AEDs can be very confusing. Each AED has unique characteristics, including spectrum of activity, cost, pharmacokinetic and pharmacodynamic properties, likelihood for dose-related side-effects and risk of serious health risks. Therefore, to the frustration of many prescribers, there is not a 'first choice' selection in specific treatment situations such as initiation in newly diagnosed patients, first add-on, women anticipating pregnancy and so on. For each of these scenarios, there may be more optimal and less optimal choices, but the final selection will depend on many patient characteristics. Table 1.3 provides pragmatic information about initiating AEDs. What follows is a rational sequence of issues that can be used to narrow down drug choices.

EPILEPSY SYNDROME

Classification of seizure type and epilepsy syndrome will be a critical issue in selecting a new AED, and should be done as a first step in selection. As noted above, some AEDs are considered 'narrow spectrum' and do not treat all seizure types. In addition, they may worsen some seizure types. For example, carbamazepine, oxcarbazepine, gabapentin, tiagabine, pregabalin and vigabatrin are most appropriate for seizures associated with partial epilepsy, and may worsen generalized seizure types such as myoclonus and absence [105–107]. Felbamate, lamotrigine, topiramate, zonisamide and levetiracetam and valproic acid are considered to be broad spectrum. They may be appropriate for most seizure types. However, as noted above, in a recent study of patients with generalized or unclassified seizures randomized to valproate, lamotrigine or topiramate, lamotrigine was found to be inferior to valproate in efficacy, leading the authors to speculate as to how broad spectrum it actually was [16]. Ethosuximide has the narrowest spectrum, and is only effective in treating absence seizures.

Often, seizures cannot be definitively classified at the time of diagnosis [108]. In the randomized study described above, 27% of patients who were entered into the study were described as unclassified [16]. If a patient cannot be classified, it is wise to choose a broad-spectrum anti-epileptic drug.

COST

It is very important to keep cost in mind, particularly for patients who have limited or no coverage for drug expenditure. Such patients may ask about use of generic substitution. These patients can be told that at present, the risks vs. benefits of using generic drugs in patients with epilepsy are only known for the older drugs. In the case of phenytoin and carbamazepine, evidence suggests that generic substitution is unwise. However, for the more expensive newer AEDs, the data do not exist, and are not likely to be available any time soon [109].

SELECTION IN NEWLY DIAGNOSED PATIENTS

Because most patients will become seizure free on initial therapy, if selected appropriately for epilepsy syndrome, and because the newly diagnosed patients are considered 'easy to treat', drugs should be selected that are most likely to be safe and well tolerated. This is particularly true because once stabilized on an effective medication, patients may be reluctant to switch for fear of further seizures, even in the presence of side-effects. For these reasons, the first drug selected often becomes a long-term choice. Issues in selection of drug therapy in newly diagnosed patients are discussed in Chapters 5 and 7.

SELECTION OF AN ADD-ON DRUG

When selecting a drug that will be added on to an existing regimen, a number of factors should be considered, including whether added benefit is foreseen, whether pharmacokinetic interactions will occur, whether compounded side-effects are likely, whether there is a risk of additional safety issues, and finally whether the drug can eventually replace the background drugs. It has not been proven that combining drugs with different mechanisms will actually increase the likelihood of seizure control. A second issue is whether the addition of a drug will lead to pharmacokinetic interactions. Interactions between old and new AEDs

Table 1.3 Suggestions for initiations of anti-epileptic drugs (AEDs)*

AED	Suggested titration	Can drug be loaded?	How is initial target dose usually selected?†	Typical initial daily target dose
Carbamazepine	Add 200 mg every 2–3 days	No	By attaining minimal serum concentration (4–6 µg/ml)	400–800 mg
Ethosuximide	500 mg/week	No	By attaining minimal serum concentration (40 µg/ml)	500–1000 mg
Felbamate	300–600 mg/week	No	By dose	1200–1800 mg
Gabapentin	300–600 mg/week	No	By dose	900–1800 mg
Lamotrigine	25 mg; initial monotherapy: 25 mg/day for 2 weeks, then 50 mg/day for 2 weeks, followed by 50-mg increases every week	No	By dose, and by attaining minimal serum concentration (4 µg/ml)	100–200 mg
Levetiracetam	250–500 mg; increase by 250–500 mg/week	Yes, i.v.	By dose	500–1500 mg
Oxcarbazepine	300–600 mg/week	No	By dose	900–1800 mg
Phenobarbital	30 mg/week	Yes, i.v. in emergency	By attaining minimal serum concentration (15 µg/ml)	60–120 mg
Phenytoin	No	Yes, 13–15 mg/kg	By attaining minimal serum concentration (10 µg/ml)	3–5 mg/kg
Primidone	125–250 mg/week	No	By attaining minimal serum concentration (8 µg/ml)	500–1000 mg
Pregabalin	75–150 mg; increase 75–150 mg/week	No	By dose	150–300 mg
Tiagabine	4 mg/week	No	By dose	16–36 mg
Topiramate	25–50 mg/week	No	By dose	100–200 mg
Valproate, valproic acid, divalproex sodium	250–500 mg/week, or 10–15 mg/kg orally daily, increasing by 5–10 mg/kg every week†	Yes, i.v.	By attaining minimal serum concentration (40–50 µg/ml)	750–1500 mg
Vigabatrin	500 mg/week	No	By dose	1000–2000 mg
Zonisamide	50 mg/week	No	By dose	100–200 mg

*This table presumes that the patient is not on a hepatic enzyme inducer such as phenytoin, phenobarbital or carbamazepine, or an enzyme inhibitor such as valproate.
†Adjustments in all patients should take individual tolerability and efficacy into account.
i.v., intravenous.

are listed in Tables 1.1 and 1.2. These potential interactions should be recognized, and doses of background drugs should be adjusted accordingly. Another type of interaction is called 'pharmacodynamic'. In this type of interaction, levels do not change, but side-effects may be greater than expected if either drug was given by itself. For example, more side-effects may be seen when combining two of the the sodium channel blockers lamotrigine, carbamazepine and phenytoin. Lamotrigine may also cause more side-effects when given with valproate, but this combination has also been noted to be favourable in terms of efficacy in some patients [52, 110]. In contrast, some of the newer drugs, such as levetiracetam, gabapentin and pregabalin, seem to be easier to add on, with fewer additive side-effects.

AEDs FOR PATIENTS WITH OTHER HEALTH CONCERNS

Some patients may be poor candidates for specific AEDs because of their past history. For example, patients who have demonstrated hypersensitivity to AEDs may have problems with more allergenic compounds. Some AEDs have a higher likelihood of cross-reacting with each other, including phenytoin, carbamazepine, phenobarbital and lamotrigine [111]. In principle, patients who are overweight should avoid carbamazepine, gabapentin, pregabalin, valproic acid and vigabatrin as these drugs tend to increase weight, although they may be warranted in some patients. Similarly, patients who are overly thin or have eating disorders may not be ideal candidates for topiramate, felbamate or zonisamide, which suppress appetite. Drugs with greater potential for psychiatric problems such as irritability, mood disorders and psychosis include levetiracetam, topiramate and vigabatrin, whereas lamotrigine, carbamazepine and valproate may stabilize mood. Use of drugs in patients with concomitant medical conditions is discussed in Chapter 13.

OTHER ISSUES IN AED USE

MONOTHERAPY VS. POLYTHERAPY

There has been a great deal of discussion in recent years relating to the question of whether monotherapy or polytherapy would be a better choice for patients who have failed their initial therapy. In fact, either option may be appropriate, and the choice will often depend on the specific situation. If the initial drug seemed to be well tolerated, and to have partial but not complete effect, then a second AED can be initiated. If complete seizure control is attained without deterioration of tolerability, the choice of whether to withdraw the first medication may not be clearcut. If, however, tolerability is poor, the first AED should be gradually withdrawn, ultimately resulting in monotherapy. Other factors may also increase the benefit of withdrawing the first AED. These include cost, likelihood of pregnancy in the future, potential for long-term side-effects (e.g. osteopenia with phenytoin therapy) and potential that the first drug may contribute to pharmacokinetic interactions. A recent study was undertaken to assess the potential risks vs. benefits of the two therapeutic strategies. In this study, patients were randomized to either add-on or sequential monotherapy. The study was stopped before full enrolment, as it became clear that neither arm would be able to demonstrate superiority to the other. However, among the 157 patients who were randomized, more discontinued as a result of dose-related side-effects and persistent seizures in the monotherapy arm than among those randomized to polytherapy, although the results were not significant [112].

Practical points for deciding to add vs. switch:

- If the patient is on a drug that is causing side-effects that interfere with quality of life, switching is advisable.
- If the patient is on a drug that could cause unwanted long-term consequences (e.g. phenytoin/osteopenia, valproate/teratogenicity in women), switching should be strongly considered.

- If the patient is on a drug that is well tolerated but ineffective, another AED can be added. Initially, the patient can be given a schedule to slowly titrate the new AED to an appropriate dose. If side-effects occur, the dose of the background AED can be reduced, or even eliminated to see if side-effects abate, before abandoning the new AED.
- If the combination of the new AED and old AED are well tolerated, and seizure control is improved (or seizure freedom obtained), a risk–benefit assessment should be made of continuing combination therapy vs. withdrawing to monotherapy.
- If a decision is made to withdraw to monotherapy, the withdrawal should be done slowly. If seizures worsen during withdrawal, reconsideration of continued polytherapy is reasonable.

USE OF SERUM LEVELS

Physicians may be confused about whether measurement of serum concentrations is important for epilepsy patients, particularly for the new AEDs. Most experts believe that it is more important to individualize dosing, and to understand the serum concentration that is optimal on an individual basis. This may mean that some individuals have optimal control and side-effect profile at a serum concentration that is outside of the recognized therapeutic norms.

Approximately 25% of patients will achieve seizure freedom below the recognized therapeutic range, and about the same number will require serum concentrations above the range to obtain the maximum seizure benefit, often with few side-effects.

Many of the new AEDs are considered to have a wide therapeutic range. The range of serum concentrations that can be beneficial varies widely from one individual to another, yet for a particular individual it may be very important to maintain serum concentrations with minimal variability. For example, one patient on lamotrigine may have excellent seizure control within a range of 2–4 mg/l, but may experience dizziness and diplopia if the level increases to 5 mg/l. Another patient, in contrast, may have breakthrough seizures if their level drops below 7 mg/l, but may tolerate levels up to 10 mg/l [45, 113].

Another area of confusion relates to timing of levels. Some AEDs have short half-lives, but nonetheless are dosed two times a day. In some cases, there is reasonably good scientific evidence that the drug has a longer duration of action in the central nervous system than would be expected based on its half-life. This has led to the common practice of dosing these drugs two times a day. It seems that other AEDs must be present at relatively constant serum concentrations throughout the day, to prevent seizure breakthroughs. Carbamazepine and phenytoin seem to fall in this category. What does this mean in terms of levels? For drugs that are dosed less frequently than their half-lives, the levels will be expected to vary substantially over the course of a day. *Thus, levels can only be compared if they are measured at the same time of day.* Take, for example, a patient who is receiving levetiracetam 1000 mg two times a day, at 8 a.m. and 8 p.m. He always gets his serum levels measured at his physician's office at the time of his appointments, 2 h after his dose. The levels would therefore be close to the peak. When measured, they are 20–25 mg/l. The patient now has a seizure at 7 p.m. and the level in the emergency room is 10 mg/l. One interpretation would be that the patient is non-compliant or the levels have dropped, but this would be incorrect. In fact, the levels were measured at trough, and are exactly where they should be. Now consider a patient on sustained-release carbamazepine, who receives 400 mg two times a day, at 8 a.m. and 8 p.m.. In this case, serum concentrations would be expected to vary very little over the course of a day, and a treating physician will have to investigate the cause of any major fluctuations. This can be very confusing for a treating physician. Nonetheless, levels can be useful if employed properly.

The following strategy may be recommended for using serum levels:

- When initiating therapy, increase doses slowly, until seizure control is achieved or side-effects occur. If seizures are controlled, obtain a serum concentration at that time. This will identify the patient's 'therapeutic optimal level'.
- Measure all levels at the same time of day, if possible. This will provide some indication of compliance, and also of variability in a given patient.
- For drugs with sustained-release formulations, or long half-lives, serum concentrations should remain within a small range (no more than 20–25% change), even if obtained at different times of day, once a steady state is achieved (e.g. phenobarbital, phenytoin (administered two times a day), Tegretol XR™ or Carbatrol™ (sustained-release carbamazepine formulations), zonisamide, Depakote ER™ (sustained-release valproate formulation), topiramate and lamotrigine (administered two times a day in patients who are not receiving enzyme-inducing AEDs). If a breakthrough seizure occurs in the setting of a low serum concentration, consider non-compliance or inappropriate dosing schedule.
- For drugs with short half-lives and no sustained-release formulation, serum concentrations should be consistent when taken at trough, but may vary by >50% if taken at other times, and should not be interpreted as indication of non-compliance (e.g. non-sustained-release valproate, gabapentin, levetiracetam, carbamazepine [administered two times a day], tiagabine and pregabalin).

AED DOSING SCHEDULES

Dosing intervals that are inappropriately long can lead to problems with both tolerability, when serum concentrations are too high, and efficacy, when they are too low [71]. This is only a problem for certain drugs, depending on whether the drug truly has a wide therapeutic window. Carbamazepine has a narrow therapeutic window because many people experience toxicity at higher serum concentrations and breakthrough seizures if the concentration is too low. For example, serum concentrations above 11 mg/l are likely to produce dizziness, ataxia and/or diplopia, whereas serum concentrations below 8 mg/l are likely to produce breakthrough seizures. Under these circumstances, the choice of dosing strategies is relatively clearcut. Dosing intervals would have to be chosen to maintain serum concentrations within, at most, a 25% band. Carbamazepine has a serum half-life of 16 h. Consider a patient who takes 1200 mg per day. If carbamazepine was dosed at 600 mg two times a day, the serum concentration might be 11 mg/l at its maximum but would fall by almost 50% between dosing intervals. If it was dosed as 400 mg three times a day, the serum concentration would fall by 25%, which is barely acceptable. This then leads to the standard practice of administering immediate-release carbamazepine once every 6 h for optimum management, in this case 300 mg four times a day (Figure 1.2). In the patient with four-times-a-day dosing, the serum concentrations would be maintained between 8 mg/l and 10 mg/l. As one can see in Figure 1.2, dosing the patient at 600 mg two times a day would make not only the troughs lower, potentially allowing for breakthrough seizures, but also the peaks higher. Thus, longer dosing intervals give a patient a double whammy, increasing the potential for breakthrough seizures as well as the potential to feel dose-related side-effects when the serum concentration reaches its peak, typically 2–3 h after dosing. This phenomenon is called 'peak-dose toxicity'. It is very common with carbamazepine, as well as with oxcarbazepine and some other short-half-life drugs. Now, imagine that the patient is being dosed with a schedule of 600 mg two times a day, feeling toxicity at the peaks and having occasional breakthrough seizures at the troughs. The physician would presume that the patient has failed a drug at maximum tolerated dose, and would move on to another anti-epileptic drug. In fact, the patient might do extremely well on carbamazepine, at the very same total daily dose, administered as 300 mg four times a day. Fortunately, in the case of carbamazepine, we now have long-acting formulations that can be administered two times a day, while maintaining very steady serum concentrations.

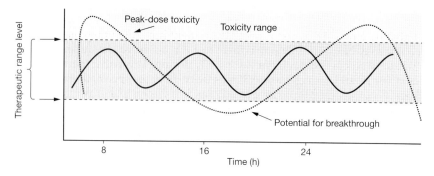

Figure 1.2 Serum levels for a patient on carbamazepine 600 mg two times a day (dashed line) vs. a patient on 400 mg three times a day. The two-times-a-day patient has higher peaks and lower troughs, leading to potential for toxicity and breakthrough seizures.

Drugs that are subject to hepatic enzyme induction by any inducers (such as phenytoin, carbamazepine, phenobarbital and primidone) may need to be dosed more frequently in the presence of those drugs because of a reduction in half-life. For example, both topiramate and lamotrigine have half-lives of 24 h when used in monotherapy or in the absence of enzyme inducers or inhibitors, but 12 h in the presence of enzyme inducers. Lamotrigine is also subject to inhibition by valproate. In the setting of valproate use, the half-life rises to 48 h, permitting once-a-day dosing if desired.

Most of the newer anti-epileptic drugs are labelled for use on a twice-daily basis. It should not, by any means, be presumed that this implies that a twice-daily schedule is optimal for every, or even any, patient. Drugs are labelled based on the way that they were tested in randomized controlled trials that led to approval. Therefore, if a drug was used twice a day in the clinical trials, this is what the label will indicate. In most cases, there is no way of knowing whether a more frequent dosing strategy would have led to better control or less side-effects. For two of the newer anti-epileptic drugs, studies were done that explored the effects of twice-daily vs. thrice-daily dosing. One study, on pregabalin, showed no difference between the two strategies, but the study was under-powered to show a statistically significant difference. There was clearly a trend towards better control and fewer side-effects with the three-times-a-day dosing. The percentage reduction in seizure frequency from baseline was 53.0% for the three-times-a-day group and 44.3% for the two-times-a-day group. A total of 19% of the three-times-a-day group withdrew due to adverse events, compared with 26% from the two-times-a-day group [94]. A study of tiagabine two times a day vs. three times a day showed similar results, although the better tolerability in the three-times-a-day group was statistically significant [114].

There is reason to believe that some drugs can be dosed less frequently than would be expected from their half-life, without fear of seizure breakthrough. Based on data from studies of suppression of photic-induced epileptic discharges, valproate and levetiracetam probably have long pharmacodynamic half-lives and can be dosed two times a day [115, 116]. In these cases, toxicity should still be considered. Although the troughs are not as great a concern, the peaks still may be. If the patient appears to be suffering from peak-dose toxicity, increasing the dosing frequency while maintaining the same total daily dose will lower the peaks, and provide better tolerability. In some cases, it may also permit higher daily doses, leading to better efficacy.

Practical suggestions for dosing of AEDs:

- When initiating a new AED, discuss with the patient how often they may be willing to take it. Some may be quite willing to adhere to a three-times-a-day regimen, whereas others will only accept once-daily or twice-daily dosing. This will impact on drug choice.
- It is reasonable to initiate most new AEDs as twice daily (or once daily for zonisamide) but if there is a problem with toxicity or efficacy, it is reasonable to ask the patient whether they would be willing to increase the dosing frequency. More frequent dosing should be considered, if possible, for gabapentin, tiagabine and pregabalin.
- Higher doses may be achievable with more frequent dosing intervals, thereby potentially improving seizure control.
- If a patient is on lamotrigine or topiramate, and a hepatic enzyme inducer is added, dosing interval may need to be shortened. This is also true if a female patient on lamotrigine is placed on an oral contraceptive, which also induces metabolism.

REFERENCES

1. Glauser T, Ben-Menachem E, Bourgeois B, Cnaan A, Chadwick D, Guerreiro C et al. ILAE treatment guidelines: evidence-based analysis of antiepileptic drug efficacy and effectiveness as initial mono-therapy for epileptic seizures and syndromes. *Epilepsia* 2006; 47:1094–1120.
2. Craig S. Phenytoin poisoning. *Neurocrit Care* 2005; 3:161–170.
3. Pack AM, Morrell MJ, Marcus R, Holloway L, Flaster E, Done S et al. Bone mass and turnover in women with epilepsy on antiepileptic drug monotherapy. *Ann Neurol* 2005; 57:252–257.
4. Brodie MJ, Richens A, Yuen AW. Double-blind comparison of lamotrigine and carbamazepine in newly diagnosed epilepsy. UK Lamotrigine/Carbamazepine Monotherapy Trial Group. *Lancet* 1995; 345:476–479.
5. Brodie MJ, Perucca E, Ryvlin P, Ben-Menachem E, Meencke HJ. Comparison of levetiracetam and controlled-release carbamazepine in newly diagnosed epilepsy. *Neurology* 2007; 68:402–408.
6. Dam M, Ekberg R, Loyning Y, Waltimo O, Jakobsen K. A double-blind study comparing oxcarbazepine and carbamazepine in patients with newly diagnosed, previously untreated epilepsy. *Epilepsy Res* 1989; 3:70–76.
7. Privitera MD, Brodie MJ, Mattson RH, Chadwick DW, Neto W, Wang S. Topiramate, carbamazepine and valproate monotherapy: double-blind comparison in newly diagnosed epilepsy. *Acta Neurol Scand* 2003; 107:165–175.
8. Benbadis SR, Tatum WO 4th, Gieron M. Idiopathic generalized epilepsy and choice of antiepileptic drugs. *Neurology* 2003; 61:1793–1795.
9. Marson AG, Al-Kharusi AM, Alwaidh M, Appleton R, Baker GA, Chadwick DW et al. The SANAD study of effectiveness of carbamazepine, gabapentin, lamotrigine, oxcarbazepine, or topiramate for treatment of partial epilepsy: an unblinded randomised controlled trial. *Lancet* 2007; 369:1000–1015.
10. Bertolino JG. Carbamazepine. What physicians should know about its hematologic effects. *Postgrad Med* 1990; 88:183–186.
11. Dong X, Leppik IE, White J, Rarick J. Hyponatremia from oxcarbazepine and carbamazepine. *Neurology* 2005; 65:1976–1978.
12. Isojarvi JI, Pakarinen AJ, Myllyla VV. Effects of carbamazepine therapy on serum sex hormone levels in male patients with epilepsy. *Epilepsia* 1988; 29:781–786.
13. Eiris J, Novo-Rodriguez MI, Del Rio M, Meseguer P, Del Rio MC, Castro-Gago M. The effects on lipid and apolipoprotein serum levels of long-term carbamazepine, valproic acid and phenobarbital therapy in children with epilepsy. *Epilepsy Res* 2000; 41:1–7.
14. Mattson RH, Cramer JA, Collins JF, Smith DB, Delgado-Escueta AV, Browne TR et al. Comparison of carbamazepine, phenobarbital, phenytoin, and primidone in partial and secondarily generalized tonic–clonic seizures. *N Engl J Med* 1985; 313:145–151.
15. Mattson RH, Cramer JA, McCutchen CB. Barbiturate-related connective tissue disorders. *Arch Intern Med* 1989; 149:911–914.
16. Marson A, Al-Kharusi A, Alwaidh M, Appleton R, Baker G, Chadwick D et al. Valproate, lamotrigine, or topiramate for generalized and unclassifiable epilepsy: results from the SANAD trial. *Lancet* 2007; 369:1016–1026.

17. Mattson RH, Cramer JA, Collins JF. A comparison of valproate with carbamazepine for the treatment of complex partial seizures and secondarily generalized tonic–clonic seizures in adults. The Department of Veterans Affairs Epilepsy Cooperative Study No. 264 Group. *N Engl J Med* 1992; 327:765–771.
18. Heller AJ, Chesterman P, Elwes RD, Crawford P, Chadwick D, Johnson AL *et al*. Phenobarbital, phenytoin, carbamazepine, or sodium valproate for newly diagnosed adult epilepsy: a randomised comparative monotherapy trial. *J Neurol Neurosurg Psychiatry* 1995; 58:44–50.
19. Richens A, Davidson DL, Cartlidge NE, Easter DJ. A multicentre comparative trial of sodium valproate and carbamazepine in adult onset epilepsy. Adult EPITEG Collaborative Group. *J Neurol Neurosurg Psychiatry* 1994; 57:682–687.
20. Verity CM, Hosking G, Easter DJ. A multicentre comparative trial of sodium valproate and carbamazepine in paediatric epilepsy. The Paediatric EPITEG Collaborative Group. *Dev Med Child Neurol* 1995; 37:97–108.
21. de Silva M, MacArdle B, McGowan M, Hughes E, Stewart J, Neville BG *et al*. Randomised comparative monotherapy trial of phenobarbital, phenytoin, carbamazepine, or sodium valproate for newly diagnosed childhood epilepsy. *Lancet* 1996; 347:709–713.
22. Christe W, Kramer G, Vigonius U, Pohlmann H, Steinhoff BJ, Brodie MJ *et al*. A double-blind controlled clinical trial: oxcarbazepine versus sodium valproate in adults with newly diagnosed epilepsy. *Epilepsy Res* 1997; 26:451–460.
23. Hodges BM, Mazur JE. Intravenous valproate in status epilepticus. *Ann Pharmacother* 2001; 35:1465–1470.
24. Ferrendelli JA. Concerns with antiepileptic drug initiation: safety, tolerability, and efficacy. *Epilepsia* 2001; 42(Suppl 4):28–30.
25. Galindo PA, Borja J, Gomez E, Mur P, Gudin M, Garcia R *et al*. Anticonvulsant drug hypersensitivity. *J Investig Allergol Clin Immunol* 2002; 12:299–304.
26. Perucca E. Pharmacological and therapeutic properties of valproate: a summary after 35 years of clinical experience. *CNS Drugs* 2002; 16:695–714.
27. Verrotti A, Trotta D, Morgese G, Chiarelli F. Valproate-induced hyperammonemic encephalopathy. *Metab Brain Dis* 2002; 17:367–373.
28. Bohles H, Sewell AC, Wenzel D. The effect of carnitine supplementation in valproate-induced hyperammonaemia. *Acta Paediatr* 1996; 85:446–449.
29. Bryant AE 3rd, Dreifuss FE. Valproic acid hepatic fatalities. III. U.S. experience since 1986. *Neurology* 1996; 46:465–469.
30. Acharya S, Bussel JB. Hematologic toxicity of sodium valproate. *J Pediatr Hematol Oncol* 2000; 22:62–65.
31. Tetzlaff JE. Intraoperative defect in haemostasis in a child receiving valproic acid. *Can J Anaesth* 1991; 38:222–224.
32. Alsdorf R, Wyszynski DF. Teratogenicity of sodium valproate. *Expert Opin Drug Saf* 2005; 4:345–353.
33. Pennell PB. 2005 AES annual course: evidence used to treat women with epilepsy. *Epilepsia* 2006; 47(Suppl 1):46–53.
34. Vajda FJ, Hitchcock A, Graham J, Solinas C, O'Brien TJ, Lander CM *et al*. Foetal malformations and seizure control: 52 months' data of the Australian Pregnancy Registry. *Eur J Neurol* 2006; 13:645–654.
35. Morrow J, Russell A, Guthrie E, Parsons L, Robertson I, Waddell R *et al*. Malformation risks of antiepileptic drugs in pregnancy: a prospective study from the UK Epilepsy and Pregnancy Register. *J Neurol Neurosurg Psychiatry* 2006; 77:193–198.
36. Meador KJ, Baker GA, Finnell RH, Kalayjian LA, Liporace JD, Loring DW *et al*. In utero antiepileptic drug exposure: fetal death and malformations. *Neurology* 2006; 67:407–412.
37. Wyszynski DF, Nambisan M, Surve T, Alsdorf RM, Smith CR, Holmes LB. Increased rate of major malformations in offspring exposed to valproate during pregnancy. *Neurology* 2005; 64:961–965.
38. Viinikainen K, Eriksson K, Monkkonen A, Aikia M, Nieminen P, Heinonen S *et al*. The effects of valproate exposure in utero on behavior and the need for educational support in school-aged children. *Epilepsy Behav* 2006; 9:636–640.
39. Adab N, Kini U, Vinten J, Ayres J, Baker G, Clayton-Smith J *et al*. The longer term outcome of children born to mothers with epilepsy. *J Neurol Neurosurg Psychiatry* 2004; 75:1575–1583.
40. Löfgren E, Mikkonen K, Tolonen U, Pakarinen A, Koivunen R, Myllyla VV *et al*. Reproductive endocrine function in women with epilepsy: the role of epilepsy type and medication. *Epilepsy Behav* 2007; 10:77–83.
41. Wallace SJ. Use of ethosuximide and valproate in the treatment of epilepsy. *Neurol Clin* 1986; 4:601–616.

42. Wheless JW, Clarke DF, Carpenter D. Treatment of pediatric epilepsy: expert opinion, 2005. *J Child Neurol* 2005; 20(Suppl 1):S1–S56; quiz S59–S60.

43. Pellock JM, Faught E, Leppik IE, Shinnar S, Zupanc ML. Felbamate: consensus of current clinical experience. *Epilepsy Res* 2006; 71:89–101.

44. Efficacy of felbamate in childhood epileptic encephalopathy (Lennox–Gastaut syndrome). The Felbamate Study Group in Lennox–Gastaut Syndrome. *N Engl J Med* 1993; 328:29–33.

45. Neels HM, Sierens AC, Naelaerts K, Scharpe SL, Hatfield GM, Lambert WE. Therapeutic drug monitoring of old and newer anti-epileptic drugs. *Clin Chem Lab Med* 2004; 42:1228–1255.

46. French JA, Kanner AM, Bautista J, Abou-Khalil B, Browne T, Harden CL *et al*. Efficacy and tolerability of the new antiepileptic drugs II: treatment of refractory epilepsy: report of the Therapeutics and Technology Assessment Subcommittee and Quality Standards Subcommittee of the American Academy of Neurology and the American Epilepsy Society. *Neurology* 2004; 62:1261–1273.

47. French JA, Kanner AM, Bautista J, Abou-Khalil B, Browne T, Harden CL *et al*. Efficacy and tolerability of the new antiepileptic drugs I: treatment of new onset epilepsy: report of the Therapeutics and Technology Assessment Subcommittee and Quality Standards Subcommittee of the American Academy of Neurology and the American Epilepsy Society. *Neurology* 2004; 62:1252–1260.

48. Steiner TJ, Dellaportas CI, Findley LJ, Gross M, Gibberd FB, Perkin GD, *et al*. Lamotrigine monotherapy in newly diagnosed untreated epilepsy: a double-blind comparison with phenytoin. *Epilepsia* 1999; 40:601–607.

49. Brodie MJ, Overstall PW, Giorgi L. Multicentre, double-blind, randomised comparison between lamotrigine and carbamazepine in elderly patients with newly diagnosed epilepsy. The UK Lamotrigine Elderly Study Group. *Epilepsy Res* 1999; 37:81–87.

50. Rowan AJ, Ramsay RE, Collins JF, Pryor F, Boardman KD, Uthman BM *et al.*; the VACSG. New onset geriatric epilepsy: a randomized study of gabapentin, lamotrigine, and carbamazepine. *Neurology* 2005; 64:1868–1873.

51. Marson A, Al-Kharusi A, Alwaidh M, Appleton R, Baker G, Chadwick D *et al*. Carbamazepine, gabapentin, lamotrigine, oxcarbazepine or topiramate for partial epilepsy: results from the SANAD trial. *Lancet* 2007; 369:1000–1015.

52. Brodie MJ, Yuen AW. Lamotrigine substitution study: evidence for synergism with sodium valproate? 105 Study Group. *Epilepsy Res* 1997; 26:423–432.

53. Perucca E. Clinical pharmacology and therapeutic use of the new antiepileptic drugs. *Fundam Clin Pharmacol* 2001; 15:405–417.

54. Hirsch LJ, Weintraub DB, Buchsbaum R, Spencer HT, Straka T, Hager M *et al*. Predictors of lamotrigine-associated rash. *Epilepsia* 2006; 47:318–322.

55. Malik S, Arif H, Hirsch LJ. Lamotrigine and its applications in the treatment of epilepsy and other neurological and psychiatric disorders. *Expert Rev Neurother* 2006; 6:1609–1627.

56. Patsalos PN, Perucca E. Clinically important drug interactions in epilepsy: interactions between antiepileptic drugs and other drugs. *Lancet Neurol* 2003; 2:473–481.

57. Fisher RS, Sachdeo RC, Pellock J, Penovich PE, Magnus L, Bernstein P. Rapid initiation of gabapentin: a randomized, controlled trial. *Neurology* 2001; 56:743–748.

58. Gidal BE, DeCerce J, Bockbrader HN, Gonzalez J, Kruger S, Pitterle ME *et al*. Gabapentin bioavailability: effect of dose and frequency of administration in adult patients with epilepsy. *Epilepsy Res* 1998; 31:91–99.

59. Patsalos PN, Perucca E. Clinically important drug interactions in epilepsy: general features and interactions between antiepileptic drugs. *Lancet Neurol* 2003; 2:347–356.

60. Asconape J, Diedrich A, DellaBadia J. Myoclonus associated with the use of gabapentin. *Epilepsia* 2000; 41:479–481.

61. Tallian KB, Nahata MC, Lo W, Tsao CY. Gabapentin associated with aggressive behavior in pediatric patients with seizures. *Epilepsia* 1996; 37:501–502.

62. Guerrini R, Parmeggiani L. Topiramate and its clinical applications in epilepsy. *Expert Opin Pharmacother* 2006; 7:811–823.

63. Banta JT, Hoffman K, Budenz DL, Ceballos E, Greenfield DS. Presumed topiramate-induced bilateral acute angle-closure glaucoma. *Am J Ophthalmol* 2001; 132:112–114.

64. Arcas J, Ferrer T, Roche MC, Martinez-Bermejo A, Lopez-Martin V. Hypohidrosis related to the administration of topiramate to children. *Epilepsia* 2001; 42:1363–1365.

65. Shorvon SD. Safety of topiramate: adverse events and relationships to dosing. *Epilepsia* 1996; 37(Suppl 2):S18–S22.

66. Bumb A, Diederich N, Beyenburg S. Adding topiramate to valproate therapy may cause reversible hepatic failure. *Epileptic Disord* 2003; 5:157–159.

67. Bill PA, Vigonius U, Pohlmann H, Guerreiro CA, Kochen S, Saffer D *et al*. A double-blind controlled clinical trial of oxcarbazepine versus phenytoin in adults with previously untreated epilepsy. *Epilepsy Res* 1997; 27:195–204.

68. Guerreiro MM, Vigonius U, Pohlmann H, de Manreza ML, Fejerman N, Antoniuk SA *et al*. A double-blind controlled clinical trial of oxcarbazepine versus phenytoin in children and adolescents with epilepsy. *Epilepsy Res* 1997; 27:205–213.

69. Kaddurah AK, Holmes GL. Possible precipitation of myoclonic seizures with oxcarbazepine. *Epilepsy Behav* 2006; 8:289–293.

70. Beydoun A. Monotherapy trials of new antiepileptic drugs. *Epilepsia* 1997; 38(Suppl 9):S21–S31.

71. Perucca E, Dulac O, Shorvon S, Tomson T. Harnessing the clinical potential of antiepileptic drug therapy: dosage optimisation. *CNS Drugs* 2001; 15:609–621.

72. Schachter SC. Oxcarbazepine: current status and clinical applications. *Expert Opin Investig Drugs* 1999; 8:1103–1112.

73. Beydoun A, Kutluay E. Oxcarbazepine. *Expert Opin Pharmacother* 2002; 3:59–71.

74. Knake S, Hamer HM, Schomburg U, Oertel WH, Rosenow F. Tiagabine-induced absence status in idiopathic generalized epilepsy. *Seizure* 1999; 8:314–317.

75. Fulton JA, Hoffman RS, Nelson LS. Tiagabine overdose: a case of status epilepticus in a non-epileptic patient. *Clin Toxicol (Phila)* 2005; 43:869–871.

76. Schachter SC. A review of the antiepileptic drug tiagabine. *Clin Neuropharmacol* 1999; 22:312–317.

77. Ettinger AB, Bernal OG, Andriola MR, Bagchi S, Flores P, Just C *et al*. Two cases of nonconvulsive status epilepticus in association with tiagabine therapy. *Epilepsia* 1999; 40:1159–1162.

78. Verdru P, Wajgt A, Delgado JS *et al*. Efficacy and safety of levetiracetam 3000 mg/d as adjunctive treatment in adolescents and adults suffering from idiopathic generalised epilepsy with myoclonic seizures. *Epilepsia* 2005; 46(Suppl 6):56.

79. Di Bonaventura C, Fattouch J, Mari F, Egeo G, Vaudano AE, Prencipe M *et al*. Clinical experience with levetiracetam in idiopathic generalized epilepsy according to different syndrome subtypes. *Epileptic Disord* 2005; 7:231–235.

80. Labate A, Colosimo E, Gambardella A, Leggio U, Ambrosio R, Quattrone A. Levetiracetam in patients with generalised epilepsy and myoclonic seizures: an open label study. *Seizure* 2006; 15:214–218.

81. French J, Arrigo C. Rapid onset of action of levetiracetam in refractory epilepsy patients. *Epilepsia* 2005; 46:324–326.

82. Betts T, Waegemans T, Crawford P. A multicentre, double-blind, randomized, parallel group study to evaluate the tolerability and efficacy of two oral doses of levetiracetam, 2000 mg daily and 4000 mg daily, without titration in patients with refractory epilepsy. *Seizure* 2000; 9:80–87.

83. Ben-Menachem E. Levetiracetam: treatment in epilepsy. *Expert Opin Pharmacother* 2003; 4:2079–2088.

84. French J, Edrich P, Cramer JA. A systematic review of the safety profile of levetiracetam: a new antiepileptic drug. *Epilepsy Res* 2001; 47:77–90.

85. Seino M. Review of zonisamide development in Japan. *Seizure* 2004; 13(Suppl 1):S2–S4.

86. Henry TR, Leppik IE, Gumnit RJ, Jacobs M. Progressive myoclonus epilepsy treated with zonisamide. *Neurology* 1988; 38:928–931.

87. Ohtahara S. Zonisamide in the management of epilepsy – Japanese experience. *Epilepsy Res* 2006; 68(Suppl 2):S25–S33.

88. Yagi K. Overview of Japanese experience-controlled and uncontrolled trials. *Seizure* 2004; 13(Suppl 1):S11–S15; discussion S16.

89. Arzimanoglou A, Rahbani A. Zonisamide for the treatment of epilepsy. *Expert Rev Neurother* 2006; 6:1283–1292.

90. Richards KC, Smith MC, Verma A. Continued use of zonisamide following development of renal calculi. *Neurology* 2005; 64:763–764.

91. Ryvlin P. Defining success in clinical trials – profiling pregabalin, the newest AED. *Eur J Neurol* 2005; 12(Suppl 4):12–21.

92. Ben-Menachem E. Pregabalin pharmacology and its relevance to clinical practice. *Epilepsia* 2004; 45(Suppl 6):13–18.

93. Elger CE, Brodie MJ, Anhut H, Lee CM, Barrett JA. Pregabalin add-on treatment in patients with partial seizures: a novel evaluation of flexible-dose and fixed-dose treatment in a double-blind, placebo-controlled study. *Epilepsia* 2005; 46:1926–1936.

94. Beydoun A, Uthman BM, Kugler AR, Greiner MJ, Knapp LE, Garofalo EA. Safety and efficacy of two pregabalin regimens for add-on treatment of partial epilepsy. *Neurology* 2005; 64:475–480.
95. Banin E, Shalev RS, Obolensky A, Neis R, Chowers I, Gross-Tsur V. Retinal function abnormalities in patients treated with vigabatrin. *Arch Ophthalmol* 2003; 121:811–816.
96. Remy C, Beaumont D. Efficacy and safety of vigabatrin in the long-term treatment of refractory epilepsy. *Br J Clin Pharmacol* 1989; 27(Suppl 1):S125–S129.
97. Kalviainen R, Aikia M, Saukkonen AM, Mervaala E, Riekkinen PJ Sr. Vigabatrin vs carbamazepine monotherapy in patients with newly diagnosed epilepsy. A randomized, controlled study. *Arch Neurol* 1995; 52:989–996.
98. Marciani MG, Maschio M, Spanedda F, Iani C, Gigli GL, Bernardi G. Development of myoclonus in patients with partial epilepsy during treatment with vigabatrin: an electroencephalographic study. *Acta Neurol Scand* 1995; 91:1–5.
99. Elterman RD, Shields WD, Mansfield KA, Nakagawa J. Randomized trial of vigabatrin in patients with infantile spasms. *Neurology* 2001; 57:1416–1421.
100. Appleton RE, Peters AC, Mumford JP, Shaw DE. Randomised, placebo-controlled study of vigabatrin as first-line treatment of infantile spasms. *Epilepsia* 1999; 40:1627–1633.
101. Vigabatrin: new indication. An advance in infantile spasms. *Prescrire Int* 1998; 7:43–44.
102. Richens A. Pharmacology and clinical pharmacology of vigabatrin. *J Child Neurol* 1991; Suppl 2:S7–S10.
103. Wheless JW, Ramsay RE, Collins SD. Vigabatrin. *Neurother* 2007; 4:163–172.
104. Ben-Menachem E. Vigabatrin. *Epilepsia* 1995; 36(Suppl 2):S95–S104.
105. Genton P, Gelisse P, Thomas P, Dravet C. Do carbamazepine and phenytoin aggravate juvenile myoclonic epilepsy? *Neurology* 2000; 55:1106–1109.
106. Gelisse P, Genton P, Kuate C, Pesenti A, Baldy-Moulinier M, Crespel A. Worsening of seizures by oxcarbazepine in juvenile idiopathic generalized epilepsies. *Epilepsia* 2004; 45:1282–1286.
107. Thomas P, Valton L, Genton P. Absence and myoclonic status epilepticus precipitated by antiepileptic drugs in idiopathic generalized epilepsy. *Brain* 2006; 129:1281–1292.
108. King MA, Newton MR, Jackson GD, Fitt GJ, Mitchell LA, Silvapulle MJ *et al.* Epileptology of the first-seizure presentation: a clinical, electroencephalographic, and magnetic resonance imaging study of 300 consecutive patients. *Lancet* 1998; 352:1007–1011.
109. Perucca E, Albani F, Capovilla G, Dalla Bernardina B, Michelucci R, Zaccara G. Recommendations of the Italian League Against Epilepsy. Working Group on Generic Products of Antiepileptic Drugs. *Epilepsia* 2006; 47:16–20.
110. Kanner AM, Frey M. Adding valproate to lamotrigine: a study of their pharmacokinetic interaction. *Neurology* 2000; 55:588–591.
111. Knowles SR, Shapiro LE, Shear NH. Anticonvulsant hypersensitivity syndrome: incidence, prevention and management. *Drug Saf* 1999; 21:489–501.
112. Beghi E, Gatti G, Tonini C, Ben-Menachem E, Chadwick DW, Nikanorova M *et al.* Adjunctive therapy versus alternative monotherapy in patients with partial epilepsy failing on a single drug: a multicentre, randomised, pragmatic controlled trial. *Epilepsy Res* 2003; 57:1–13.
113. Johannessen SI. Can pharmacokinetic variability be controlled for the patient's benefit? The place of TDM for new AEDs. *Ther Drug Monit* 2005; 27:710–713.
114. Biraben A, Beaussart M, Josien E, Pestre M, Savet JF, Schaff JL *et al.* Comparison of twice- and three times daily tiagabine for the adjunctive treatment of partial seizures in refractory patients with epilepsy: an open label, randomised, parallel-group study. *Epileptic Disord* 2001; 3:91–100.
115. Rowan AJ, Binnie CD, Warfield CA, Meinardi H, Meijer JW. The delayed effect of sodium valproate on the photoconvulsive response in man. *Epilepsia* 1979; 20:61–68.
116. Kasteleijn-Nolst Trenite DG, Marescaux C, Stodieck S, Edelbroek PM, Oosting J. Photosensitive epilepsy: a model to study the effects of antiepileptic drugs. Evaluation of the piracetam analogue, levetiracetam. *Epilepsy Res* 1996; 25:225–230.
117. French JA, Gidal BE. Antiepileptic drug interactions. *Epilepsia* 2000; 41(Suppl 8):S30–S36.

2

Overview of therapeutics in epilepsy: epilepsy surgery

Deana M. Gazzola, Chad Carlson, Philippe Ryvlin, Vijay M. Thadani, John Taylor, Sylvain Rheims

INTRODUCTION

Of the estimated 50–60 million individuals suffering from epilepsy worldwide, approximately 20–30% are medically refractory [1, 2]. For some in this population, epilepsy surgery is the best treatment option. The exact prevalence of surgical candidates is currently unknown but is thought to approximate 4.5% of all patients with epilepsy [3]. This would suggest that there are 2.3 million potential surgical candidates worldwide. Yet a 1996 retrospective analysis charted the number of epilepsy surgeries performed over the preceding decade at 100 of the most active epilepsy centres worldwide, and tallied only 3992 cases, suggesting surgery is under-utilized [4]. In addition, a recent study which analysed time to epilepsy surgery showed that a large number of patients have surgery 20 years or more after onset of epilepsy [5]. While this is at least partly due to delayed development of refractory seizures, other factors such as the fear of post-operative deficits, and the less than optimal rate of long-term post-operative seizure freedom (approximately 65% in temporal lobe epilepsy after 5 or more years), probably play a role [6].

It is the general sentiment of these authors that surgery should be considered early in the treatment of medically refractory patients. The reasons for this are multiple. Some studies suggest that a longer duration of epilepsy prior to surgery is associated with a lower chance of post-operative seizure freedom, although other studies have contradicted this point [7–9]. Another important consideration is the significant number of seizure-related deaths and injuries that could be avoided with earlier treatment.

In one study, the rate of death in chronic medically refractory patients was shown to be more than double that seen in age-matched controls [10]. The greatest mortality occurred

Deana M. Gazzola, MD, Assistant Professor, NYU Comprehensive Epilepsy Center, Department of Neurology, NYU School of Medicine, New York, USA

Chad Carlson, MD, Assistant Professor, NYU Comprehensive Epilepsy Center, New York, USA

Philippe Ryvlin, MD, PhD, Institut Des Epilepsies de l'Enfant et de l'adolescent, Hospices Civils de Lyon, Université Claude Bernard Lyon 1, Lyon, France

Vijay M. Thadani, MD, Section of Neurology, Dartmouth Hitchcock Medical Center/Dartmouth Medical School, Lebanon, New Hampshire, USA

John Taylor, DO, Section of Neurology, Dartmouth Hitchcock Medical Center/Dartmouth Medical School, Lebanon, New Hampshire, USA

Sylvain Rheims, MD, Institut Des Epilepsies de l'Enfant et de l'adolescent, Hospices Civils de Lyon, Université Claude Bernard Lyon 1, Lyon, France

in patients aged 30 years or younger. Sudden unexpected death in epilepsy (SUDEP) is one explanation for increased mortality in patients with epilepsy compared with the general population. In fact, it is the most common epilepsy-related cause of premature death [6]. The annual incidence of SUDEP ranges from 0 to 10 in 1000 patients, and the highest incidence is seen in surgical candidates [6].

GOALS OF SURGERY

The ultimate goal of epilepsy surgery is to improve both seizure control and patient quality of life. While there have not been many randomized controlled trials (RCTs) comparing medical management with surgical management due to ethical reasons, one head-to-head comparison performed in Canada did show significantly improved seizure control and quality of life in the surgical group compared with the medically managed group [11]. Unfortunately, there is currently a lack of evidence-based guidelines on how to approach the pre-surgical work-up. As a result, some of the recommendations presented in this chapter are based on opinion and personal practice style.

DEFINITION OF TERMS

Before proceeding, some terms should be defined. *Ictal focus* refers to the area of brain, either cortex or deeper structures, in which the ictal activity originates. *Epileptogenic zone* (EZ) refers to the minimum amount of brain tissue that should be resected to render the patient seizure free. This includes the ictal focus, as well as surrounding areas that generate interictal discharges (*irritative zone*) [3]. The term *lesional epilepsy* refers to epilepsy that can be attributed to a focal brain abnormality such as a tumour. The term *symptomatic epilepsy* is often used in conjunction with the term lesional as it implies the underlying lesion is causing the patient's symptoms. Appropriately, *non-lesional epilepsy* does not have a focal correlate visible on neuroimaging, although often one assumes there is an underlying microscopic abnormality not visible to the naked eye. These cases are often referred to as *cryptogenic*, as the aetiology and pathological process are unknown. *Extra-temporal* refers to ictal foci that originate in lobes other than the temporal lobe. And lastly, *neocortical* refers to ictal foci that originate in the hemispheric cortex in contrast to deeper, more *mesial* structures such as the hippocampus or amygdala. The latter two terms are often used in the setting of *temporal lobe epilepsy* (TLE).

THE PRE-SURGICAL WORK-UP

A very basic principle that remains to this day the cornerstone of epilepsy surgery is localization of the ictal focus, followed by complete resection of the EZ.

The advances in epilepsy surgery and its survival across the centuries are largely attributable to the deliberate and conscientious medical practices of its forefathers. The development of modern imaging and recording devices also greatly contributed to progress in the field. A formal process now exists when considering a patient for epilepsy surgery. The basic components of the pre-surgical evaluation, while not formally standardized across epilepsy centres, will be discussed below. A patient case, presented in parallel, will highlight a typical work-up in a stepwise fashion.

Patient AB is a 22-year-old male with a 14-year history of seizures. His outpatient neurologist has referred him to an epilepsy centre for pre-surgical evaluation. AB has tried and failed two anti-epileptic drugs (AEDs). His seizures occur once a month and he finds them disabling. He is currently unable to drive, and has recently lost his job. When asked about his seizures, he describes a 'strange noise' that he often hears 5–10s prior to seizure onset. After this, he believes he stares and has difficulty speaking. He cannot recall details because he has no recollection of his seizures.

PATIENT SELECTION

Certain criteria should be met when considering a patient for epilepsy surgery. Of course, the patient needs to understand the objective of the evaluation and should desire surgical treatment. The seizures generally should be perceived by the patient as disabling and have a negative impact on quality of life. Seizure frequency and severity, AED side-effects, impact on employment and finances, and the patient's subjective rating of disability all influence this assessment. However, one must also present a balanced, objective view of the surgical risk–benefit ratio to ensure that the patient has realistic expectations.

In general, the patient should have been tried on and failed two AEDs. Once a patient has failed two drugs, the likelihood of achieving sustained seizure freedom with any other medical treatment is less than 5% [12]. Therefore, waiting to consider surgery until more AEDs are exhausted is not necessary, so long as the AEDs were appropriately selected and managed.

Lastly, the patient's epilepsy syndrome should be appropriate for surgery. The most typical and appropriate candidate is the patient with localization-related partial epilepsy and a single ictal focus. Patients with other epilepsy types are potential surgical candidates, including multifocal epilepsies, particularly when one's goal is palliative treatment. Generally speaking, idiopathic primary generalized epilepsies do not make good surgical cases, although there are exceptions. Overall, the eligibility criteria required to enter a pre-surgical evaluation should be relatively liberal provided the patient is medically refractory and suffers from disabling seizures.

Based on the above criteria, AB could be a good surgical candidate. He is considered refractory as he has failed two AEDs, his seizures are probably partial onset given his associated aura and semiology, and he views them as disabling and desires surgery.

PRE-SURGICAL TESTING

The primary aim of the pre-surgical evaluation is to identify the EZ, which includes the ictal focus and any surrounding irritative zones. The identification of co-existing eloquent (functional) cortex is also essential. Some of these regions may overlap, and all figure into determining the extent of resection. Different modalities (scalp-electroencephalography, magnetoencephalography [MEG], subdural grids) may differ in the precise localization of the EZ. For this reason, rather than relying on one single method of analysis, findings from multiple modalities are compared and together used to identify the EZ. Some of these investigations can be considered mandatory parts of the pre-surgical evaluation, while others are used to provide additional information, particularly when localization is uncertain. The basic steps of the pre-surgical work-up, as well as the various investigatory tests, will be discussed below.

STEP ONE: HISTORY

A *detailed interview* of the patient and parents, relatives or friends who have witnessed the seizure is an important part of the pre-surgical evaluation. This interview should recapitulate all relevant past history and provide the most detailed description of the patient's seizure(s). Past history, particularly that pertaining to perinatal injury, febrile convulsions, meningitis or encephalitis, severe brain trauma, or any other cerebral insult will often provide some clues regarding aetiology and the prognosis of epilepsy surgery. For instance, a history of febrile seizures is frequently associated with a mesial temporal lobe focus, and these patients are often excellent surgical candidates [11, 13, 14]. Conversely, history of herpes virus encephalitis is more likely to result in bilateral or multi-focal epilepsy not amenable to successful surgical treatment.

Family history of epilepsy and other neurological disorders should also be ascertained. This information helps to identify specific syndromes such as autosomal dominant nocturnal frontal lobe epilepsy or a *forme fruste* of tuberous sclerosis.

One of the most reliable localizers of an ictal focus is a patient description of a stereotyped aura [15, 16]. For example, a rising epigastric sensation, déjà vu and a dreamy state strongly suggest seizure onset in the temporal lobe. However, one must remember one caveat: the aura might not indicate the area of initial seizure onset in all cases. Rather, in some situations these symptoms may occur after propagation of seizure activity from a clinically silent cortical area not readily detectable by surface electroencephalography. A description of what occurs during the seizure itself, the seizure semiology, along with a description of post-ictal language abilities can also assist with seizure lateralization. Descriptions of unilateral ictal motor manifestations can also be helpful but are, at times, misleading. The best semiological information comes from direct video-electroencephalography observations, as bystander and family reports may be contradictory, particularly with regard to the side of motor manifestation or head and eye deviation.

STEP TWO: PHYSICAL EXAMINATION

A *physical examination* may provide useful information, including subtle asymmetry of deep tendon reflexes or unilateral weakness, which could help to lateralize the seizure focus. In addition, certain skin abnormalities could suggest the presence of an underlying cortical malformation disorder such as tuberous sclerosis.

> More history is gathered from family members present at the appointment. AB's seizures begin with behavioural and speech arrest, during which he stares quietly. He then remains non-verbal and unresponsive. No automatisms are noted. He is always confused post-ictally, with garbled speech, but returns to baseline after 15 minutes. Every 2–3 months he has a generalized convulsion. He has no known epilepsy risk factors, no known family history of epilepsy, and he is otherwise healthy. His physical examination is completely normal. The semiological description of behavioural arrest and language impairment suggests that AB's seizures lateralize to the left hemisphere and might localize to the temporal region. The auditory aura he experiences suggests the seizures are neocortical in origin. Aetiology remains unknown.

STEP THREE: MANDATORY INVESTIGATIONS

The following are considered *mandatory investigations* at most major epilepsy centres, and each will be discussed separately.

Magnetic Resonance Imaging

High-resolution magnetic resonance imaging (MRI) can be very helpful in detecting epileptogenic structural lesions. According to the American Academy of Neurology guidelines for evaluation of a first unprovoked seizure, brain imaging with computerized tomography (CT) or MRI is recommended and was given a Level B classification [17]. Of course, the EZ might extend beyond the visible region of abnormality. The quality of the MRI has a major impact on its sensitivity, and should be performed using an 'epilepsy protocol'. This protocol uses thin-slice thickness through the temporal lobes in the coronal plane. MRI performed using an epilepsy protocol and reviewed by neuroradiologists with expertise in the field of epilepsy surgery has the highest detection rate of underlying epileptogenic structural abnormalities [18]. Certain sequences should also be performed: three-dimensional T1-weighted images as well as T2 and fluid-attenuated inversion recovery (FLAIR) sequences are essential and standard; gradient echo sequences can detect small cavernomas [19, 20]; and gadolinium should be used when a tumour is suspected.

With increasing magnet strength, improved identification of pathology has been observed. A recent prospective study showed that experienced review of 3-tesla MRI studies resulted in the detection of new lesions in 65% of previously MRI-negative studies [21]. This is significant because multiple studies have shown that patients with a detectable focal lesion on neuroimaging are more likely to be seizure free post-surgically compared with those who have negative imaging [22, 23].

A number of non-conventional MRI sequences and data analysis have also been used in patients with seemingly cryptogenic refractory partial epilepsy, including double inversion recovery, magnetization transfer ratio, T2-mapping, fast FLAIR-based T2 measurement and voxel-based morphometry [24–27]. Most of these techniques do not readily detect focal abnormalities on initial visual analysis and require the use of statistical parametric mapping to demonstrate significant findings. Their clinical utility is currently unknown and their use is largely investigational at this time.

Electroencephalography

Interictal electroencephalography recordings often demonstrate epileptiform discharges in patients with refractory epilepsy. Interictal discharges provide important information for lateralization and localization of the seizure focus, although in a minority of cases they can be falsely localizing. In TLE, the presence of unilateral anterior temporal spikes is a strong predictor of post-operative seizure freedom [28, 29]. In contrast, bitemporal spikes are associated with poorer prognosis, although they do not preclude a successful outcome so long as they occur predominantly on the side to be resected [30]. Resection of a focal epileptogenic brain lesion in infants and children with multi-focal or generalized epileptiform discharges can result in seizure freedom and overall improvement [31]. A similar positive outcome can be seen in patients with tuberous sclerosis [32, 33]. In addition, specific electroencephalogram (EEG) patterns can provide clues about pathology. For example, focal fast rhythmic epileptiform discharges on surface EEG are associated with focal cortical dysplasias [34].

AB had a brain MRI with epilepsy protocol performed, the results of which were normal. A routine EEG showed mild focal slowing in the left temporal region, which suggests the presence of focal cortical dysfunction.

Video-electroencephalography Monitoring

Prolonged video-electroencephalography monitoring, in the majority of surgical candidates, plays an essential role in the pre-surgical evaluation. An optimal session should capture several of the patient's typical seizures. The video recording, along with direct observation by the nurse and/or physician during the seizure, can allow improved characterization of the seizure semiology. Post-ictal deficits, such as the Todd's phenomenon, can also be characterized in the inpatient setting, allowing for improved localization and lateralization.

The typical admission varies from several days to several weeks, largely dependent on how quickly the patient has several seizures for characterization. The number of seizures required depends on the number of distinct seizure types the patient has and how easily these are localized and lateralized upon review. Patients with unilateral interictal spikes and a single seizure type may require two or three seizures, whereas patients with multi-focal discharges and multiple distinct seizure types may require two or three seizures of each type. In order to facilitate rapid, but safe, capture of seizures, the patient's AEDs are weaned off after admission. Provocation techniques such as sleep deprivation, exercise, photic stimulation and hyperventilation can be employed to further increase the likelihood of capturing seizures. Seizure precautions are enforced in the epilepsy monitoring unit, particularly for patients on reduced or discontinued medications.

Ictal EEG often provides valuable lateralizing and localizing information in TLE, although results can be variable with extra-temporal seizures [35]. Characterization of the earliest ictal rhythms associated with the seizure identifies the ictal onset zone. In some patients, the ictal onset is seen following clear behavioural changes, demonstrating that the ictal onset was not captured on scalp EEG. In other patients, the ictal onset is characterized by a bilateral pattern and lateralization is not possible. Patients with prominent motor manifestations may have muscle and/or movement artefacts which confound lateralization. In these poorly localized or lateralized cases, invasive intracranial monitoring may be necessary.

AB undergoes prolonged video-electroencephalography monitoring. After 2 days of monitoring, intermittent spikes with a broad field, covering the left anterior temporal, left mid-temporal, and left parasagittal regions are seen. The highest spike amplitude occurs in the mid-temporal region. He has two typical complex partial seizures, electrographically characterized by rhythmic delta and theta activity over the left temporal and parasagittal regions (Figure 2.1). Based on these findings, AB's seizures clearly lateralize to the left hemisphere. The EZ likely localizes to the left temporal lobe, considering the seizure semiology and amplitude of the interictal discharges. However, the broad field of the interictal discharges, coupled with the ictal pattern which involves the parasagittal region, suggests a more extensive EZ.

Neuropsychological Testing

A comprehensive cognitive and psychiatric evaluation is an important part of the pre-surgical evaluation. For instance, verbal memory impairment is often seen in the setting of left TLE, and findings on neuropsychological testing can help to lateralize and localize the EZ. The predictive value for lateralization and localization of the epileptogenic focus depends, at least in part, on the criteria utilized and the measures employed. When combined with other modalities such as electroencephalography and MRI, neuropsychological testing has been shown to slightly increase the rate of correct EZ lateralization from 93% to 95% [36].

In addition, neuropsychological testing can be used to predict post-surgical verbal memory function, although findings have been somewhat controversial. Previous findings have suggested that patients with left mesial temporal sclerosis (MTS) are at low risk for

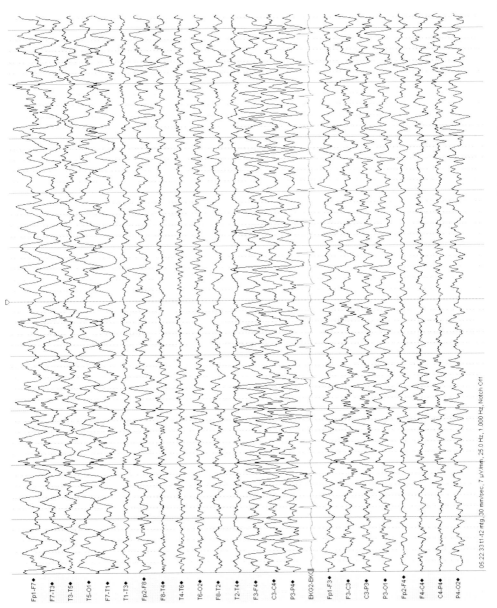

Figure 2.1 Electroencephalogram of Patient AB exhibiting rhythmic sharply contoured delta and theta activity over the left temporal and parasagittal areas.

developing worsened verbal memory impairment following dominant left anterior temporal lobectomy (ATL) [37]. However, more recent findings suggest that normal baseline verbal memory function prior to ATL, or selective amygdalo-hippocampectomy, might actually increase the risk of post-surgical deterioration in MTS patients [38, 39].

Psychiatric Issues

Overall, the prevalence of psychiatric disorders in patients referred for epilepsy surgery is high [40, 41]. One study analysed psychopathology in patients prior to and following ATL [40]. A DSM-IIIR diagnosis (depression, anxiety and organic/personality disorder being most common) was present in 65% of patients before surgery. New psychiatric problems arose in 31% of patients in the months following surgery; however, in the group as a whole the severity of psychiatric symptoms was lower 6 months post-operatively compared with baseline [40]. Another multicentre study analysed pre- and post-operative results of patients' Beck Psychiatric Symptoms Scales, and found significant improvement in patient depression and anxiety scores post-surgically [42]. This was particularly true for those patients who became seizure free. These findings suggest that ATL is associated with some positive effect on neuropsychological function.

Psychiatric disorders do not preclude a patient from epilepsy surgery, as illustrated by one study of US veterans demonstrating uniform post-surgical results in patients with and without psychiatric illness, although larger studies are needed [43]. Patients with baseline psychopathology can benefit from psychological surveillance, monitoring for any decline or improvement in function post-operatively. Early psychiatric evaluation can also help to identify patients who are at risk for post-ictal psychosis, which can be difficult to manage. Such patients can be placed on anti-psychotic medication prophylactically when admitted for video-electroencephalography.

Intracarotid Amytal (Wada) Test

The intracarotid amytal or Wada test is used to determine language lateralization and assess memory function prior to surgery [44]. The Wada is performed by placing a catheter in the femoral artery and advancing it to the internal carotid artery (ICA). An anaesthetic agent (most commonly amobarbital) is injected to anaesthetize one cerebral hemisphere and assess function of the contralateral, non-anaesthetized hemisphere. The exact paradigm for testing varies from centre to centre. Many centres utilize clinical criteria (e.g. contralateral hemiplegia) for establishing an adequate injection whereas others will utilize a combination of clinical testing and continuous EEG. Assessment of both language and memory also varies amongst centres. Most paradigms involve presentation of a series of pictures, objects or words during hemispheric anaesthesia followed by recall and recognition testing after a complete return to baseline [45].

The Wada remains the gold standard in determining language and memory laterality. Studies have found that patients with a hemispheric memory deficit ipsilateral to the seizure focus on the Wada have an increased probability of being seizure free post-surgically [46]. However, there are risks associated with the test, including carotid dissection (0.7%), cerebral infarction, arterial spasm with potential transient deficits and transient femoral neuropathy [45, 47]. The Wada is also limited by other factors. Testing procedures are not standardized, making it difficult to compare test results from one epilepsy centre to another. Variation in patient vascular anatomy and cross-filling patterns can lead to misinterpretation of results, thus cerebral angiography is routinely performed prior to injection of anaesthetic [48]. Likewise, insufficient administration of anaesthetic can give falsely lateralizing results. Lastly, the limited supply of amobarbital and the invasive nature of the test make the Wada costly and inefficient.

Alternatives to the Wada Test

Because of these associated risks and limitations, alternative methods to determine language dominance are being investigated, some of which include MEG, functional MRI (fMRI) and repetitive transcranial magnetic stimulation [43, 49–51]. More study and refinement of the latter techniques, however, will be needed before they can supplant the Wada.

AB undergoes a neuropsychological assessment, which reveals normal general cognitive ability (full scale intelligence quotient [IQ] = 104), with mild verbal memory impairment. He also has a Wada test which lateralizes language to the left hemisphere. On testing of left-hemispheric memory (right ICA injection), AB correctly recalls 11 out of 12 objects, and on right-hemispheric testing (left ICA injection), he correctly recalls 12 out of 12 objects. Memory is equally good bilaterally, suggesting AB could have memory impairment following unilateral ATL if hippocampectomy is included. The finding of intact memory function bilaterally also supports the notion of a neocortical focus. Neuropsychological testing reveals mildly impaired verbal (but not visual) memory, which would suggest mild dysfunction of the left temporal region.

STEP FOUR: MULTI-DISCIPLINARY CONFERENCE

Before proceeding any further, most major epilepsy centres will have a multi-disciplinary conference (MDC), during which all of the pre-surgical data is reviewed. Experts from all disciplines attend, including epilepsy, neurosurgery, neuroradiology and neuropsychology. The purpose of the MDC is to review, in a uniform setting, all clinical, radiological and electrophysiological data pertaining to the patient's epilepsy. Following this review, the group makes a recommendation on the surgical treatment option(s) available, which the primary epileptologist and neurosurgeon will discuss with the patient. In addition, non-surgical options and further diagnostic testing are recommended for some patients.

AB is presented at the MDC. It is the consensus of the group that his seizure focus lateralizes to the left hemisphere, and likely localizes to the left temporal neocortex based on semiology and the Wada results. However, the broad field of interictal discharges and early ictal involvement of the parasagittal region raises the possibility of more extensive cortical involvement. In addition, AB's Wada test suggests he is left language dominant. It is recommended that AB have a supplemental test such as an MEG to help better localize the EZ, and then undergo invasive intracranial monitoring during which language mapping can be performed. These steps are discussed in detail below.

STEP FIVE: ADDITIONAL INVESTIGATIONS

Additional investigations are typically performed when scalp video-electroencephalography monitoring is unable to lateralize or well-localize the EZ. If the patient requires more invasive intracranial monitoring, these studies are performed prior to implantation to help guide subdural electrode placement.

Magnetoencephalography

Magnetoencephalography (MEG) is a relatively new imaging modality used at select epilepsy centres. It measures magnetic fields generated by electrical dipoles tangentially oriented to the cortical surface.

Numerous studies have identified an excellent correlation between MEG localizations and seizure onsets. A prospective study involving 49 patients comparing magnetic source imaging (MSI) and the intracranial EEG in epilepsy surgery identified a positive predictive value of the MSI for seizure localization of 82%. When comparison included surgical outcome, the positive predictive value was 90% [52].

In addition to epileptogenic foci, MEG can also localize sensory cortex, motor cortex, visual cortex and map language function. This information can be of great importance when trying to anticipate deficits from a proposed resection, and can be used as an adjunct to invasive cortical mapping.

Functional Neuroimaging

There are limited useful data on the different modalities used in functional neuroimaging. The studies that have analysed these modalities are quite heterogeneous, leading one group to recommend that formal RCTs be performed to assess utility [53]. Because of the complexity of functional neuroimaging studies, they are often compared with findings on MRI. In patients with normal brain MRIs, functional neuroimaging might reveal abnormalities, although there is a possibility that these could be falsely localizing. As a result, functional neuroimaging tends to be reserved for those patients with unknown EZ localization.

Positron emission tomography (PET) has utilized several types of ligands over the last 25 years, the most common being [18F]-fluorodeoxyglucose (FDG). Brain accumulation of FDG reflects regional glucose metabolism. Focal hypometabolism on FDG-PET has been shown to correlate with seizure foci [54]. In contrast, epileptogenic tubers have demonstrated increased uptake of α-methyl-L-tryptophan [55]. A meta-analysis was performed by Willmann *et al.* [56] to determine whether findings on PET had any value in predicting post-surgical outcome in TLE cases. They found that ipsilateral PET hypometabolism was associated with good surgical outcome (positive predictive value of 86%) [56]. However, in patients with a normal MRI scan, the predictive value for good outcome was 80%, and in patients with non-localizing ictal scalp-electroencephalography, predictive value was only 72% [56]. One can conclude that the presence of ipsilateral PET hypometabolism may predict good post-surgical outcome in refractory TLE cases, but does not add diagnostic value when the EZ is already localized by ictal scalp-electroencephalography [56].

For an *ictal single photon emission computer tomography* (SPECT), the patient is injected with a radioactive tracer during a seizure. The best imaging is obtained when the injection is made within seconds of seizure onset. Ictal SPECT typically demonstrates focal hyperperfusion in brain regions involved in seizure activity. Temporal and extra-temporal seizure foci with or without structural lesions can be identified and confirmed with intracranial electroencephalography (iEEG) studies, and when the findings on ictal SPECT and iEEG are concordant, there is a greater chance of a positive surgical outcome [57]. Ictal SPECT imaging can be further enhanced by performing computerized subtraction of interictal findings from ictal findings, and co-registering on MRI (SISCOM). SISCOM may be most helpful in those patients who suffer from focal epilepsy but have normal MRI findings, and in those patients with extensive focal cortical dysplasia [58, 59]. However, if one considers intracranial electroencephalography the gold standard, ictal SPECT can give misleading information. In one study, ictal SPECT incorrectly lateralized the EZ in 25% of cases, and in an additional 13% of cases, localization was incorrect [57].

Functional MRI (fMRI) relies on the principle that increased neuronal activity is associated with regional increases in cerebral blood flow [60]. There is a relative increase in the ratio of oxygenated to deoxygenated blood, which results in a change in MRI signal [60]. Employing these principles, fMRI can localize motor, sensory and language cortex. It can anatomically localize cortical speech regions such as Broca's and Wernicke's areas [61]. Functional MRI is also a promising technique for predicting outcome in post-surgical patients [62]. Overall, fMRI is viewed as a reliable technique for lateralization and localization of language function [60], and serves as a good adjunct in the pre-surgical evaluation.

Magnetic resonance spectroscopy measures the relative amounts of N-acetyl aspartate (NAA), choline and creatine present in different regions of the brain and expresses the values as ratios. NAA is a neuronal compound that is reduced in gliotic scars, and choline and creatine are found in glia. Abnormal NAA:choline and NAA:creatine ratios are also associated with regions of abnormal metabolism and MTS, and have been shown to correlate with epileptogenic foci. In one study, magnetic resonance spectroscopy imaging localized the EZ to the correct lobe (as defined by surface electroencephalography) in 65% of patients with neocortical epilepsy [63].

AB undergoes an MEG study, the results of which are presented in Figure 2.2. A single population of interictal epileptiform discharges is detected in the left anterior temporal lobe. This finding suggests that AB's epileptogenic zone is primarily localized to the left anterior temporal lobe, and is less likely to extend extra-temporally. Subdural implantation will be focused on the anterior temporal region using a grid, with additional extra-temporal coverage of the parasagittal region using subdural strips. Depth electrodes will also be placed in the left hippocampus to evaluate the pattern of ictal spread.

STEP SIX: INTRACRANIAL ELECTROENCEPHALOGRAPHY

There are no set criteria used to decide whether or not invasive recordings should be performed, and in many cases it is not considered mandatory. In general, extra-temporal cases are implanted with intracranial electrodes more frequently than temporal lobe cases. Localization of the EZ can be determined in approximately 70–80% of implanted patients with extra-temporal epilepsy [35]. In the case of AB above, the presence of a broader ictal onset on video-electroencephalography, ipsilateral hemispheric language dominance and no memory asymmetry on Wada memory testing make the use of intracranial electrodes

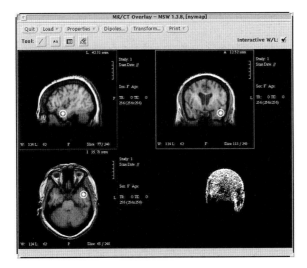

Figure 2.2 Magnetic source image of Patient AB, illustrating the single population of interictal discharges in the left anterior temporal region (circled white dots).

an important part of diagnosis. When proceeding with intracranial monitoring, the precise site of the epileptogenic focus is usually uncertain. As a result, considerable thought and planning are required prior to implantation, aiming for optimal yield in data, while putting the patient at the most minimal risk possible.

Invasive recordings with subdural electrodes are extremely helpful in accurately localizing cortical surface epileptogenic regions [64]. Most major epilepsy centres in North America use grids, strips and depth electrodes, or a combination thereof. The extent to which the brain is covered by electrodes varies by case. For example, if one cannot lateralize the seizure focus prior to implantation then a liberal and symmetric array of electrode coverage should be used. Often bilateral strip placement is performed in this setting, as shown in Figure 2.3. Conversely, a subdural grid is typically placed when the EZ has already been lateralized and partially localized, as the grid's design focuses a high density of electrodes over a particular region of interest. For example, if one is certain the seizure focus localizes to right frontal neocortex, a selective grid can be used to further define the EZ (Figure 2.4). Strips can be added to extend coverage to other suspicious cortical areas, or to cover less accessible regions such as interhemispheric or subtemporal cortex. Grids can also be used to map motor, sensory, language and visual cortical function, thus avoiding excision of eloquent cortex [64].

Subdural electrodes placed on the cortical surface may not correctly localize epileptiform activity arising from deeper generators such as the hippocampus [65, 66]. This limitation is partly overcome by using intracerebral depth electrodes, which have the ability to sample deep areas of the brain [65, 67]. Depth electrodes can also be placed intralesionally, such as in a tuber, to help identify the ictal generator [64, 68].

Major complications of intracranial EEG include infection, haematoma, transient neurological deficits and herniation from cerebral oedema, but the rate of occurrence is low, at 1–2% [37]. More minor post-operative morbidities include headache, nausea, vomiting, fever and meningismus. Some centres use steroids to avoid post-operative morbidity; however, this is a controversial topic [69, 70].

AB undergoes intracranial implantation as planned. Interictal discharges were most frequently seen in the grid region covering the anterior temporal lobe. Three typical seizures were recorded, all emanating from four grid electrodes covering the left anterior temporal lobe, shown in Figure 2.5. Ictal activity progressed to the left hippocampal depth electrodes after 15 s. Language mapping was performed, demarcating the areas of language function, which were posterior and inferior to the region of ictal onset. A tailored resection of the left anterior temporal lobe was performed. Considering the slow progression to the hippocampus and the patient's preserved memory function ipsilateral to the lesion, the amygdala and hippocampus were not resected. Following surgery, AB was seizure free and had no deficits. Pathology results demonstrated microscopic focal cortical dysplasia. This case illustrates the utility of intracranial monitoring. Mapping of language, sensory, motor and even visual function enables individualized tailored resections to be performed in patients, avoiding post-surgical deficits.

The basic steps of a pre-surgical evaluation, as discussed in the preceding sections of this chapter, are illustrated in a flow diagram in Figure 2.6 for the reader's convenience and reference. The next section of this chapter will cover different types of epilepsy surgery.

EPILEPSY SURGERY

Each of the major categories of epilepsy surgery will be discussed in detail in this section. We will begin with the most common surgical epilepsy diagnosis, TLE, which was illustrated by the case of AB.

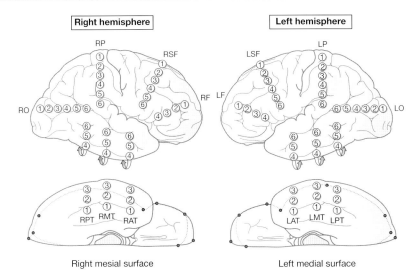

Figure 2.3 Illustration of a typical bilateral subdural strip array. LAT, left anterior temporal; LMT, left medial temporal; LPT, left posterior temporal; LO, left occipital; LP, left parietal; LSF, left superior frontal; LF, left frontal; RAT, right anterior temporal; RMT, right medial temporal; RPT, right posterior temporal; RF, right frontal; RSF, right superior frontal; RP, right parietal; RO, right occipital. The temporal electrodes fold under the temporal lobe and are continued on the mesial surface.

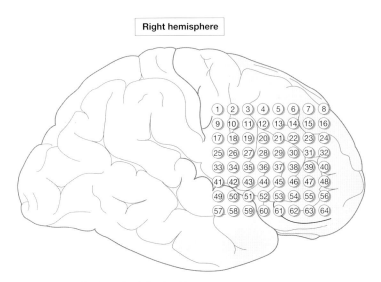

Figure 2.4 Illustration of a right frontal subdural grid.

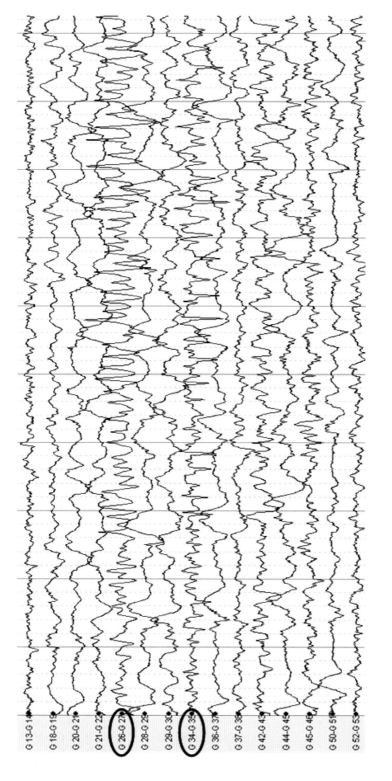

Figure 2.5 Portion of Patient AB's intracranial tracing, which focuses on the grid electrodes. Ictal onset is seen to occur primarily in four grid electrodes (G26, G27, G34 and G35), which are circled above. These electrodes were anatomically grouped and positioned over the anterior temporal region, posterior and inferior to eloquent language cortex.

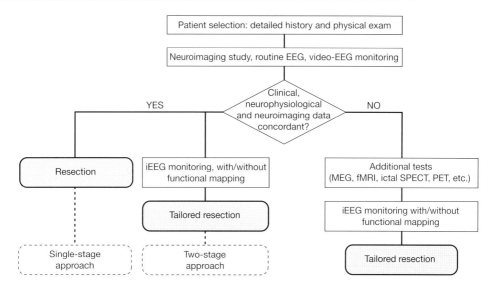

Figure 2.6 Flow chart illustrating the progression through a standard pre-surgical evaluation. First, one uses patient history and epilepsy classification to select proper candidates. Second, neuroimaging studies, routine electroencephalography and video-electroencephalography monitoring are performed. At this point, a decision is made on how to proceed based on the concordance of the data. There are three options. If data are concordant, one can proceed with either a single-stage resection or, alternatively, intracranial electroencephalography (iEEG) monitoring followed by tailored resection (two-stage surgery). If data are not concordant, additional testing can be performed and then followed by iEEG monitoring and tailored resection if appropriate.

TEMPORAL LOBE SURGERY

TLE is the most common surgical epilepsy diagnosis, and is secondary to various underlying pathologies. There are two major types of TLE: mesial (which is most commonly associated with hippocampal sclerosis) and neocortical. The surgical approach to both types of TLE is usually identical, involving a standard ATL with amygdalo-hippocampectomy (AH). When there is high risk of memory impairment, the mesial structures can be spared. Some centres advocate an isolated AH instead of the standard ATL. However, the two resections usually accompany one another, based on the reasoning that over years of seizure activity, neural networks develop between cortex and hippocampus. These networks serve little function other than ictal genesis, therefore the entire unit (ATL and AH) is removed.

The different types of TLE will be discussed below.

Mesial Temporal Lobe Epilepsy

The typical seizure localizing to the mesial temporal lobe has a characteristic semiology and electrographic pattern. The patient often describes an aura characterized by autonomic features, such as a rising epigastric sensation, a flushed feeling, tachycardia or diaphoresis. The patient may stare quietly, have oral and hand automatisms, and may have dystonic posturing of an extremity. Some patients may attempt to interact with their environment, albeit inappropriately. Electrographically, classically, one sees a pattern of sharply contoured rhythmic theta activity during ictus.

Patients with mesial temporal lobe epilepsy (mTLE) can often undergo single-stage temporal resections without intracranial monitoring. Stereotactic radiosurgery using a gamma knife is an alternative to the conventional ATL with AH for the treatment of mTLE.

Focal radiation of hippocampal seizure focus has led to remission in some cases, and one can avoid a craniotomy. However, the long-term results are at present uncertain, and seizure cessation is not instantaneous. Rather, seizures wind down over a period of months [71].

Neocortical Temporal Lobe Epilepsy

Semiologically, patient auras often involve lateral cortical regions resulting in auditory or psychic phenomena. As in mTLE, oral and hand automatisms can be seen. Semiologically, neocortical TLE seizures are often fairly bland in nature, and it is often only after ictal activity has spread to other regions that symptoms develop [72]. Post-ictally the patient is confused, perhaps with impairment of language function depending on hemispheric dominance. The aetiology of neocortical TLE can be secondary to focal cortical dysplasia, trauma or tumours, but it is frequently cryptogenic in nature with normal neuroimaging. Compared with mTLE, electrographic findings in neocortical cases are more abundant, with increased incidence of epileptiform activity and ipsilateral slow waves [72]. There is sometimes still a need for invasive monitoring due to poor localization on surface electroencephalography. In addition, the use of a staged invasive approach with cortical mapping may be utilized due to the proximity of the EZ to language cortex.

'Other' TLE Syndromes

There are certain TLE syndromes which prove a challenge in seizure focus localization. These include:

(i)   Bilateral TLE. Seizures recorded on surface electroencephalography arise independently from left and right temporal lobes. In one study, bilateral interictal temporal spikes were detected in up to 42% of patients with unilateral hippocampal sclerosis [73]. These patients may be surgical candidates, but require invasive monitoring using bilateral hippocampal depth electrodes and subdural strips. It is essential to determine whether the patient has independent seizures arising from both temporal lobes, or simply has bilateral interictal discharges with unilateral seizure onset. If independent bitemporal onset is confirmed, the chance of complete seizure freedom is low, but seizure reduction is possible.
(ii) 'Pseudo-temporal' lobe epilepsy. Interictal discharges appear to arise from the temporal lobe but actually come from other regions with atypically oriented dipoles.
(iii) 'Temporal plus' seizures. The ictal focus involves a complex epileptogenic network beyond the limits of the temporal lobe, possibly involving neighbouring structures [74]. It has been shown that epilepsy patients with temporal plus seizures are less likely to become seizure free following a simple ATL, but have better outcomes when an ATL is performed with additional extra-temporal resection [74].

TLE Surgical Outcomes

Generally speaking, long-term seizure remission is greater in patients with TLE compared with non-TLE (extra-temporal) surgical groups, with seizure-free rates consistently ranging from 50% to 70% [75–77].

In addition, the type of TLE probably plays a role in outcome. Some studies have compared mTLE outcomes with neocortical TLE outcomes. While some have shown no difference between the two groups [78–80], other studies have documented a more favourable 1-year post-operative outcome in patients with mTLE vs. neocortical TLE [81]. The presence of hippocampal sclerosis on MRI and the absence of generalized seizures seem to correlate with good 2-year post-operative outcomes in patients with mTLE [80].

While seizure frequency is an important indicator of surgical success, quality of life is the outcome ultimately impacted and hopefully improved. Post-operative seizure control and quality of life tend to be better in patients younger than 45 years compared with older patients [82, 83]. In addition, older age at surgery seems predictive of a stronger decline in verbal memory following dominant hemisphere surgery [39]. The risks of major complications of surgery might also be higher in patients older than 35 years of age [84].

EXTRA-TEMPORAL SURGERY

The delineation of the extra-temporal ictal focus can be challenging. Scalp-electroencephalography is often non-localizing and at times falsely localizes the ictal focus [85]. As a result, intracranial electroencephalography monitoring is usually necessary, after which focal tailored resections are performed based on localization of the EZ and functional mapping results.

Extra-temporal epilepsy is commonly divided into two subgroups: lesional and non-lesional. Each differs in surgical approach and carries its own prognosis.

Extra-temporal Epilepsy: Symptomatic, Lesional

Symptomatic, lesional cases of extra-temporal epilepsy are often associated with better outcome and tend to be more amenable to surgery compared with non-lesional cases, although the underlying nature of the lesion is an important variable. The complete removal of a well-delineated lesion can be effective treatment provided there is good concordance between the site of the lesion, the clinical semiology of the seizures and the electrophysiological data. A complete lesionectomy, which includes resection of margins, has a higher chance of achieving seizure freedom post-operatively [35]. Partial lesionectomy is less likely to result in seizure freedom [86]. Always of major concern is whether surgery can be performed without causing significant neurological deficits. A post-operative deficit is deemed acceptable in some cases, such as when there is a significant baseline impairment caused by the lesion; the patient is willing to risk a minor deficit such as sensory loss as a trade-off for better seizure control; or surgery is being performed as an extraordinary measure in a declining patient. It is important to maintain an open dialogue during all phases of the pre-surgical evaluation to ensure the patient fully understands both the potentially positive and negative outcomes of surgery.

Intracranial EEG may be required to define the border and localization of the EZ in relation to the lesion, and to define surrounding eloquent cortex. A large proportion of patients with cortical malformations have foci in the frontal or peri-rolandic regions, and the epileptogenic area is frequently larger than the visually identified lesion. The decision to perform invasive monitoring in lesional cases should be based on the anatomy, electrophysiology and clinical data, with an understanding of the limitations and risks of the evaluation.

Extra-temporal Epilepsy: Cryptogenic, Non-Lesional

Extra-temporal non-lesional epilepsy can be quite challenging to treat surgically. With respect to seizure focus localization, the use of intracranial electroencephalography is often critical. Electrode placement is typically guided by the ictal semiology, scalp-electroencephalography interictal and ictal patterns, and data from other investigations such as MEG. The likelihood of achieving seizure freedom following focal resection is somewhat lower if imaging is normal [23]. Despite these challenges, good results are attainable, making surgical treatment worthwhile for many patients.

PALLIATIVE SURGERY

Corpus Callosotomy

In some cases, the seizure focus is unable to be localized or is deemed unresectable due to the presence of bilateral or broad hemispheric discharges, or proximity to eloquent cortex. In these situations, and in those cases where the seizure exhibits rapid contralateral spread, a corpus callosotomy can be considered. Callosotomy often prevents secondary generalization of focal seizures, and can be successfully used to prevent drop attacks [87].

Callosotomy can be performed by completely severing the corpus callosum, or by sectioning only the anterior two-thirds. Transient disturbances of language, as well as disturbances of coordination on one side of the body are not uncommon post-operative complications. It is standard thinking that complete resection is more likely to result in dysfunction. As a result, the convention at many epilepsy centres is to perform an initial anterior division of the callosum. If necessary, the remaining posterior one-third may be divided; however, the morbidity associated with a second surgery concerns many neurosurgeons [88].

FUTURE DIRECTIONS IN EPILEPSY THERAPY

Chronic electrical stimulation of the cerebellum was attempted over 40 years ago as a treatment for epilepsy. More recently, chronic deep brain stimulation of the anterior nucleus of the thalamus and the subthalamic nucleus has been used in both focal and generalized forms of epilepsy. Most methods have involved continuous or intermittent stimulation, regardless of the presence or absence of ictal activity (open-loop systems). Research is currently focused on the development of an intelligent, closed-loop device that can detect seizure onset and then deliver counter-shock discharges. Preliminary studies have shown that such a device is feasible and potentially beneficial [89]. The NeuroPace Responsive Neurostimulator system™ is one such closed-loop neurostimulator [90, 91]. The device demonstrated excellent safety and tolerability in a recent feasibility trial, and there was preliminary evidence of efficacy [91]. A randomized, double-blinded, multicentre clinical trial was recently completed, the results of which were pending prior to this chapter's publication [91].

The major advantage of stimulating devices over resection is the potential to spare eloquent cortex. They are not without their own risk, however. Deep brain stimulation is associated with a 5% risk of complication, primarily infection and haemorrhage [92]. Another innovative alternative to implantable neurostimulators is intracranial drug delivery, a process currently undergoing development. Using a neuroprosthesis to deliver γ-aminobutyric acid (GABA) epidurally in rats, John et al. [93] have been able to terminate ictal activity, although large amounts of γ-aminobutyric acid were required. Similar results were obtained when utilizing the AED pentobarbital [94]. Such results are promising, and projects aimed at developing a device for use in human subjects are currently under way.

SURGICAL RISK, COMPLICATIONS AND BENEFITS

Unfortunately, many patients receive misinformation about the dangers of epilepsy surgery, dissuading them from seeking evaluation. In actuality, the death rate from epilepsy surgery is about 1%, with anterior temporal lobectomy having a lower mortality (<1%) than hemispherectomy [95]. In a recent report by Engel et al. [77], 2 out of 556 patients (0.4%) from seven centres died within a month of surgery, but deaths were unrelated to the surgical procedure. The risk of death related to surgery is likely to be lower than that related to sudden unexpected death in epilepsy (SUDEP), which is estimated to be 0.35 to 4.5 per 1000 patient years, depending on patient profile [96]. One could therefore argue that the risk of surgery is less than the risk of continued, medically refractory epilepsy. Beyond overt mortality, continued seizures have been associated with cognitive decline over time in TLE [97].

Potential surgical complications include infection, cerebral haemorrhage, subdural haematoma and neurological deficits. There is also evidence that epilepsy surgery can precipitate psychiatric disturbances and worsen anxiety and depression in some patients [77]. However, other contradictory findings have documented a post-operative improvement in depression, suggesting that more research in this area is needed [42]. One large literature review was performed by the Quality Standards Subcommittee of the American Academy of Neurology in 2003 [77], and assessed the overall outcome of epilepsy surgery. Surgical complications were tallied in a total of 556 patients from seven centres. A total of 6% of patients experienced neurological deficits (3% transient and 3% permanent) [77]. Post-operative infections were documented in 5% of patients, and hydrocephalus was described in three cases of large resections. A separate series of three papers which included 219 patients discussed post-operative cognitive and behavioural changes [77, 98–100]. Disturbances were described in 6% of patients and were transient in at least 3% and predominantly related to persistence of seizures [77, 98–100]. Ultimately, the risk of morbidity in epilepsy surgery depends on the specifics of the particular surgery planned for each patient. Risks cannot be realistically estimated until the results of EEG monitoring, neuroimaging and neuropsychological testing are known.

In chronically refractory patients who do not undergo surgery, only 5–14% will achieve seizure remission [101]. Epilepsy surgery offers a better chance of obtaining seizure freedom in many cases, and in the aforementioned Engel *et al.* study [77] seizure reduction correlated with improved quality of life. In one Class I trial, patients who underwent surgery had improved quality of life after 1 year compared with patients who were treated with medication alone [77]. A trend towards better social function was also seen in patients in the Class I trial, and in several Class IV trials (evidence from uncontrolled studies, case series, case reports or expert opinion), with improvement in employment and activities of daily living [77]. Lastly, there is an overall reduction of long-term medical costs for patients who undergo epilepsy surgery [102].

CONCLUSION

Epilepsy surgery may not be appropriate for all patients, but should be considered early in the treatment course of medically refractory patients for maximal potential benefit. Epilepsy surgery offers the optimal chance of seizure freedom for many patients. Ultimately, alternatives to resective therapy may provide similar rates of seizure freedom without the potential complications of resective surgery. Until that time, continued improvements in localization methods and resective techniques should improve the treatment options for patients with medically refractory epilepsy.

REFERENCES

1. Dichter MA, Brodie MJ. New antiepileptic drugs. *Drug Therapy* 1996; 334:1583–1590.
2. Kwan P, Brodie MJ. Refractory epilepsy: a progressive, intractable but preventable condition? *Seizure* 2002; 11:77–84.
3. Rosenow F, Luders H. Presurgical evaluation of epilepsy. *Brain* 2001; 124:1683–1700.
4. Engel J Jr. Surgery for seizures. *N Engl J Med* 1996; 334:647–652.
5. Berg AT, Langfitt J, Shinnar S *et al.* How long does it take for partial epilepsy to become intractable? *Neurology* 2003; 60:186–190.
6. Tellez-Zenteno JF, Ronquillo LH, Wiebe S. Sudden unexpected death in epilepsy: evidence-based analysis of incidence and risk factors. *Epilepsy Res* 2005; 65:101–115.
7. Eliashiv SD, Dewar S, Wainwright I *et al.* Long-term follow-up after temporal lobe resection for lesions associated with chronic seizures. *Neurology* 1997; 48:1383–1388.
8. Foldvary N, Nashold B, Mascha E *et al.* Seizure outcome after temporal lobectomy for temporal lobe epilepsy: a Kaplan–Meier survival analysis. *Neurology* 2000; 54:630–634.

9. Yoon HH, Kwon HL, Mattson RH *et al.* Long-term seizure outcome in patients initially seizure-free after resective epilepsy surgery. *Neurology* 2003; 61:445–450.

10. Mohanraj R, Norrie J, Stephen LJ *et al.* Mortality in adults with newly diagnosed and chronic epilepsy: a retrospective comparative study. *Lancet Neurol* 2006; 5:481–487.

11. Wiebe S, Blume WT, Girvin JP *et al.* A randomized, controlled trial of surgery for temporal-lobe epilepsy. *N Engl J Med* 2001; 345:311–318.

12. Kwan P, Brodie MJ. Early identification of refractory epilepsy. *N Engl J Med* 2000; 342:314–319.

13. VanLandingham KE, Heinz ER, Cavazos JE, *et al.* Magnetic resonance imaging evidence of hippocampal injury after prolonged focal febrile convulsions. *Ann Neurol* 1998; 43:413–426.

14. Shinnar S. Febrile seizures and mesial temporal sclerosis. *Epilepsy Currents* 2003; 3:115–118.

15. Loddenkemper T, Kotagal P. Lateralizing signs during seizures in focal epilepsy. *Epilepsy Behav* 2005; 7:1–17.

16. So EL. Value and limitations of seizure semiology in localizing seizure onset. *J Clin Neurophysiol* 2006; 23:353–357.

17. Krumholz A, Wiebe S, Gronseth G *et al.* Practice parameter: evaluating an apparent unprovoked first seizure in adults (an evidence-based review): report of the Quality Standards Subcommittee of the American Academy of Neurology and the American Epilepsy Society. *Neurology* 2007; 69:1996–2007.

18. Von Oertzen J, Urbach H, Jungbluth S *et al.* Standard magnetic resonance imaging is inadequate for patients with refractory focal epilepsy. *J Neurol Neurosurg Psychiatry* 2002; 73: 643–647.

19. LaBauge P, Laberge S, Brunereau L *et al.* Hereditary cerebral cavernous angiomas: clinical and genetic features in 57 French families. *Lancet* 1998; 352:1892–1897.

20. Brunereau L, Leveque C, Bertrand P *et al.* Familial form of cerebral cavernous malformations: evaluation of gradient-spin echo (GRASE) imaging in lesion detection and characterization at 1.5 T. *Neuroradiology* 2001; 43:973–979.

21. Knake S, Triantafyllou C, Wald LL *et al.* 3T phased array MRI improves the presurgical evaluation in focal epilepsies: a prospective study. *Neurology* 2005; 65:1026–1031.

22. Chapman K, Wyllie E, Najm I *et al.* Seizure outcome after epilepsy surgery in patients with normal preoperative MRI. *J Neurol Neurosurg Psychiatry* 2005; 76:710–713.

23. Yun CH, Lee SK, Lee SY *et al.* Prognostic factors in neocortical epilepsy surgery: multivariate analysis. *Epilepsia* 2006; 47: 574–579.

24. Rugg-Gunn FJ, Eriksson SH, Boulby PA *et al.* Magnetization transfer imaging in focal epilepsy. *Neurology* 2003; 60:1638–1645.

25. Boulby PA, Symms MR, Barker GJ. Optimized interleaved whole-brain 3D double inversion recovery (DIR) sequence for imaging the neocortex. *Magn Reson Med* 2004; 51:1181–1186.

26. Rugg-Gunn FJ, Boulby PA, Symms MR *et al.* Whole-brain T2 mapping demonstrates occult abnormalities in focal epilepsy. *Neurology* 2005; 64: 318–325.

27. Salmenpera TM, Symms MR, Rugg-Gunn FJ *et al.* Evaluation of quantitative magnetic resonance imaging contrasts in MRI-negative refractory focal epilepsy. *Epilepsia* 2007; 48: 229–237.

28. Barry E, Sussman NM, O'Connor MJ *et al.* Presurgical electroencephalographic patterns and outcome from anterior temporal lobectomy. *Arch Neurol* 1992; 49: 21–27.

29. Holmes MD, Kutsy RL, Ojemann GA *et al.* Interictal, unifocal spikes in refractory extratemporal epilepsy predict ictal origin and postsurgical outcome. *Clinical Neurophysiology* 2000; 111:1802–1808.

30. Holmes MD, Miles AN, Dodrill CB *et al.* Identifying potential surgical candidates in patients with evidence of bitemporal epilepsy. *Epilepsia* 2003; 44:1075–1079.

31. Wyllie E, Lachhwani DK, Gupta A *et al.* Successful surgery for epilepsy due to early brain lesions despite generalized EEG findings. *Neurology* 2007; 69:389–397.

32. Avellino AM, Berger MS, Rostomily RC *et al.* Surgical management and seizure outcome in patients with tuberous sclerosis. *J Neurosurg* 1997; 87:391–396.

33. Weiner HL, Carlson C, Ridgway EB *et al.* Epilepsy surgery in young children with tuberous sclerosis: results of a novel approach. *Pediatrics* 2006; 117:1494–1502.

34. Kuruvilla A, Flink R. Focal fast rhythmic epileptiform discharges on scalp EEG in a patient with cortical dysplasia. *Seizure* 2002; 11:330–334.

35. Siegel AM. Presurgical evaluation and surgical treatment of medically refractory epilepsy. *Neurosurg Rev* 2004; 27:1–21.

36. Moser DJ, Bauer RM, Gilmore RL *et al.* Electroencephalographic, volumetric, and neuropsychological indicators of seizure focus lateralization in temporal lobe epilepsy. *Arch Neurol* 2000; 57:707–712.

37. Seidenberg M, Wyler AR, Hermann B *et al.* Neuropsychological outcome following anterior temporal lobectomy in patients with and without the syndrome of mesial temporal lobe epilepsy. *Neuropsychology* 1998; 12:303–316.
38. Gleissner U, Helmstaedter C, Schramm J *et al.* Memory outcome after selective amygdalohippocampectomy: a study in 140 patients with temporal lobe epilepsy. *Epilepsia* 2002; 43:87–95.
39. LoGalbo A, Sawrie S, Roth DL *et al.* Verbal memory outcome in patients with normal preoperative verbal memory and left mesial temporal sclerosis. *Epilepsy Behav* 2005; 6:337–341.
40. Glosser G, Zwil AS, Glosser DS *et al.* Psychiatric aspects of temporal lobe epilepsy before and after anterior temporal lobectomy. *J Neurol Neurosurg Psychiatry* 2000; 68:53–58.
41. De Toffol B. Psychopathology in medically refractory partial seizures. *Rev Neurol (Paris)* 2004; 160:5S288–300.
42. Devinsky O, Barr WB, Vickrey BG *et al.* Changes in depression and anxiety after resective surgery for epilepsy. *Neurology* 2005; 65:1744–1749.
43. Maganti R, Rutecki P, Bell B *et al.* Epilepsy surgery outcome among US veterans. *Epilepsy Behav* 2003; 4:723–728.
44. Wada J, Rasmussen T. Intracarotid injection of sodium amytal for the lateralization of cerebral speech dominance. 1960. *J Neurosurg* 2007; 106:1117–1133.
45. Abou-Khalil B. An update on determination of language dominance in screening for epilepsy surgery: the Wada test and newer noninvasive alternatives. *Epilepsia* 2007; 48:442–455.
46. Sperling MR, Saykin AJ, Glosser G *et al.* Predictors of outcome after anterior temporal lobectomy: the intracarotid amobarbital test. *Neurology* 1994; 44:2325–2330.
47. Loddenkemper T, Morris HH 3rd, Perl J 2nd. Carotid artery dissection after the intracarotid amobarbital test. *Neurology* 2002; 59:1797–1798.
48. Silfvenius H, Fagerlund M, Saisa J *et al.* Carotid angiography in conjunction with amytal testing of epilepsy patients. *Brain Cogn* 1997; 33:33–49.
49. Papanicolaou AC, Simos PG, Castillo EM *et al.* Magnetocephalography: a noninvasive alternative to the Wada procedure. *J Neurosurg* 2004; 100:867–876.
50. Benke T, Koylu B, Visani P *et al.* Language lateralization in temporal lobe epilepsy: a comparison between fMRI and the Wada test. *Epilepsia* 2006; 47:1308–1319.
51. Kamada K, Sawamura Y, Takeuchi F *et al.* Expressive and receptive language areas determined by a non-invasive reliable method using functional magnetic resonance imaging and magnetoencephalography. *Neurosurgery* 2007; 60:296–306.
52. Knowlton RC, Elgavish R, Howell J *et al.* Magnetic source imaging versus intracranial electroencephalogram in epilepsy surgery: a prospective study. *Ann Neurol* 2006; 59:835–842.
53. Whiting P, Gupta R, Burch J *et al.* A systematic review of the effectiveness and cost-effectiveness of neuroimaging assessments used to visualise the seizure focus in people with refractory epilepsy being considered for surgery. *Health Technol Assess* 2006; 10:1–250, iii–iv.
54. Theodore WH, Sato S, Kufta CV *et al.* FDG-positron emission tomography and invasive EEG: seizure focus detection and surgical outcome. *Epilepsia* 1997; 38:81–86.
55. Mauguiere F, Ryvlin P. The role of PET in presurgical assessment of partial epilepsies. *Epileptic Disord* 2004; 6:193–215.
56. Willmann O, Wennberg R, May T *et al.* The contribution of 18F-FDG PET in preoperative epilepsy surgery evaluation for patients with temporal lobe epilepsy. A meta-analysis. *Seizure* 2007; 16:509–520.
57. Thadani VM, Siegel A, Lewis P *et al.* Validation of ictal single photon emission computed tomography with depth encephalography and epilepsy surgery. *Neurosurg Rev* 2004; 27:27–33.
58. O'Brien TJ, So EL, Mullan BP *et al.* Subtraction peri-ictal SPECT is predictive of extratemporal epilepsy surgery outcome. *Neurology* 2000; 55:1668–1677.
59. O'Brien TJ, So EL, Cascino GD *et al.* Subtraction SPECT coregistered to MRI in focal malformations of cortical development: localization of the epileptogenic zone in epilepsy surgery candidates. *Epilepsia* 2004; 45:367–376.
60. Gaillard WD. Metabolic and functional neuroimaging. In: Wyllie E (ed.) *The Treatment of Epilepsy: Principles and Practice.* 4th edition. Philadelphia: Lippincott Williams and Wilkins, 2006, pp. 1047–1048, 1053.
61. Gaillard WD, Balsamo L, Xu B *et al.* Language dominance in partial epilepsy patients identified with an fMRI reading task. *Neurology* 2002; 59:256–265.
62. Powell HWR, Richardson MP, Symms MR *et al.* Preoperative fMRI predicts memory decline following anterior temporal lobe resection. *J Neurol Neurosurg Psychiatry* 2007; doi:10.1136/jnnp.2007.115139.

63. Mueller SG, Laxer KD, Cashdollar N *et al.* Identification of abnormal neuronal metabolism outside the seizure focus in temporal lobe epilepsy. *Epilepsia* 2004; 45:355–366.

64. Nair DR, Burgess R, McIntyre CC *et al.* Chronic subdural electrodes in the management of epilepsy. *Clinical Neurophysiology* 2007; doi:10.1016/j.clinph.2007.09.117.

65. Sperling MR, O'Connor MJ. Comparison of depth and subdural electrodes in recording temporal lobe seizures. *Neurology* 1989; 39:1497–1504.

66. Eisenschenk S, Gilmore RL, Cibula JE *et al.* Lateralization of temporal lobe foci: depth versus subdural electrodes. *Clinical Neurophysiology* 2001; 112:836–844.

67. Spencer SS, Spencer DD, Williamson PD *et al.* Combined depth and subdural electrode investigation in uncontrolled epilepsy. *Neurology* 1990; 40:74–79.

68. Aghakhani Y, Kinay D, Gotman J *et al.* The role of periventricular nodular heterotopia in epileptogenesis. *Brain* 2005; 128:641–651.

69. Sahjpaul RL, Mahon J, Wiebe S. Dexamethasone for morbidity after subdural electrode insertion – a randomized controlled trial. *Can J Neurol Sci* 2003; 30: 340–348.

70. Araki T, Otsubo H, Makino Y *et al.* Efficacy of dexamethasone on cerebral swelling and seizures during subdural grid EEG recording in children. *Epilepsia* 2006; 47:176–180.

71. Regis J, Rey M, Bartolomei F *et al.* Gamma knife surgery in mesial temporal lobe epilepsy: a prospective multicenter study. *Epilepsia* 2004; 45:504–515.

72. O'Brien TJ, Kilpatrick C, Murrie V *et al.* Temporal lobe epilepsy caused by mesial temporal sclerosis and temporal neocortical lesions. *Brain* 1996; 119:2133–2141.

73. Hamer HM, Najm I, Mohamed A *et al.* Interictal epileptiform discharges in temporal lobe epilepsy due to hippocampal sclerosis versus medial temporal lobe tumors. *Epilepsia* 1999; 40:1261–1268.

74. Ryvlin P, Kahane P. The hidden causes of surgery-resistant temporal lobe epilepsy: extratemporal or temporal plus? *Curr Opin Neurol* 2005; 18:125–127.

75. Tellez-Zenteno JF, Dhar R, Wiebe S. Long-term seizure outcomes following epilepsy surgery: a systematic review and meta-analysis. *Brain* 2005; 128:1188–1198.

76. McIntosh AM, Kalnins RM, Mitchell LA *et al.* Temporal lobectomy: long-term seizure outcome, late recurrence and risks for seizure recurrence. *Brain* 2004; 127:2018–2030.

77. Engel J Jr, Wiebe S, French J *et al.* Practice parameter: temporal lobe and localized neocortical resections for epilepsy: report of the Quality Standards Subcommittee of the American Academy of Neurology, in association with the American Epilepsy Society and the American Association of Neurological Surgeons. *Neurology* 2003; 60:538–547.

78. Burgerman RS, Sperling MR, French JA *et al.* Comparison of mesial versus neocortical onset temporal lobe seizures: neurodiagnostic findings and surgical outcome. *Epilepsia* 1995; 36:662–670.

79. Jung WY, Pacia SV, Devinsky R. Neocortical temporal lobe epilepsy: intracranial EEG features and surgical outcome. *J Clin Neurophysiol* 1999; 16:419–425.

80. Spencer SS, Berg AT, Vickrey BG *et al.* Predicting long-term seizure outcome after resective epilepsy surgery: the multicenter study. *Neurology* 2005; 65:912–918.

81. Paglioli E, Palmini A, da Costa JC *et al.* Survival analysis of the surgical outcome of temporal lobe epilepsy due to hippocampal sclerosis. *Epilepsia* 2004; 45:1383–1391.

82. Mihara T, Inoue Y, Matsuda K *et al.* Recommendation of early surgery from the viewpoint of daily quality of life. *Epilepsia* 1996; 37:S33–S36.

83. Sirven JI, Malamut BL, O'Connor MJ *et al.* Temporal lobectomy outcome in older versus younger adults. *Neurology* 2000; 54:2166–2170.

84. Rydenhag B, Silander HC. Complications of epilepsy surgery after 654 procedures in Sweden, September 1990–1995: a multicenter study based on the Swedish National Epilepsy Surgery Register. *Neurosurgery* 2001; 49:51–57.

85. Aghakhani Y, Rosati A, Olivier A *et al.* The predictive localizing value of tonic limbposturing in supplementary sensorimotor seizures. *Neurology* 2004; 62:2256–2261.

86. Nolan MA, Sakuta R, Chuang N *et al.* Dysembryoplastic neuroepithelial tumors in childhood: long-term outcome and prognostic features. *Neurology* 2004; 62:2270–2276.

87. Rathore C, Abraham M, Rao RM *et al.* Outcome after corpus callosotomy in children with injurious drop attacks and severe mental retardation. *Brain Dev* 2007; 29:577–585.

88. Rahimi SY, Park YD, Witcher MR *et al.* Corpus callosotomy for treatment of pediatric epilepsy in the modern area. *Pediatr Neurosurg* 2007; 43:202–208.

89. Kossoff EH, Ritzl EK, Politsky JM *et al.* Effect of an external responsive neurostimulator on seizures and electrographic discharges during subdural electrode monitoring. *Epilepsia* 2004; 45:1560–1567.

90. Morrell M. Brain stimulation for epilepsy: can scheduled or responsive neurostimulation stop seizures? *Curr Opin Neurol* 2006; 19:164–168.

91. Sun FT, Morrell MJ, Wharen RE Jr. Responsive cortical stimulation for the treatment of epilepsy. *Neurotherapeutics* 2008; 5:68–74.

92. Theodore WH, Fisher RS. Brain stimulation for epilepsy. *Lancet Neurol* 2004; 3:111–118.

93. John JE, Baptiste SL, Sheffield LG *et al.* Transmeningeal delivery of GABA to control neocortical seizures in rats. *Epilepsy Res* 2007; 75:10–17.

94. Ludvig N, Kuzniecky RI, Baptiste SL *et al.* Epidural pentobarbital delivery can prevent locally induced neocortical seizures in rats: the prospect of transmeningeal pharmacotherapy for intractable focal epilepsy. *Epilepsia* 2006; 47:1792–1802.

95. Pilcher W, Roberts D, Flanigin H *et al.* Complications of epilepsy surgery. In: Engel J (ed.) *Surgical Treatment of Epilepsies*. 2nd edn. New York: Raven Press, 1993, pp. 565–581.

96. Racoosin JA, Feeney J, Burkhart G *et al.* Mortality in antiepileptic drug development programs. *Neurology* 2001; 56:514–519.

97. Jokeit H, Ebner A. Long term effects of refractory temporal lobe epilepsy on cognitive abilities: a cross sectional study. *J Neurol Neurosurg Psychiatry* 1999; 67:44–50.

98. Holloway KL, Corrie WS, Wingkun EC *et al.* Epilepsy surgery: removing the thorn from the lion's paw. *South Med J* 1995; 88:619–625.

99. Kilpatrick C, Cook M, Kaye A *et al.* Non-invasive investigations successfully select patients for temporal lobe surgery. *J Neurol Neurosurg Psychiatry* 1997; 63:327–333.

100. C:son Silander H, Blom S, Malmgren K, *et al.* Surgical treatment for epilepsy: a retrospective Swedish multicenter study. *Acta Neurol Scand* 1997; 95:321–330.

101. Callaghan BC, Anand K, Hesdorffer D *et al.* Likelihood of seizure remission in an adult population with refractory epilepsy. *Ann Neurol* 2007; 62:382–389.

102. Boon P, D'Have M, Van Walleghem P *et al.* Direct medical costs of refractory epilepsy incurred by three different treatment modalities: a prospective assessment. *Epilepsia* 2002; 43:96–102.

3

Neurostimulation for the treatment of epilepsy – vagus nerve stimulation

Elinor Ben-Menachem

INTRODUCTION

Neurostimulation is not a new idea and it is not reserved for epilepsy alone. Today, neurostimulation is used in many areas such as pain, bladder regulation, control of tremor and epilepsy. The new main methods of neurostimulation for epilepsy that have been tested in a wider group of patients are deep brain stimulation (DBS) and vagus nerve stimulation (VNS). The only procedure that is approved as an effective treatment for epilepsy is vagus nerve stimulation and now more than 50 000 people have been operated on and treated with it for epilepsy. Although DBS has been in clinical evaluation for over 30 years, it is still not an accepted method of treatment for patients with refractory epilepsy and is still under evaluation. One of the main reasons for this is that it has been unclear if DBS has a significant anti-epileptic effect; there is no consensus as to what depth the electrodes should be implanted, there is a higher risk for bleeding and infection during the procedure, and there have been too few patients and too few adequate trials to be able to make a clear judgement, as in the case of VNS.

VAGUS NERVE STIMULATION

The first, although crude and external, vagus nerve stimulator was actually a creation of J. L. Corning in the 1880s [1], who observed a reduction in seizures in his patients using his methodology. The purpose was to achieve a reduction in seizures by reducing cerebral blood flow through cardio-inhibitory vagal stimulation. VNS was, however, forgotten as a useful anti-seizure therapy until Zabara [2, 3, 4] began to seriously analyse the effect of stimulation in chemically-induced seizures in dogs. The results were dramatic and the development has now advanced to an accepted and registered form of treatment for epilepsy and depression worldwide.

Data demonstrating that peripheral stimulation of the vagus nerve has been found to influence the brain and cause marked changes in the electroencephalogram (EEG) have been described previously [5–10]. Later, it was shown that VNS could inhibit seizures in the maximal electroshock (MES) and pentylenetetrazol (PTZ) models in rats [11] and in monkeys [12].

Elinor Ben-Menachem, MD, PhD, Professor of Neurosciences, Institute of Clinical Neurosciences, Sahlgrenska Academy at Göteborg University, Göteborg, Sweden

The first trials in humans were published in 1990 [13, 14] and then in 1993 [15]. A total of 16 patients with refractory partial-onset seizures were implanted and given intermittent stimulation of a 30-s train of impulses (ON) every 5 min (OFF). Because of the positive results of these pilot studies, double-blind, low-dose placebo-controlled trials were performed to further elucidate the efficacy of VNS in partial seizures [16, 17].

ANATOMY

Studies in cats have shown that the vagus nerve consists of 80% afferent fibres, projecting from the viscera to the nucleus tractus solitarius (NTS) [18]. Afferent fibres provide parasympathetic innervation to the lungs, heart and gastrointestinal tract and also innervate the voluntary muscles in the larynx and pharynx. There is an asymmetrical innervation to the heart, with the right vagus nerve (VN) innervating the sinoatrial node and the left innervating the atrioventricular node, at least in dogs. In dogs, when the right VN is stimulated, bradycardia is elicited more so than when the left VN is stimulated [19]. This is the rationale for implanting the VNS on the left side of the neck and not the right side. There are, however, some reports of successful stimulation of the right vagus nerve in humans [20]. Afferent fibres from receptors in the lungs, heart, aorta, gastrointestinal tract and aortic chemoreceptors, as well as a small group of afferent fibres from the concha of the ear, have their cell bodies in the nodose and jugular ganglia and project to the NTS as well as to the medial reticular formation in the medulla, the dorsal medial nucleus (DMN), area postrema and nucleus cunneatus. From the NTS, there are synaptic connections to higher centres in the brain as the hypothalamus, dorsal raphe, nucleus ambiguus, the DMN of the vagus nerve, amygdala and the thalamus, which in turn projects to the insular cortex [21]. Positron emission tomography (PET) and functional magnetic resonance imaging (fMRI) studies in humans with VNS have confirmed the influence of the VN on higher brain structures and thus provides a rationale for why VNS elicits an anti-convulsive effect. The main conclusions from these studies are that the thalamus is consistently involved, and that there are profound changes in the brain blood flow during VNS which correspond to anatomical synaptic projections. Using fMRI, it was found that the areas of significant activation in response to VNS were bilateral orbitofrontal and parieto-occipital cortex, the left temporal cortex and left amygdala [22–26]. Besides these specific areas, there was a general diffuse increase in brain activity.

The VN in the neck is enclosed in the carotid sheath. In the mid-cervical area the superior laryngeal nerve branches off at the carotid bifurcation. This nerve is secondarily stimulated during VNS and can give rise to a feeling of tightness or even pain in the throat area. The recurrent laryngeal nerve travels alongside the VN, and it will also be affected by stimulation of the VN, causing vibration of the left vocal cord during stimulation and subsequently complaints of hoarseness during ON times or even a snoring sound during sleep. This is the main site for complaints during stimulation.

MECHANISM OF ACTION

The mechanism of action of VNS is unknown. Cerebrospinal fluid (CSF) studies in humans have indicated changes in a number of amino acids and neurotransmitters, especially the amino acid ethanolamine, which is a sign of increased turnover of membrane components [27]. Perhaps this is an indication of an increased amino acid turnover in a more general sense as is also inferred by the observation of an increase in neuronal *fos* expression in the medulla vagal areas, the locus coeruleus, thalamic and hypothalamic nuclei, amygdala, and cingulated and retrosplenial cortex in rats with VNS compared with controls [28].

Another clue is that in rats, when noradrenaline was depleted by 6-hydroxydopamine infusion into the locus coeruleus, the seizure suppressive effect of VNS was abolished [29].

In summary, current information suggests that VNS activates neuronal networks in the thalamus and other limbic structures and that noradrenaline may mediate the anti-seizure activity of VNS but still the mechanism of action is not clear.

THE DEVICE AND IMPLANTATION

The stimulation device is a pacemaker which is implanted under the left clavicle. Two stimulating electrodes are placed around the left VN in the neck distal to the branching of the recurrent laryngeal nerve. The operation is carried out under either local or general anaesthesia and takes about 1–2 h. The patient can go home the same day.

After the operation, the VNS can be turned on by use of a computer and program wand, either immediately or the next day. Some centres prefer to allow the patient to heal for 1–2 weeks before turning the device on. Usually one starts by giving a current of 0.25 mA and gradually increases in 0.25-mA increments to 1.25–2 mA over a period of several weeks. Other parameters include: frequency (Hz) – the usual setting is 20–30 Hz, because animal studies have shown the best effect to be in the range of 10–60 Hz [4, 11]; pulse width (250–500 µs); and time on (usually 30 s) and time off (usually 3–5 min). The time on and off can be changed and many use rapid cycling of 7 s on and 0.2 s off, thereby increasing the amount of stimulation time given daily. However, there is no hard evidence to suggest that one of the different time parameters is better than the others [30]. Even the amount of current can vary from individual to individual, with some having better effect at higher currents (>2 mA) and others better effect with lower currents (0.75–1.75 mA).

EFFICACY IN EPILEPSY

Randomized 'Placebo-Controlled' Double-Blind Studies

Two pivotal studies have been conducted in order to determine whether VNS really does have an anti-seizure effect. These two trials also served as the main evidence for approval for the US and European regulatory boards for use in patients with refractory partial-onset seizures.

The first study (E03) [16] was an international multicentre trial. A total of 114 patients over the age of 12 completed the prospective baseline phase of the study. All had more than six partial-onset seizures monthly before implantation despite anti-epileptic drug (AED) therapy. One hundred and thirteen patients were implanted and then randomized to one of two groups. One group received 30 s of VNS every 5 min and the other group received 30 s of VNS every 90 min. After 3 months of treatment (no changes in the AEDs were allowed), there was a 24.5% decrease in seizures in the frequent stimulation group compared with 6.1% in the infrequent stimulation group. This was statistically significant ($P = 0.01$). Thirty-one per cent of the frequent stimulation group had >50% seizure reduction compared with 13% in the infrequent stimulation group.

The next study (E05) [17] was a multicentre US-based trial, in which 199 refractory partial-onset seizure patients were implanted and followed for 3 months. A total of 103 patients were in the infrequent stimulation group and 95 were in the frequent stimulation group with similar stimulation parameters as for the E03 study. After 3 months of stimulation there was a 28% decrease in seizures in the frequent stimulation group and a 15% decrease in the infrequent stimulation group. The difference between the groups was significant at $P = 0.039$. Between-group comparisons for 50% responders was not significant (23.4% vs. 15.7%). However, the high-stimulation group was more likely to achieve a 75% seizure reduction than the low-stimulation group (10.6% vs. 2%).

Seizure severity is very difficult to measure in a clinical trial. Anecdotally, many patients report an improvement in seizure severity or duration, even in the absence of improvement as measured by seizure frequency.

Acute Seizure Interruption

After implantation, every patient is given a magnet, which can be worn on a wristband, or clipped to a belt. Magnet current, pulse width and duration of stimulation can be set independently from the intermittent automatic stimulation. Patients are instructed to place the magnet against the chest, against the battery pack, and count off 2 s. This will trigger the VNS to stimulate. The magnet should then be removed from the chest, since keeping the magnet on the chest will prevent the device from triggering. Typical magnet stimulations last between 30 and 60 s. Many patients report that seizures can be aborted with the magnet. If the patient is unable to use the magnet because they have no warning before becoming incapacitated, a family member or spouse can use the magnet. There are no controlled data of any kind to confirm that magnet stimulation is effective, but there are numerous anecdotal reports of benefit. The magnet function seems to be useful in about 30% of patients [31]. Patients who believe the magnet is beneficial in aborting seizures also report an increased feeling of control over their condition, which can be psychologically empowering.

Long-Term Follow-Up Studies

There have been many reports of long-term follow-up studies, most retrospective studies reporting from a single-centre patient population with results almost identical to the studies mentioned below. Two major prospective long-term follow-up studies have assessed the change in seizure frequency and tolerability from the end of the clinical trials for up to 1 year (E05 study [32]) and up to 3 years (E01–E05 studies [33]).

In the 12-month follow-up from the E05 study, 195 patients were followed from the time they ended the double-blind phase and went into the open-label follow-up phase of the trial. In the analysis with the last visit carried forward, by 3 months after the end of the double-blind trial patients had a 34% median seizure reduction and by the end of the year it was up to 45%. Thirty-four per cent had a >50% seizure reduction and 20% had a >75% seizure reduction. The current stimulation was around 1.75 mA at the end of the year.

In the E01–E05 studies, a total of 440 patients were followed for up to 3 years. Seizure reduction decreased from baseline to 3 months into the follow-up phase and then at 2 years, after which it reached a plateau. Twenty-three per cent of patients had a >50% seizure reduction at 3 months, 37% at 1 year, 43% at 2 years and 43% at 3 years. Side-effects decreased progressively during the 3-year follow-up.

Children

One VNS study, the E04 [34], was a paediatric prospective open-safety study of VNS and included 60 children aged between 3 and 18 years. Sixteen of the patients were under 12 years of age. In this study, patients with various types of refractory seizures were included, even some with primary generalized seizures (27%). By 3 months of stimulation, there was a 23% median seizure decrease. At 6 months it was 42% ($n = 46$). By 1 year the decrease was 34% ($n = 51$) and at 18 months it was 42% ($n = 46$). There was no association between improvement and seizure type.

In a large, six-centre, albeit retrospective, study with 95 children [35], there was an average seizure reduction of 36.1% at 3 months and 44.7% at 6 months.

In yet another large six-centre retrospective study, 50 patients with Lennox–Gastaut syndrome were evaluated at baseline and then at 3 and 6 months after implantation. Median age at implantation was 13 years but there were even 2-year-olds participating. Sixty per cent had IQs under 70, 36% had tried the ketogenic diet and five had had callosotomies previously. The median seizure reduction at 3 months ($n = 43$) was 58.2% and at 6 months was 57.9% ($n = 24$). By 6 months there was a >50% decrease in 58% of patients. Drop attacks were reduced at 3 months by 55% and at 6 months by 88%. In the five patients with callosotomies, seizures were reduced by 73% at 3 months and 69% at 6 months [36]. Other smaller studies have reported similar results [37, 38].

Smaller Studies of Special Groups

There have been numerous case reports of VNS in different types of epilepsy such as tuberous sclerosis [39], status epilepticus [40], epilepsy associated with hamartomas [41], infantile spasms and progressive myoclonic epilepsy of Unverricht–Lundborg type [42]. All report good efficacy and low frequency of side-effects.

The efficacy of VNS now seems to be established for focal-onset seizure types and there is evidence that it has efficacy for other seizure types as well. Therefore, VNS can be considered to be a broad-spectrum treatment. It seems to be effective in the most refractory focal-onset seizure patients, even in those who have already undergone epilepsy surgery. Improvement is not immediate but tends to increase over 18–24 months of treatment. Most studies cited above report subjective improvements in various quality-of-life measures while on VNS. More objective studies also report improvements in mood [43–45], memory [46, 47] and quality of life measured by the Quality of Life in Epilepsy Inventory [48, 49].

SAFETY AND TOLERABILITY

Acute Side-Effects

The majority of acute complications of the VNS implantation have been common infections, vocal cord pareses, lower facial weakness, and in a few cases, bradycardia and asystole.

Post-operative infections occur in 3–6% of patients. Most often, these have been treated with oral antibiotics and rarely have the generator or electrodes been removed because of this complication. In the E05 study, however, infection leading to device removal occurred in 3 of 198 patients (1.5%). Left cord paralysis occurred in one patient in the E03 study but resolved when the device was removed. In the E05 study, reversible left-cord paralysis was reported in two patients.

Lower facial weakness was reported in the E05 study in two patients and in one in the E03 study. This was probably because of high surgical incisions when connecting the electrodes to the VN. This side-effect, as well as infection risk, has become very rare with the improvement of surgical techniques.

Tatum *et al.* [50] reported four patients who experienced ventricular asystole during testing of the device during implantation. Asconapé *et al.* [51] reported one patient where this occurred. No asystolic events have occurred outside the operating room, and patients have been able to use the VNS post-operatively. The occurrence rate of this adverse event is estimated to be one in 875 cases, or 0.1%. Possible reasons could be abnormal electrode placement, indirect stimulation of the cervical cardiac nerves, technical malfunction of the device, polarity reversal of the leads by the surgeon or an idiosyncratic reaction. Even the occurrence of this adverse event seems to have declined as a result of the awareness of the surgeons [52].

CHRONIC ADVERSE EVENTS

The most common adverse events are stimulus-related coughing, throat pain and hoarseness. All tend to improve with time [33]. In the E03 study, only voice alternation (37.2%), hoarseness (37.2%) and throat pain (11%) were reported in more than 10% of patients. However, in the E05 study [18], voice alternation was reported in 66.3% of patients on high stimulation and 30% on low stimulation, cough in 45% on high stimulation and 42% on low, throat pain in 28.1% on high stimulation, dyspnoea in 25%, vomiting and paraesthesias in 17.9% and infection in 11.6%. The symptoms were judged mild or moderate and rarely required adjustment of the stimulation parameters. No changes in autonomic function tests such as blood pressure, heart rate, Holter monitor measures, lung function tests or blood chemistry were noted in the E05 study. A method to decrease the above side-effects is to slowly titrate up the stimulation intensity by, for example, 0.25 mA weekly or every other week.

LONG-TERM TOLERABILITY

There have been several long-term follow-up reports [32, 33, 53]. In the 12-month long-term follow-up data for the E05 study [33], 195 patients were included. No cardiac events or changes as in relative risk variability were seen in the 12-month follow-up. Pulmonary function tests and blood chemistries were unchanged from baseline. A total of 97.8% of the adverse events were reported as mild to moderate and were reversible with a reduction in stimulation parameters. Noteworthy is the lack of central nervous system (CNS) or cognitive side-effects.

In the 3-year follow-up of all patients in E01–E05 [33], paraesthesias, cough and hoarseness reports decreased with time. Dyspnoea was the most common adverse event reported at 3 years (3.2%). Three serious events of respiratory difficulties and three of hoarseness were reported. The other serious adverse events were one accidental death, four sudden, unexpected, unexplained deaths in epilepsy, one thrombocytopenia, one aspiration pneumonia, one renal failure and one pneumonia/sepsis. No changes in Holter monitor or lung function tests or blood chemistries that could be attributed to VNS were ever noted.

In summary, side-effects are mainly stimulation related, reversible and tend to decrease over time. They are usually mild to moderate and seldom require that the device be explanted. No idiosyncratic side-effects have ever been reported. Most adverse events are predictable and related to stimulation parameters. CNS side-effects such as tiredness, psychomotor slowing, irritation and nervousness have not been frequently reported and they do not stand out as major side-effects of VNS.

A number of reports of sleep-disordered breathing and sleep apnoea with VNS have appeared. These problems have been seen in adults as well as children. Excessive daytime sleepiness after VNS implantation should be explored with polysomnography, if possible. Continuous positive airway pressure or turning the device off at night may solve the problems [54–56].

LONG-TERM MANAGEMENT OF VNS

Once a patient has been stabilized on therapy, it is recommended that patients with VNS have their device interrogated by a physician trained in VNS assessment approximately every 3–6 months. This serves two purposes. One is to ensure lead connection is intact. Lead breakage, although rare, has been reported, particularly after trauma in the location of the leads. If lead breakage is suspected, usually noted by a marked increase in device impedance, a chest X-ray can be performed to look for lead integrity. The second purpose is to look for a battery end-of-life message, indicating that the battery needs to be replaced. Over time, as they get used to the device, patients may also tolerate increases in voltage to which they were intolerant initially.

If a patient complains of pain or problems with the device, they should be brought in for an immediate visit. If there is a need to turn off the device until a visit can be arranged, the patient can be told to tape the magnet to their chest. This will stop the device from stimulating, until the magnet is removed.

END OF BATTERY LIFE

One relative disadvantage of VNS therapy is that the lithium–titanium battery has a finite life span, and needs to be replaced. An end-of-life indicator is now built into the device, so that patients and physicians will be signalled during routine device checks if a battery replacement is required. This indicator will begin to display an end-of-battery-life message approximately 6 months before the battery is completely expended. Battery replacement should be performed before the battery is expended, as there are several case reports of seizure relapse or exacerbation after battery expiration. Battery replacement requires surgery with general anaesthesia, but only involves a small incision in the chest, and minimal recovery. Fortunately, over time VNS has been incrementally improved, leading to smaller devices with longer battery life. At the time of writing, with model 102, average battery life is between 3 and 8 years. Battery life is longer or shorter in given individuals, depending on the frequency and intensity of stimulation and the number of magnet-triggered stimulations.

Magnetic Resonance Imaging

There are some issues with magnetic resonance imaging (MRI) in patients with implanted devices, and VNS is no exception. Patients with VN stimulator implantation are not able to undergo imaging of the chest, breast or abdomen [57]. MRI of the brain can be done, but only on machines that conform to a specific standard. Only a transmit–receive head coil should be employed. The device must also be turned off before MRI is performed. It is wise to check with your own hospital or local MRI team to assess safety of imaging, as requirements may change as new machines are put into use.

Cost

VNS placement has a significant upfront cost, in terms of both surgery and the cost of the device itself. Requirements for reimbursement vary from country to country. In some countries, it is necessary to justify implantation by documenting that medication has failed. This is not necessary in other countries. Cost–benefit analyses have indicated that VNS may actually be cost effective when compared with the use of an additional anti-epileptic drug over the long term, which is often the alternative [58].

The Place of VNS Therapy in the Treatment of Epilepsy

When should the VNS be used? There is now solid evidence that VNS is an effective treatment for patients with partial-onset seizures, as discussed above [59, 60]. Then there are large open-label studies with long-term follow-up indicating a broad spectrum of activity in most seizure types. Currently, VNS is being implanted in patients with refractory seizures who cannot have resective surgery or who have had surgery with poor results. It may be a good alternative for non-compliant patients, as well as patients who do not tolerate anti-epileptic drugs well. In fact, most paediatric neurologists and neurosurgeons would also agree that VNS should be offered to patients before considering a callosotomy as VNS is less invasive, has fewer side-effects and seems to have good efficacy in this patient group. Prospective comparative studies to anti-epileptic drugs need to be done to provide evidence for efficacy in less refractory patients or those with new-onset seizures [61].

CONCLUSION

Currently, VNS is the only approved neuromodulating therapy for use in patients with refractory epilepsy. It is no longer considered an unusual or dangerous therapy but it is still used almost exclusively for refractory epilepsy patients and still has not been generally accepted for use as a first-line or even second-line therapy. However, compared with the new AEDs, VNS has similar efficacy results in clinical trials and in many epilepsy syndromes, but the long-term efficacy results are even more positive, with continued improvement in seizure reduction for up to 2 years. Two of the major reasons for not using VNS early are that it is a surgical procedure, and that its safety during MRI procedures, especially using 3-tesla, is not yet elucidated. The safety profile of VNS is very favourable and the side-effects are totally different from those seen with AEDs. The most important aspects are that there are no pharmacological considerations and cognitive and sedative side-effects are not reported or may even improve, and it is safe for all age groups. Side-effects are restricted to local irritation, hoarseness, coughing and, in a few cases, swallowing difficulties when the stimulator was ON, but these tend to disappear with time and can be modulated with device adjustment. No idiosyncratic side-effects have emerged nor have there been any reports of teratogenicity as a result of VNS. Compliance is guaranteed. The cost of the implantation of the VNS, when spread over 8 years (battery length), is actually less than the cost of using one new AED over an 8-year period, and real savings on hospital costs due to seizures can be expected [58]. DBS is another exciting possibility but the high level of invasiveness and low patient numbers in clinical studies are major concerns and limitations for classifying these procedures as standard treatments. Today, after 60 years of clinical trials and treatment reports, DBS still needs to be subjected to the same rigorous clinical evaluations as other therapies in order to determine if it is a viable treatment modality for patients with refractory epilepsy. Some controlled studies are, however, ongoing.

REFERENCES

1. Lanska DJ. J. L. Corning and vagal nerve stimulation for seizures in the 1880s. *Neurology* 2002; 58:452–459.
2. Zabara J. Peripheral control of hypersynchronous discharge in epilepsy (abstract). *Electroencephalogr Clin Neurophysiol* 1985; 61:S162.
3. Zabara J. Time course of seizure control to brief repetitive stimuli (abstract). *Epilepsia* 1985; 26:518.
4. Zabara J. Inhibition of experimental seizures in canines by repetitive stimulation. *Epilepsia* 1992; 33:1005–1012.
5. Bailey P, Bremer F. A sensory cortical representation of the vagus nerve. *J Neurophysiol* 1938; 1:405–412.
6. Zanchetti A, Wang SC, Moruzzi G. The effect of vagal stimulation on the EEG pattern of the cat. *Electroencephalogr Clin Neurophysiol* 1952; 4:357–461.
7. Chase MH, Sterman MB, Clemente CD. Cortical and subcortical patterns of response to afferent vagal stimulation. *Exper Neurol* 1966; 16:36–49.
8. Chase MH, Nakamura Y, Clemente CD *et al*. Afferent vagal stimulation: neurographic correlates of induced EEG synchronization and desynchronization. *Brain Res* 1967; 5:236–249.
9. Stoica I, Tudor I. Effects of vagus afferents on strychnine focus of coronal gyrus. *Rev Roum Neurol* 1967; 4:287–295.
10. Stoica I, Tudor I. Vagal trunk stimulation influences on epileptic spiking focus. *Rev Roum Neurol* 1968; 5:203–210.
11. Woodbury DM, Woodbury JW. Effects of vagal stimulation on experimentally induced seizures in rats. *Epilepsia* 1990; 31(Suppl 2):S7–S19.
12. Lockard JS, Congdon WC, DuCharme LL. Feasibility and safety of vagal stimulation: the monkey model. *Epilepsia* 1990; 31(Suppl 2):S20–S26.
13. Penry JK, Dean JC, Prevention of intractable partial seizures by intermittent vagal stimulation in humans: preliminary results. *Epilepsia* 1990; 31(Suppl):S40–S43.
14. Uthman BM, Wilder BJ, Hammond EJ *et al*. Efficacy and safety of vagus nerve stimulation patients with complex partial seizures. *Epilepsia* 1990; 31(Suppl 2):S44–S50.
15. Uthman BM, Wilder BJ, Penry JK *et al*. Treatment of epilepsy by stimulation of the vagus nerve. *Neurology* 1993; 43:1338–1345.
16. Ben-Menachem E, Manon-Espaillat R, Ristanovic R *et al*. Vagus nerve stimulation for treatment of partial seizures. 1. A controlled study of effect on seizures. *Epilepsia* 1994; 35:616–626.
17. Handforth A, DeGiorgio CM, Schachter SC *et al*. Vagus nerve stimulation therapy for partial-onset seizures. A randomized active-control trial. *Neurology* 1998; 51:48–55.

18. Foley JO, DuBois F. Quantitative studies of the vagus nerve in the cat. I. The ratio of sensory to motor fibers. *J Comp Neurol* 1937; 67:49–97.
19. Randall WC, Ardell JL. Differential innervation of the heart. In: Sipes D, Jalife J (eds) *Cardiac Electrophysiology and Arrhythmias*. New York: Grune and Strattin, 1985, pp. 137–144.
20. McGregor A, Wheless J, Baumgartner J *et al*. Right-sided vagus nerve stimulation as a treatment for refractory epilepsy in humans. *Epilepsia* 2005; 36:91–96.
21. Rutecki P. Anatomical, physiological, and theoretical basis for the antiepileptic effect of vagus nerve stimulation. *Epilepsia* 1990; 31(Suppl 2):S1–S6.
22. Ko D, Heck C, Grafton S *et al*. Vagus nerve stimulation activates central nervous system structures in epileptic patients during PET H215O blood flow imaging. *Neurosurgery* 1996; 39:426–430.
23. Henry TR, Votaw JR, Bakay RAE *et al*. Acute blood flow changes and efficacy of vagus nerve stimulation in partial epilepsy. *Neurology* 1999; 52:1166–1173.
24. Henry TR, Bakay RAE, Votaw JR *et al*. Blood flow alterations induced by therapeutic vagus nerve stimulation in partial epilepsy 1: acute effects at high and low levels of stimulation. *Epilepsia* 1998; 39:983–990.
25. Bohning DE, Lomarev MP, Denslow S *et al*. Feasibility of vagus nerve stimulation-synchronized bloods oxygenation level-dependent functional MRI. *Investigative Radiology* 2001; 36:470–479.
26. Henry TR, Bakay RA, Pennell PB *et al*. Brain blood-flow alterations induced by therapeutic vagus nerve stimulation in partial epilepsy: II. prolonged effects at high and low levels of stimulation. *Epilepsia* 2004; 45:1064–1070.
27. Ben-Menachem E, Hamberger A, Hedner T *et al*. Effects of vagus nerve stimulation on amino acids and other metabolites in the CSF of patients with partial seizures. *Epilepsy Res* 1995; 20:221–227.
28. Naritoku DK, Terry WJ, Helfert RH. Regional induction of fos immunoreactivity in the brain by anticonvulsant stimulation of the vagus nerve. *Epilepsy Res* 1995; 22:53–62.
29. Krahl SF, Clark KB, Smith DC *et al*. Locus coeruleus lesions suppress the seizure attenuating effects of vagus nerve stimulation. *Epilesia* 1998; 39:709–714.
30. DeGiorgio C, Heck C, Bunch S *et al*. Vagus nerve stimulation for epilepsy: randomized comparison of three stimulation paradigms. *Neurology* 2005; 65:317–319.
31. Morris GL 3rd. A retrospective analysis of the effects of magnet-activated stimulation in conjunction with vagus nerve stimulation therapy. *Epilepsy Behav* 2003; 4:740–745.
32. DeGiorgio CM, Schachter SC, Handforth A *et al*. Prospective long-term study of vagus nerve stimulation for the treatment of refractory seizures. *Epilepsia* 2000; 41:1195–1200.
33. Morris GL, Mueller WM; the Vagus Nerve Stimulation Study Group E01–E05. Long-term treatment with vagus nerve stimulation in patients with refractory epilepsy. *Neurology* 1999; 53:1731–1735.
34. Murphy JV; the Pediatric VNS Study Group. Left vagal nerve stimulation in children with medically refractory epilepsy. *J Pediatr* 1999; 134:563–566.
35. Helmers SL, Wheless JW, Frost M *et al*. Vagus nerve stimulation therapy in pediatric patients with refractory epilepsy: retrospective study. *J Child Neurol* 2001; 16:843–848.
36. Frost M, Gates J, Helmers SL *et al*. Vagus nerve stimulation in children with refractory seizures associated with Lennox–Gastaut syndrome. *Epilepsia* 2001; 42:1148–1152.
37. Majorie HJM, Berfelo W, Aldenkamp AP *et al*. Vagus nerve stimulation in children with therapy-resistant epilepsy diagnosed as Lennox–Gastaut syndrome. Clinical results, neuropsychological effects and cost-effectiveness. *J Clin Neurophys* 2001; 18:419–428.
38. Lundgren J, Åmark P, Blennow G *et al*. Vagus nerve stimulation in 16 children with refractory epilepsy. *Epilepsia* 1998; 39:809–813.
39. Parain D, Penniello MJ, Berquen P *et al*. Vagal nerve stimulation in tuberous sclerosis complex patients. *Pediatr Neurol* 2001; 25:213–216.
40. Winston KR, Levisohn P, Miller BR *et al*. Vagal nerve stimulation for status epilepticus. *Pediatr Neurosurg* 2001; 34:190–192.
41. Murphy JV, Wheless JW, Schmoll CM. Left vagal nerve stimulation in six patients with hypothalamic hamartomas. *Pediatr Neurol* 2000; 23:167–168.
42. Smith B, Shatz R, Elisevich K *et al*. Effects of vagus nerve stimulation on progressive myoclonus epilepsy of Unverricht–Lundborg type. *Epilepsia* 2000; 41:1046–1048.
43. Harden CL, Pulver MC, Ravdin LD *et al*. A pilot study of mood in epilepsy patients treated with vagus nerve stimulation. *Epilepsy Behav* 2000; 1:93–99.
44. Elger G, Hoppe C, Falkai P *et al*. Vagus nerve stimulation is associated with mood improvements in epilepsy patients. *Epilepsy Behav* 2000; 42:203–210.

45. Nemeroff CB, Mayberg HS, Krahl SE *et al.*VNS therapy in treatment-resistant depression: clinical evidence and putative neurobiological mechanisms. *Neuropsychopharmacology* 2006; 31:1345–1355.
46. Clark KB, Naritoku DK, Smith DC *et al.* Enhanced recognition memory following vagus nerve stimulation in human subjects. *Nature Neuroscience* 1999; 2:94–98.
47. Ghacibeh GA, Shenker JI, Shenal B *et al.* The influence of vagus nerve stimulation on memory. *Cogn Behav Neurol* 2006; 19:119–122.
48. Cramer JA. Exploration of changes in health-related quality of life after 3 months of vagus nerve stimulation. *Epilepsy Behav* 2001; 2:460–465.
49. Hallbook T, Lundgren J, Blennow G *et al.* Long term effects on epileptiform activity with vagus nerve stimulation in children. *Seizure* 2005; 14:527–533.
50. Tatum WO, Moore DB, Stecker MM *et al.* Ventricular asystole during vagus nerve stimulation for epilepsy in humans. *Neurology* 2000; 52:1267–1269.
51. Asconapé JJ, Moore DD, Zipes DP *et al.* Bradycardia and asystole with the use of vagus nerve stimulation for the treatment of epilepsy: a rare complication of intraoperative device testing. *Epilepsia* 1999; 40:1452–1454.
52. Ali II, Pirzada NA, Kanjwal Y *et al.* Complete heart block with ventricular asystole during left vagus nerve stimulation for epilepsy. *Epilepsy Behav* 2004; 5:768–771.
53. Ben-Menachem E, Hellström K, Waldton C *et al.* Evaluation of refractory epilepsy treated with vagus nerve stimulation for up to 5 years. *Neurology* 1999; 52:1265–1267.
54. Marzec M, Edwards J, Sagher O *et al.* Effects of vagus nerve stimulation on sleep-related breathing in epilepsy patients. *Epilepsia* 2003; 44:930–935.
55. Holmes MD, Chang M, Kapur V. Sleep apnea and excessive daytime somnolence induced by vagal nerve stimulation. *Neurology* 2003; 61:1126–1129.
56. Khurana DS, Reumann M, Hobdell EF *et al.* Vagus nerve stimulation in children with refractory epilepsy: unusual complications and relationship to sleep-disordered breathing. *Childs Nerv Syst* 2007; 23:1309–1312.
57. Benbadis SR, Nyhenhuis J, Tatum WO *et al.* MRI of the brain is safe in patients implanted with the vagus nerve stimulator. *Seizure* 2001; 10:512–515.
58. Ben-Menachem E, Hellstrom K, Verstappen D. Analysis of direct hospital costs before and 18 months after treatment with vagus nerve stimulation therapy in 43 patients. *Neurology* 2002; 59(Suppl 4):S44–S47.
59. Privitera MD, Welty TE, Ficker DM *et al.* Vagus nerve stimulation for partial seizures. *Cochrane Database Syst Rev* 2002 (1): CD002896 Review.
60. Fisher RS, Krauss GL, Ramsay E *et al.* Assessment of vagus nerve stimulation for epilepsy: report of the Therapeutics and Technology Assessment Subcommittee of the American Academy of Neurology. *Neurology* 1997; 49:293–297.
61. Cramer J, Ben-Menachem E, French J. Treatment options for refractory epilepsy: new medications and vagal nerve stimulation. *Epilepsy Res* 2001; 47:17–25.

Section II

Childhood epilepsy

4

Treatment of severe epilepsies with onset under 2 years of age

Christin M. Eltze, J. Helen Cross

INTRODUCTION

The incidence of childhood epilepsy is highest in the first year of life [1, 2]. Most published series document poor long-term outcome with continuing seizures and neurodevelopmental impairment in 40–60% [3–8]. Structural brain abnormalities are common, seen in 42–60%, and aetiologies encompass a wide spectrum of developmental brain malformations, acquired brain injuries, and genetic and metabolic conditions. Despite the previously reported poor clinical outcome, there are infants whose epilepsy takes a more benign course. Several idiopathic epilepsy syndromes have been delineated and are now included in the recently proposed international classifications [9, 10]. These have in common absence of structural brain abnormalities, spontaneous seizure remission or responsiveness to first-line anti-epileptic medication and normal neurodevelopmental progress of most children. The underlying aetiology of these idiopathic forms is most likely genetic. Mutations in genes encoding ion channels have been found in some syndromes (Table 4.1).

A catastrophic course with medication-resistant seizures and severe impairment of developmental progress is characteristic of other neonatal/infantile epilepsy syndromes (Table 4.2). With the exception of one (malignant migrating partial seizures in infancy), these are categorized under epileptic encephalopathies, a new concept in which epileptiform abnormalities are understood to contribute significantly to progressive cerebral dysfunction in addition to the underlying aetiology. Seizure activity may have a negative impact on the immature brain, with impairment of neurodevelopment and cognitive function in later life. Emerging evidence to support this hypothesis includes the clinical observation of fluctuating developmental progress and cognitive function associated with seizure severity in humans as well as studies on animal models [11–13]. Thus, optimized diagnostic and therapeutic strategies that result in improved seizure control could have a significant impact on cognitive outcome in this age group.

Because of the heterogeneity of aetiologies, clinical course and outcomes in this early group, epilepsy management is challenging. This is compounded by diagnostic difficulties: a significant proportion of infants with normal brain imaging can not be categorized

Christin M. Eltze, MSc, MD, MRCPH, University College London Institute of Child Health and Great Ormond Street Hospital for Children NHS Trust, London, UK

J. Helen Cross, MB, ChB, PhD, FRCP, FRCPCH, University College London Institute of Child Health and Great Ormond Street Hospital for Children NHS Trust, London, UK

Table 4.1 Epilepsy syndromes with onset in the first 2 years of life, with good outcome in majority of patients

	Age of onset	Seizure types	Interictal EEG	Chromosomal loci; genes
Benign neonatal seizures [121]				
Non-familial	1–7 days	Focal clonic/apnoeas	Normal or focal/multi-focal abnormalities, discontinuous, 'theta pointu alternant' pattern	20; KCNQ2
Familial (autosomal dominant)	2–3 days	Diffuse tonic, probable focal		8; KCNQ3
Benign neonatal infantile seizures [122]*				
Autosomal dominant	Mean 11 weeks ± 9 weeks†	Focal, secondarily generalized	Normal or focal abnormalities	2; SCN2A
Benign infantile seizures [123–125]				
Non-familial	3–20 months (majority <12 months)	Focal	Normal	16 [126], 19
Familial (autosomal dominant)	4–8 months			1; ATP1A2 [127]
Benign myoclonic epilepsy in infancy [128, 129]	6 months to 3 years	Myoclonic Reflex myoclonus	Normal Ictal EEG: generalized spike or polyspike and wave discharges	Unknown

*Not included in recent ILAE classification proposal [9]; †onset from neonatal period up to 13 months [130].
EEG, electroencephalogram

Table 4.2 Epilepsy syndromes with onset in the first 2 years of life, with poor outcome in majority of patients

	Age of onset	Seizure types	Interictal EEG	Other characteristics
Early infantile epileptic encephalopathy (Ohtahara syndrome) [128, 129]	Birth to 3 months	Tonic spasms, focal, rarely myoclonus	Suppression–burst pattern (in waking and sleep)	Aetiology: predominantly structural brain abnormalities, developmental brain malformations; transition to West syndrome at 3–6 months of age
Severe myoclonic encephalopathy [131]	Birth to 28 days	Myoclonic, focal, tonic spasms (later)	Suppression–burst pattern (enhanced or only in sleep)	Aetiology: unknown, or metabolic disorders
Malignant partial seizures in infancy [102, 103]	First year of life, birth to 7 months	Focal (large variety of motor and autonomic manifestations), occur in clusters	Multi-focal spikes. Ictal: continuous but shifting epileptiform activity from one region to another and from one hemisphere to the other	No structural brain abnormalities
West syndrome [44]	Birth to 5 years, majority in first 12 months (peak 3–7 months)	Spasms, focal seizures antecedent or concomitantly in one-third	Hypsarrhythmia	Aetiology: wide spectrum. Structural brain abnormalities, metabolic disorders, chromosomal abnormalities or unknown
SMEI (Dravet syndrome) [76]	Within first year	Initially, atypical febrile convulsions (prolonged, unilateral clonic seizures). Subsequently, tonic, tonic–clonic, myoclonus, focal	Initially, normal. Subsequently, generalized, focal and multi-focal abnormalities	Genetic aetiology: chromosome 5q31-q33, SCN1A mutation in 35–85% of patients [77, 133]; chromosome 2q24, GABR2, γ2 subunit of GABA receptor in two patients with SMEI

EEG, electroencephalogram; GABA, γ-aminobutyric acid; GABR, γ-aminobutyric receptor; SCN, severe congenital neutropenia; SMEI, severe myoclonic epilepsy in infancy.

under the current international epilepsy syndrome classification, and the diagnosis of a benign syndrome is often impossible at the onset [14]. Seizures in this age group may be difficult to recognize because of subtle manifestations such as hypotonia, simple staring, mild convulsive movements or autonomic features including flushing, pallor and peri-oral cyanosis. Typical generalized tonic–clonic seizures are rare. More commonly, focal seizures with head and eye deviation, tonic posturing with uni- or bilateral involvement and clonic movements are observed. Seizures that clinically appear to be generalized frequently have focal ictal electroencephalogram (EEG) correlates [15, 16]. In the differential diagnosis, a number of paroxysmal non-epileptogenic attacks have to be considered (Table 4.3). A video recording of the events supplied by carers can be very helpful in this context and video-electroencephalography (EEG) may be necessary in addition to the standard EEG recording (awake and sleep states).

Once the diagnosis of epilepsy is confirmed, an adequately staged diagnostic work-up is important to guide therapeutic interventions. This should include optimized magnetic resonance imaging (MRI) for all young children under 2 years [17]. Symptomatic focal epilepsies with hemispheric or focal lesions can be amenable to epilepsy surgery. Especially for infants with medication-resistant seizures, neurological signs and neurodevelopmental impairment, who have no structural brain abnormalities on the magnetic resonance (MR) scan, neurometabolic and genetic investigations should be considered as detailed in Table 4.4.

In the following paragraphs, we will address the therapeutic options for infants younger than 2 years old presenting with severe medication-resistant epilepsies. These include a trial of vitamin supplementation, pharmacological treatment, ketogenic diet and epilepsy surgery.

VITAMIN SUPPLEMENTATION

A number of treatable metabolic disorders, including vitamin-responsive conditions, present with medically resistant seizures in the first year of life [18]. Response to empirical treatment may have to guide further investigative work-up. Two examples are described in detail whilst other disorders are also listed in Table 4.5.

DISORDERS OF VITAMIN B6 METABOLISM

Pyridoxal 5′-phosphate (PLP) is the B6 vitamer, which has co-factor activity and acts with several enzymes that are involved in the metabolism of neurotransmitters (e.g. dopamine, serotonin, glutamate and γ-aminobutyric acid [GABA]). Progress in the understanding of

Table 4.3 Non-epileptogenic paroxysmal disorders in infancy

Syncopes	Reflex anoxic syncope
	Cyanotic breath holding
	Vasovagal/vagovagal syncope
	Cardiogenic (e.g. long Q–T syndrome)
Other paroxysmal disorders	Sandifer syndrome (gastro-oesophageal reflux)
	Benign sleep myoclonus
	Benign myoclonus in infancy
	Hyperekplexia
	Paroxysmal movement disorders
	Benign paroxysmal torticollis in infancy
	Benign paroxysmal tonic upwards gaze
	Parasomnias: night terrors, sleep walking, etc.

Table 4.4 Investigations in infants with epilepsy

Core investigations	Woods light examination (renal ultrasound, cardiac echo) Magnetic resonance imaging EEG (sleep and awake recording)
Infants with difficult-to-treat epilepsy	Full blood count with differential blood film Urea & electrolytes Liver function tests Serum lactate/pyruvate Ammonia Acylcarnitine profile, free carnitine Biotinidase Pre-prandial glucose CSF/blood ratio (abnormal ≤ 0.45) Urate Plasma very-long-chain fatty acids Plasma amino acids Chromosomes Urinary organic acids Urinary sulphites
Further tests to consider	Lysosomal enzymes Copper, caeruloplasmin Transferin isoelectric focusing (congenital disorders of glycolization) Urine oligosaccharides, mucopolysaccharides CSF: amino acids (including CSF/plasma glycine ratio); lactate; biogenic amines Molecular genetics: DNA – *SCN1A* mutation, *ARX* mutation [134, 135], *CDKL5* mutation [136], *POLG* mutation [137, 138], mitochondrial deletions (MELAS, MERRF, etc.) Muscle biopsy: respiratory chain enzymes

CSF, cerebrospinal fluid; DNA, deoxyribonucleic acid; EEG, electroencephalogram; MELAS, mitochondrial encephalomyopathy, lactic acidosis and stroke-like episodes; MERRF, myoclonic epilepsy with ragged red fibres.

disorders caused by deficiency of cerebral PLP has been made recently. Increased consumption of PLP through inactivation or defects of its biosynthesis in liver and brain involving pyridox(am)ine phosphate oxidase underlie two disorders with infantile presentations [19, 20].

Pyridoxine-dependent Epilepsy

A mutation of the aldehyde dehydrogenase (ALDH) *7A1* gene on chromosome 5q31 encoding antiquitin (α-aminoadipic semialdehyde dehydrogenase) has recently been discovered as a major cause of pyridoxine-dependent epilepsy [21]. Dysfunction of the enzyme antiquitin, which is part of the pipecolic pathway of lysine catabolism, results in accumulation of a metabolite (L-Δ1-piperideine-6-carboxylate) that condenses with PLP and inactivates the co-factor. A lead to the discovery of this phenomenon was the observation of raised pipecolic acid in the cerebrospinal fluid (CSF) of patients with pyridoxine-dependent epilepsy prior to treatment and the decrease following pyridoxine supplementation [19, 22]. Measurement of urinary α-aminoadipic semialdehyde, another accumulating metabolite in the above-mentioned pathway, has been suggested as a biomarker for pyridoxine-dependent epilepsy [20]. The typical clinical presentation of this disorder is in the first days of life with intractable, often multiple, seizure types and encephalopathy, observed

Table 4.5 Treatable metabolic epileptic encephalopathies

Condition	Clinical manifestations	Investigations	Treatment
Disorders of vitamin B6 metabolism			
Pyridoxine-dependent epilepsy	Early-onset multiple seizure types, encephalopathy, hyperalertness, irritability, abnormal cry, startle	Urinary α-aminoadipic semialdehyde Mutation analysis aldehyde dehydrogenase 7A1 gene 5q31	Initially (early onset form): pyridoxine 100 mg i.v.; maintenance treatment: 15 mg/kg/day orally (higher doses may be required) [20]
Pyridoxamine phosphate oxidase deficiency	Premature delivery, fetal distress, metabolic acidosis, seizure onset within 12 h of delivery	CSF biogenic monoamine neurotransmitter metabolites	Pyridoxal phosphate 40 mg/kg/day
Folinic acid responsive seizures	Neonatal-onset seizures, frequent status epilepticus, developmental delay	CSF biogenic monoamine neurotransmitter metabolites	Folinic acid
Biotinidase deficiency	Myoclonic seizures, infantile spasms, hypotonia, ataxia, developmental impairment, optic atrophy, sensorineuronal hearing loss, alopecia, conjunctivitis, skin rash	Enzyme essay	Biotin 5–20 mg/day [18]
Holocarboxylase deficiency		Activity of mitochondrial carboxylases of cultured fibroblasts or in leucocytes following biotin supplementation	
Serine deficiency syndromes (3-phophoglycerate deficiency)	Seizures: tonic–clonic, myoclonic, infantile spasms. Developmental arrest, congenital microcephaly	Plasma/CSF amino acids	L-serine 400–600 mg/kg/day [139] (reduction of seizures, improvement of MR imaging findings, little developmental progress)
Glucose transporter-1 deficiency syndromes [140]	Seizures (cyanotic, drop attacks, abnormal eye movements), developmental delay; movement disorder: ataxia, dystonia, pyramidal tract signs	Glucose CSF/blood ratio ≤0.45 (following 4–6-h fast). Glucose uptake into erythrocytes. Mutation analysis, GLUT1 gene (1p35–p13.3)	Ketogenic diet
Creatine deficiency disorders: GAMT*	Various seizures: infantile spasms, atypical absences, astatic seizures, GTC, developmental arrest, movement disorder, severe language impairment	Plasma/urine creatinine (low), MR spectroscopy (low creatinine peak), urinary guanidinoacatic acid (increased)	Creatine replacement: 0.5–2 g/kg/day [141]. Diet: arginine restricted, ornithine supplemented

*Guanidinoacetate methyltransferase.
CSF, cerebrospinal fluid; GTC, generalized tonic–clonic; MR, magnetic resonance.

in one-third of cases, with hyperalertness, irritability, abnormal cry or startle. Additional systemic features that can mimic sepsis are abdominal distension, vomiting, hypothermia, respiratory distress and metabolic acidosis. Associated cerebral malformations have been described and include hypoplasia of the posterior part of the corpus callosum, cerebellar hypoplasia, focal cortical dysplasia and hydrocephalus [23]. The EEG is commonly grossly abnormal and a 'burst suppression' pattern is often seen [24]. Infants show a prompt response to 100-mg pyridoxine given intravenously. Close cardiorespiratory monitoring during the first injection is recommended as apnoea and cardiovascular instability with isoelectric EEG can occur. More commonly, children may show cerebral depression with hypotonia and sleepiness. The late-onset form presents up to the age of 3 years and is not associated with encephalopathy or structural brain abnormalities. There may be a partial response to anti-epileptic medication initially but seizures eventually became intractable. Seizures respond to 100mg/day pyridoxine orally within 1–2 days and lifelong supplementation with 15mg/kg/day up to 500mg is necessary [20]. Untreated cases develop severe motor disorder with sensory impairments. The outcome is variable in treated cases and worse motor, cognitive and language functions are associated with early onset of the condition [23].

Pyridox(am)ine Phosphate Oxidase (PNPO) Deficiency

A defect in the enzyme that oxidizes phosphorylated pyridoxine and pyridoxamine to form PLP in liver and brain has been reported in five neonates of three families presenting with an epileptic encephalopathy that showed no or incomplete response to pyridoxine. One of these neonates responded to treatment with pyridoxal phosphate (10mg/kg by nasogastric tube given 6-hourly) at the age of 2 weeks. All neonates were born prematurely, had signs of fetal distress (one requiring intubation post delivery), metabolic acidosis was common and the seizure onset was in the first 12h of life. The EEG demonstrated a suppression–burst pattern that was reversed in the neonate treated with PLP. Cerebral depression with hypotonia and unresponsiveness was observed in this neonate following the first dose [25]. All patients had a similar pattern of biochemical changes, implicating a dysfunction of the PLP-dependent enzymes including aromatic L-amino-acid decarboxylase: low CSF concentrations of homovanillic acid (dopamine metabolite) and 5-hydroxyindolacetic acid (serotonin metabolite), raised CSF methoxytyrosine, threonine and glycine. Subsequently, homozygous mutations in the *PNPO* gene situated on chromosome 17q21 were found with expression studies demonstrating null activity or marked reduced activity of pyridox(am)ine phosphate oxidase [26].

The condition was fatal in four neonates and the infant that was treated with PLP had a severe dystonic motor disorder, global developmental delay and acquired microcephaly at 2 years and 8 months. These patients may represent the severe end of the phenotypic spectrum. Recently, six children with PNPO deficiency and atypical biochemical findings were reported: two who received treatment within the first month of life showed normal development or moderate psychomotor retardation thereafter, whereas four with no or late treatment died or showed severe psychomotor delay [27].

Wang *et al.* report response of medically intractable seizures to PLP in 11 of 94 children with epilepsy of unknown aetiology [28]. Seizure onset was in the first year of life in 10 patients and at 15 months in one patient. Six patients presented with infantile spasms. Five of the 11 PLP responders could be successfully controlled with pyridoxine, whilst six required PLP. Unfortunately, biochemical data from CSF and urine were not available for this cohort. PLP and pyridoxine may have other anti-epileptic properties independently from the mechanisms described above that may contribute to improvement of seizure control as adjunct to conventional anti-epileptic treatment [20].

PLP has a role in the empirical treatment of neonatal-onset epileptic encephalopathies and should be the next step after intravenous (i.v.) pyridoxine (PLP 100mg). In addition, there is a wider indication for drug-resistant epilepsy with unknown aetiology, especially early-onset forms including West syndrome. PLP doses of 10–50 mg/kg/day have been used. Other disorders of vitamin B6 metabolism that are associated with milder types of epilepsy have been described [19, 20].

Folinic Acid-Responsive Seizures

This condition was discovered by coincidence. A 6-month-old patient with neonatal-onset, medication-resistant and pyridoxine-unresponsive epilepsy became seizure free after folinic acid was commenced because of a misunderstanding [29]. Since then, further cases have been reported in the literature [30–33]. High-performance liquid chromatography, used to measure neurotransmitter metabolites, revealed an unknown compound which is a marker for this disorder. This compound decreased on treatment with folinic acid [30]. CSF neopterin, 5-methyltetrahydrofolate and dopamine, as well as serotonine metaobolites, were normal. Although the described patients presented breakthrough seizures and frequent episodes of status epilepticus on treatment with folinic acid, seizure control was regained with increased doses. The children exhibited global developmental delay, despite seizure control. MRI showed diffuse cerebral atrophy, cerebellar atrophy or signal abnormalities in the white matter. Although the underlying pathomechanism is unknown, this appears to be an autosomal recessive inherited condition, as some of the index cases had siblings that died with intractable neonatal-onset seizures [34]. Empirical treatment with folinic acid (2–5 mg/kg/day orally) should therefore be considered in neonatal-onset seizures that are unresponsive to pyridoxine and pyridoxal phosphate.

PHARMACOLOGICAL TREATMENT

GENERAL PRINCIPLES

Both conventional and newer anti-epileptic drugs (AEDs) are used in infants. Specific pharmacokinetic characteristics in infants, such as slower gastrointestinal absorption, higher volumes of distribution and shorter clearance periods, require adjustment of anti-epileptic drug doses. The dose of carbamazepine may have to be increased to 30–50 mg/kg/day compared with older children (15–35 mg/kg/day) [35]. The non-linear pharmacokinetic profile of phenytoin imposes a challenge in this age group, especially when the drug is given orally with subsequent insufficient plasma levels or toxicity. Phenobarbital and valproate have linear pharmacokinetic characteristics and are less problematic to use in this age group [35]. Valproate, however, interferes with mitochondrial function (β-fatty acid oxidation) and can uncover inborn errors of metabolism, such as mitochondrial cytopathies [36]. Hepatotoxic encephalopathies have been reported in infants under the age of 2 years; commonly in children with severe epilepsy, neurological abnormalities and severe developmental impairment [15]. Valproate should be avoided in infants with abnormal liver function and multi-organ failure, polytherapy or in those where the exact aetiology is unclear [37]. It may otherwise be quite effective in children with cerebral malformations. Benzodiazepines, such as clonazepam and nitrazepam, cause somnolence, hypotonia with increased secretion of saliva and subsequent risk of aspiration.

Most data from anti-epileptic drug trials are available from children with infantile spasms but there is a paucity of data from randomized controlled trials for other infantile epilepsy syndromes as well as for newer AEDs. The majority of studies have open-label uncontrolled designs and there are no comparative trials with conventional anti-epileptic drugs. In the following section, the pharmacological treatment of specific epilepsy syndromes will be discussed.

INFANTILE SPASMS AND WEST SYNDROME

Natural or synthetic adrenocorticotropic hormone (ACTH), glucocorticosteroids and vigabatrin (VGB) are the main pharmacological agents currently suggested for the treatment of infantile spasms (IS). In addition, conventional and newer anti-epileptic drugs, as well as vitamin B6, are used. There is no agreement which agent should be commenced first line. Protocols differ in dosing regimes as well as duration of treatment courses, depending on geographical area and availability of these agents. VGB is not licensed in the US, natural ACTH has been replaced by synthetic ACTH in some European countries and Japan, and different types of oral steroids are in use. Despite a large number of published trials investigating efficacy and tolerability of VGB, glucocorticosteroids, ACTH and other anti-epileptic drugs for the treatment of ISs, only limited conclusions can be drawn due to differences in design and treatment protocols as well as poor overall quality of most randomized studies [38, 39]. Two systematic literature reviews have been published recently: (i) the practice parameter for the medical treatment of infantile spasms of the American Academy of Neurology (AAN) and the Child Neurology Society based on a review that included 159 articles (published between 1966 and May 2002) classified into four levels of evidence (Class I: prospective randomized controlled trial with masked outcome assessment; Class II: prospective matched group cohort study in representative population with masked outcome assessment; Class III: all other controlled trials, including natural history controls or patients serving as own controls; Class IV: uncontrolled studies, case series, case reports or expert opinion) [39] and (ii) a Cochrane review in the UK that included 11 randomized controlled trials [38].

ACTH and Oral Steroids

Hormonal therapy in the form of ACTH has been used for the treatment of infantile spasms for more than 40 years. It is thought to reduce corticotropin-releasing hormone (CRH) through its action on cerebral melanocortin receptors [40]. There is evidence from animal rodent models that CRH has epileptogenic properties in the immature brain. CRH is also increased in patients with infantile spasms [41]. Another suggested mode of action is the modulation of neurocorticosteroids that act on $GABA_A$ receptors [42].

The AAN practice parameter concluded that ACTH is probably effective for the short treatment of IS and resolution of hypsarrhythmia [39]. The proportion of patients experiencing cessation of spasms, usually within 2 weeks of treatment, varied between 42% and 87% in five randomized trials (one class II and four class III trials). The total duration of treatment ranged from 4 to 12 weeks (highest dose 2 to 6 weeks) and relapses occurred in 15–33%. There was insufficient evidence to recommend an optimum dose. One class I [43] and one class III trial [44] comparing low-dose against high-dose regimes revealed no significant differences: Hrachovy et al. 1994 compared $150\,IU/m^2/day$ with $20–30\,IU/m^2/day$ (natural ACTH) and Yanagaki et al. 1999, $1\,IU/kg/day$ with $0.2\,IU/kg/day$ (synthetic ACTH). Dosing regimes for ACTH vary according to country, with starting doses of $10–20\,IU/day$ (synthetic ACTH) used in Japan to $150\,IU/m^2/day$, more commonly $40\,IU/day$ for 1–2 months in the US [45].

With respect to oral glucocorticosteroids the AAN review concludes that there is insufficient evidence for efficacy of oral steroids in the treatment of IS. One class II and several class III trials showed cessation of spasms in <42% of patients at doses of 2 mg/kg/day. Two studies (Baram et al., 1996; Hrachovy et al., 1983) compared ACTH with prednisolone (2 mg/kg/day). Whilst Baram et al. showed superiority of ACTH vs. prednisolone using a high-dose regime (150 units/m²/day), Hrachovy et al. failed to show a difference with lower doses of ACTH (20–30 units/day). In the Cochrane review, results from the two studies were combined showing a responder rate of 67% for ACTH compared with 31% for prednisolone (Peto odds ratio 4.2, 95% confidence interval [CI] 1.4–12.4). The authors concluded that treatment with ACTH was superior to low-dose prednisolone (2 mg/kg/day).

The common reported adverse effects associated with ACTH treatment and oral steroids are hypertension, irritability, infection and cerebral atrophy. Hypertension and cerebral atrophy were more common with higher doses of ACTH [39]. In addition, longer duration of ACTH treatment was associated with cardiomyopathy [46]. A number of retrospective studies, as well as an open-label prospective comparative study from Japan, suggest that lower doses of synthetic ACTH (doses ranging from 0.2 to 1.28 IU/kg/day) are better tolerated than and as effective as higher doses [44, 47]. A total of 51 out of 106 patients were seizure free at follow-up (98 patients were followed >2 years) in one retrospective series [48]. Cessation of spasms and resolution of hypsarrhythmia was reported in 17 out of 27 (55%) patients treated with 0.2 IU/kg/day for 2–3 weeks [49]. Of the 27 patients that were followed up for >12 months, 13 (48%) remained in remission, including one patient who received a second 2-week treatment course of synthetic ACTH at higher dose (1 IU/kg/day). Cryptogenic ISs show better responses compared with symptomatic cases that may require higher doses [48, 50].

Vigabatrin

Vigabatrin (VGB) increases availability of the inhibitory neurotransmitter γ-aminobutyric acid (GABA) by binding irreversibly to its degrading enzyme, GABA transaminase. Because it is only minimally metabolized and almost entirely eliminated by renal secretion, there is no induction of hepatic enzymes and interaction with other anti-epileptic drugs. Efficacy of VGB for the treatment in IS has been shown in a number of studies. The AAN review identified three controlled trials (one class I, two class III), including one randomized placebo-controlled trial, and 11 class IV studies. In the three controlled studies, 22–44% of symptomatic IS and 27–55% of idiopathic IS responded with relapse rates ranging from 8% to 20%. Higher doses of VGB (100–150 mg/kg/day) appear to be more effective for seizure cessation and resolution of hypsarrhythmia. However, Mackay *et al.* were unable to determine dose dependency from nine prospective trials with various dosing regimes because the number of patients was too small [39]. Patients with IS associated with tuberous sclerosis (TS) show particularly good responses to VGB. In their systematic review, Mackay *et al.* pooled data from seven studies (two class III and five class IV) showing remission of spasms in 41 (91%) out of 45 patients [39]. Another small trial comparing VGB with hydrocortisone, which included only patients with TS, found 100% responder in the VGB group ($n = 11$) vs. 4 out of 11 (45%) in the hydrocortisone group [51].

Adverse effects include sedation, irritability, insomnia and hypotonia leading to withdrawal in 0–6% [39]. Of more concern are irreversible concentric visual field defects that occur in up to 43% of patients [52–54]. Whether these effects are dose dependent and cumulative over time or are the result of an idiosyncratic drug reaction is a controversial topic [52, 55, 56]. The evaluation of visual fields is difficult in infants. Although alternative assessment methods that are tolerated by young children have been developed, at present no recommendations can be made with respect to frequency and methods used for evaluation [57, 58, 39].

Vigabatrin vs. ACTH or Prednisolone

A recently published multicentre randomized controlled trial compared effectiveness of tetracosactide (synthetic ACTH: 0.5 mg [40 IU] on alternate days for 2 weeks, increased to 0.75 mg [60 IU] on alternate days if seizure control had not been achieved after 1 week), prednisolone (10 mg four times per day for 2 weeks, increasing to 20 mg three times per day if seizures were not controlled after 1 week) and VGB (maximum dose 150 mg/kg/day) for the short-term treatment of cryptogenic and symptomatic IS. After 2 weeks, patients allocated to prednisolone or tetracosactide received a reducing dose of prednisolone (reduction by 10 mg every 5 days or, if on a higher dose of prednisolone, reduction to 40 mg, 20 mg and 10 mg every 5 days). Patients with TS were excluded, presuming VGB to be more effective in TS [59].

Cessation of spasms on days 13 and 14 was more likely with hormonal treatments – 78% of patients enrolled to prednisolone and tetracosactide vs. 54% in the VGB group were spasm free (difference 19%, 95% CI 1–36, $P = 0.045$). The early superior effect of corticosteroids was not maintained in the long term. The study was under-powered to establish difference or equivalency between prednisolone and tetracosactide. At follow-up after 12 or 13 months, there was no difference between the treatment groups with respect to proportion of patients with absence of spasms (80 out of 106, 75%) and patients seizure free (60 out of 106, 57%) [60]. The neurodevelopmental outcome was assessed using the Vineland Adaptive Behaviour Scale (VABS), a survey questionnaire that is completed through an interview with carers. The VABS composite score in the subgroup of patients with no aetiology was higher in the hormone-treatment group (difference 9.3, 95% CI 1.3–17.3; $P = 0.025$) at 14 months' follow-up compared with the VGB group. Five children had died during the follow-up: one child with *Staphylococcus aureus* septicaemia on day 15 of prednisolone treatment and four children died later from other causes (Leigh's disease, aspiration pneumonia and epileptic encephalopathy).

Other Agents

Sodium valproate (VPA), benzodiazepines (nitrazepam, clonazepam), topiramate (TPM), zonisamide (ZNS) and high-dose pyridoxal-phosphate have been used for the treatment of IS. The majority of studies are uncontrolled retrospective or prospective case series providing insufficient evidence for their efficacy [39]. One controlled study compared nitrazepam with ACTH [61]. The reported outcome measure, however, was reduction rather than cessation of spasms. The proportion of subjects showing >50 % reduction of spasms in the short term was higher in the nitrazepam group. However, relapse rates, effects on EEG and long-term outcome are not reported [38]. Although suppression of spasms and improvement of EEG abnormalities can be achieved with benzodiazepines such as nitrazepam and clonazepam, unwanted effects such as hypotonia and increase of secretions with risk of aspirations limits their use in clinical practice [46]. Sodium VPA, often used in higher doses (27 mg/kg/day to 100 mg/kg/day or 100–200 mg/kg/day), suppressed spasms in 70–90% of patients with relapses in 23% of cases. Thrombocytopenia has been observed in several studies [39].

A small pilot study showed that TPM (doses 8–25 mg/kg/day) suppressed spasms in 5 of 11 (45%) young children, who did not respond to other anti-epileptic drugs. One child relapsed (20%) and after 18 months, four (36%) remained seizure free. Adverse effects were irritability, sleep disturbance, rapid breathing and unsteadiness. Data from recent case series are more disappointing, showing cessation of spasms in 0–20% in the short term [62, 63], in 16% (9 out of 54) after long-term follow-up [64] and around one-third of patients showed >50% seizure reduction [62, 63]. The mean doses of TPM were lower in two of these studies (4.7 mg/kg/day and 5.2 mg/kg/day) [63, 64]. The most common reported side-effects included irritability, weight loss and anorexia. In addition, clinically symptomatic metabolic acidosis has been reported recently in case series of infants and toddlers [65].

A number of Japanese case series report cessation of spasms after treatment with ZNS in 20–38% (doses 4–13 mg/kg/day) [66]. The proportion of responders was higher amongst cryptogenic IS. Over one-third of patients relapsed as documented in two studies with long-term follow-up [67, 68]. A recent study reported cessation of spasms and resolution of hypsarrhythmia in 6 of 23 (26%) children with symptomatic IS. Children who were refractory to ZNS failed also to respond to VBT and ACTH [69].

Around 30 of 216 (15%) of patients with IS went into remission following treatment with high-dose PLP (30–50 mg/kg/day). This was more likely to occur with cryptogenic cases. Twenty per cent relapsed (all symptomatic IS) within 10 months after initial suppression of spasms [70]. The efficacy of sulthiam ([STM], doses 5–10 mg/kg/day) has also been investigated in a multicentre randomized placebo-controlled trial that included 30 symptomatic and seven cryptogenic IS patients. All patients were started on pyridoxine 3 days prior to and continued treatment during the 6-day double-blind period. Six of 20 (30%) patients in the treatment group responded (cessation of spasms and resolution of hypsarrhythmia) and none in the placebo group ($n = 17$). The three TS patients in the treatment group failed to respond. Somnolence was more commonly observed in the treatment group (4 out of 20 [20%] vs. 1 out of 17 [6%]). None of the responders relapsed during the follow-up period (6–32 months, mean 16 months) [71]. The ketogenic diet is a further option in resistant cases and will be discussed later in this chapter.

Further data are required to make evidence-based recommendations on the treatment of infantile spasms. The choice remains between steroids and vigabatrin as first-line therapy and this may be influenced by the aetiology, and preference of the caring physician with the parents. Synthetic ACTH and oral steroids appear to be most efficacious in short-term control only of infantile spasms without TS but are associated with significant side-effects. Data from retrospective series suggest that a greater time lag between appropriate treatment and remission of spasms [72–74] or more recently longer duration of hysparrhythmia [75], is associated with a more unfavourable developmental/cognitive outcome. However, there is a lack of data from prospective longitudinal studies that use appropriate standardized methods for the neurodevelopmental evaluation, to support the view that early aggressive treatment would achieve a better cognitive outcome independently from the underlying aetiology. The choice of the most appropriate treatment has to be made for each patient in discussion with the parents under consideration of the individual clinical circumstances and adverse effects.

SEVERE MYOCLONIC EPILEPSY IN INFANCY (DRAVET SYNDROME)

Severe myoclonic epilepsy in infancy (SMEI), first described by Dravet, is an early-onset epilepsy syndrome with catastrophic course and poor seizure as well as cognitive outcome. Onset is in the first year of life. Developmentally normal infants present with atypical febrile convulsions (focal features, prolonged) and episodes of febrile as well as afebrile status epilepticus. The occurrence of afebrile multiple type seizures including myoclonus from the second year of life onwards is accompanied by developmental plateauing or regression. Whilst the interictal EEG is initially normal, later in the course with expression of afebrile seizures generalized, multi-focal and focal epileptiform abnormalities are seen. Photosensitivity has been observed in up to 42% of patients and has been recognized in the first year of life. Increase in body temperature to over 38°C by fever and probably also bathing in hot water are potent triggers of seizures in this syndrome [76]. Over 70% of patients presenting with the typical features were found to have a mutation in the gene encoding the α-subunit of a neuronal voltage-gated sodium channel, *SCN1A* [77]. However, detection rates for *SCN1A* mutations vary between 35% and 85% [78–80]. Patients with atypical and borderline variants have also *SCN1A* mutations and are likely to present part of the phenotypical spectrum. SMEI, perhaps under-reported, is a rare diagnosis and an incidence estimated at 1 in 40000 life births has been reported [81]. The majority of the published information relating to anti-epileptic drug treatment in this patient group is derived from case series and open-label uncontrolled studies with few exceptions. Pharmacological control of seizures is difficult and temporary improvement can be achieved with VPA, benzodiazepines and phenobarbital [76]. Carbamazepine and lamotrigine should be avoided as these can aggravate seizures [76, 82]. Phenytoin has been reported to induce movement disorders in patients with SMEI and may have in combination with VPA an increased risk of hepatic failure [83, 84].

Stiripentol (STP), in combination with VPA and clobazam, was useful in controlling convulsive seizures in children with SMEI over the age of 3 years. Chiron *et al.* conducted a randomized placebo-controlled trial that showed a significantly higher proportion of responders (>50% reduction of clonic or tonic–clonic seizures) during the 2 months double-blinded period in the treatment group (71%) compared with the placebo group (5%) [85]. In addition, the total number of clonic or tonic–clonic seizures was significantly reduced in the treatment group, in which 9 out of 21 patients (43%) became seizure free. None of the patients in the placebo group became seizure free. In the subsequent open-label period, patients were treated with 50–100 mg/kg/day STP. Long-term outcome data of a retrospective cohort ($n = 46$), published by the same group, showed that after a mean follow-up of 2.9 years, 65% of patients still had more than 50% seizure reduction [86]. Seizure duration and number of episodes of status epilepticus were reduced. The most frequent side-effects were loss of appetite (25%), weight loss (17%), insomnia (13%), somnolence (13%) and ataxia (13%). STP inhibits the hepatic p450 cytochrome enzymes and slows degradation of dependent anti-epileptic drugs. A broad anti-epileptic effect of STP has been demonstrated in animal models (pentetrazole and supramaximal shock models) [87]. Although its mode of action is still under investigation, *in vitro* studies demonstrated interference with GABA-ergic transmission, especially increased opening duration of GABA$_A$ channels [88]. However, it remains unclear as to whether the anti-epileptic benefit seen is directly from STP or from the enhancement of metabolites of comedication.

TPM may also be effective in this patient group. Two small controlled open-label studies that enrolled patients aged between 2 and 22 years showed similar results with 55% of responders (>50% seizure reduction) and 16% of patients becoming seizure free. TPM doses ranged from 3 to 10 mg/kg/day [89, 90]. In a further open-label multicentre study enrolling patients with intractable epilepsy under the age of 2 years, two out of six infants with SMEI demonstrated >50% seizure reduction [91].

Zonisamide and potassium bromide are other agents that have been used in SMEI and atypical or borderline variants (no atypical absence seizures, myoclonic seizures less frequent) with some effect [76, 92, 93]. Potassium bromide was less effective for absence and myoclonic seizures, but reduced occurrence of generalized tonic–clonic seizures by >50% in 8 out of 22 (36%) patients after 12 months of treatment. SMEI borderline patients required higher doses (mean doses 101 mg/kg/day) compared with the SMEI group (58 mg/kg/day).

Some authors advocate early and aggressive treatment of seizures with a view that this will lead to optimized developmental outcome, following the premise that this is an epileptic encephalopathy. There are anecdotal data to suggest this may be the case, although the role of the genotype in outcome is also not fully determined. Sankar *et al.* propose the following strategy: sodium VPA, as first-line anti-epileptic medication, should be commenced following the first febrile or afebrile status epilepticus or when a second febrile or afebrile seizure occurs within a month [94]. In addition, regular use of anti-pyretic medication during febrile illnesses and medication for acute treatment at the onset of convulsive seizures, such as rectal diazepam or buccal midazolam, is advocated at this stage. With onset of afebrile seizures, especially with associated impairment of developmental progress, STP adjunctive to VPA and clobazam or TPM with VPA is suggested. The ketogenic diet can also be considered. As third-line anti-epileptic medication, ethosuximide, levetiracetam or zonisamide are proposed for myoclonias and ethosuximide for atypical absences/non-convulsive states.

OTHER INFANCY-ONSET EPILEPSY SYNDROMES WITH CATASTROPHIC COURSE

Ohtahara syndrome, or early infantile epileptic encephalopathy (EIEE) and early myoclonic encephalopathy (EME), are rare syndromes presenting in the neonatal period or early infancy and have most characteristically a suppression–burst pattern on the EEG. Although at the onset, tonic spasms and partial seizures are the main seizure types of EIEE, EME presents with fragmentary, erratic myoclonias as well as partial seizures. Structural brain abnormalities appear to be more common in EIEE, while the aetiology in EME is frequently obscure, or inborn errors of metabolism have been reported [95]. Some EIEE cases show a characteristic evolution to West and Lennox–Gastaut syndromes as patients become older, suggesting that EIEE is an age-dependent epileptic encephalopathy. There is considerable overlap between EIEE and EME, which is reviewed by some authors as different manifestations on the same spectrum of one condition [96]. In both syndromes, seizures are resistant to pharmacological treatment and motor as well as cognitive outcomes are poor. In EIEE, treatment with ACTH before 3 months of age achieves poor results. Cryptogenic cases may respond to ACTH following transition to West syndrome [96]. Zonisamide has been reported to have been effective in four patients with EIEE, and recently a case responding to high-dose phenobarbital (serum levels 60–100 mg/dl) has also been reported [97–99]. Vigabatrin has been effective in infants with focal cortical dysplasia and may therefore be considered in patients with symptomatic EIEE [100, 101].

Malignant migrating partial seizures in infancy have only recently been included in the international syndrome classifications under symptomatic (or probably symptomatic) focal epilepsies [9, 102]. Polymorphic treatment-resistant seizures with focal characteristics start between the first week and 7 months of age. Seizures occur in clusters that are associated with cognitive and motor deterioration. The ictal EEG is characteristic, with continuous shifting activity from one region to another and from one hemisphere to the other. The long-term outcome is poor, with some patients developing secondary microcephaly. Patients with uncontrollable seizures have a high risk of mortality in the first year with respiratory complications. Limited developmental progress may be observed in patients whose seizure disorder can be brought under control. Neuroimaging reveals normal findings [103]. It remains unclear as to whether this is a single condition or a syndromic manifestation of multiple aetiologies. Information on treatment is limited. Conventional anti-epileptic drugs and corticosteroids appear to be ineffective [102]. Vigabatrin and carbamazepine may worsen seizures [103]. Bromide has been effective in two reported cases and levetiracetam in one reported case, resistant to other anti-epileptic agents [104, 105].

THE KETOGENIC DIET

The ketogenic diet has been used in the treatment of epilepsy for almost 100 years. This is a high-fat diet, designed to mimic the effects on starvation in the production of ketones. Several studies have shown benefit in older children with drug-resistant epilepsy, in the use of both the classical diet (where the diet is based on the ratio of long-chain fat to carbohydrate including protein) [106] and the medium-chain triglyceride diet [107]. Criticism has been directed at the high dietetic resource required, and the unpalatability of the diet, but neither should be consideration to non-use. The availability of liquid preparation in the use of either diet (medium-chain triglyceride emulsion or liquigen with which a formula can be made up, or Ketocal™, a complete formula of 4:1 ratio [SHS International Ltd – Nutricia Clinical Care]) allows availability to a younger population, as well as those with gastrostomy feeding.

Limited data are available with regard to its use in infants. Many of the recent studies include the very young but numbers are small and results not specifically reported for this age group. Where present, however, data suggest this age group may be more responsive than the older population. Nordli *et al.* reported on 32 patients aged under 2 years who had been placed on the ketogenic diet for the treatment of epilepsy, four of whom had a progressive disorder [108]. Six (6 out of 32, 19.4%) became seizure free, 11 (35.5%) had a greater than 50% reduction in seizures and 14 (45.2%) had no worthwhile improvement. Of 17 with infantile spasms, six (35.3%) became seizure free and six (35.3%) had a greater than 50% reduction in seizures. Five developed complications; these included one each with severe vomiting, renal stone, gastro-oesphageal bleed (thought to be an erosive oesophagitis from a nasogastric tube), hyperlipidaemia, and ulcerative colitis. All complications were reversible and occurred in patients who had begun on the diet after 12 months of age. Kossoff *et al.*, reporting on the efficacy in children with tuberous sclerosis, included one patient in their study under the age of 12 months with focal seizures, who became seizure free on the diet.

A further study reported specifically on its use in children with infantile spasms [109]. At 3, 6, 9 and 12 months, 38%, 39%, 53% and 46% respectively of the 23 patients on the diet were >90% improved, with three seizure free at 12 months. Only 13 out of 23 children remained on the diet at 12 months.

Traditionally, there has been concern about early side-effects from the diet. It cannot be regarded as a natural treatment as children will be subject to side-effects just as with any other anti-convulsant. It should, therefore, only be considered at the very least as second line in the management of the epilepsy. There remains a theoretical concern about a risk of hypoglycaemia on initiation, but this appears to be unproven in clinical practice. Children in this age group are more likely to be prone to hyperketosis that may present with similar symptomatology at the onset of the diet, and of course may be resolved with similar treatment. There is no reason, however, why glucose homeostasis should not be maintained in the absence of a metabolic disease, which of course requires exclusion prior to initiation. This aside, there are certain metabolic diseases for which this would be a treatment, such as glucose transporter defects. Vomiting as the result of gastro-oesophageal reflux may be aggravated, as fat delays gastric emptying.

One question is what length of time children should remain on the diet. The risk of complications and long-term effects remain key to this. The risk of renal stones has been shown to be higher in the younger population [110] and, therefore, such children should be monitored for this. There is also evidence of increasing deviation of z scores, with regard to linear growth with age, particularly marked in those children initiated on the diet under 2 years of age [111]. Careful consideration of risks vs. benefits needs to be given in each individual case, and particularly the need with regard to epilepsy syndrome for longer-term treatment.

EPILEPSY SURGERY

The prognosis for epilepsy presenting under the age of 2 years remains poor for both seizure control and neurodevelopmental progress. Where children present with catastrophic epilepsy in the first 2 years of life, evidence of lateralization or localization should be sought to determine whether surgical resection in the management may be considered. The reverse situation may also be applied: all children presenting with epilepsy with a unilateral lesion as a likely cause should be referred to an epilepsy programme for consideration of surgery, in view of the risk of an epileptic encephalopathy and probable poor response to medical treatment. Children presenting for surgery at this age are likely to have similar seizure outcome to older children [112, 113], dependent on the underlying pathology, and the premise is that by terminating seizures at a younger age there is an improved neurodevelopmental outcome.

Surgery is now established in infants presenting with West syndrome, the result of a lateralized brain lesion. In one series of children presenting with lateralized spasms and evidence of lateralization on EEG, surgical intervention with resection of unilateral abnormal tissue (usually as a multi-lobar resection or hemispherectomy), whether detected on FDG-positron emission tomography or magnetic resonance imaging, led to 56% of patients being seizure free [114]. This was associated with an apparent improved developmental outcome as measured by Vineland Adaptive Behaviour Scales up to 2 years post surgery [115] as compared with medical series. Subsequent analysis of a further cohort has revealed an improved developmental outcome the shorter the duration of spasms prior to surgery [116].

The majority of procedures involve hemidisconnection or lobar resection, mainly for cerebral malformations, a pathology responsible for three-quarters of the surgical population in this age group [117]. Seizure outcome appears as good as the older population, with 48–75% seizure free dependent on the series [113, 117–119], with a substantial number showing worthwhile improvement. More difficult to determine in any series of children in this age group has been longitudinal evidence of improved developmental outcome following surgery and the relationship to seizure outcome. There is a lack of standardized measures that enables longitudinal follow-up of such children, and in particular comparator groups in whom surgery has not been performed. Studies therefore rely on parental report, which often refers to such parameters as increased awareness rather than definitive developmental gains [113]. In the very least, series suggest maintenance of developmental or intelligence quotient, which suggest a maintained developmental trajectory post-operatively, whereas in those who continue with seizures a slowed trajectory may be presumed, leading to a widening of the gap between individuals and their peers and therefore an apparent drop in IQ [120]. Further longitudinal studies are required to clarify this.

SUMMARY

Epilepsy with onset under the age of 2 years remains a challenge to management. Despite increasing data in certain well-defined epilepsy syndromes, there remains a paucity of studies of anti-epileptic use in this age group. There is no question that early onset of epilepsy in general has a poor prognosis for seizure and developmental outcome; there is limited evidence that early aggressive management of seizures may improve outcome. This aside, children with epilepsy as the result of unilateral or focal brain lesions should be referred early for surgical evaluation.

ACKNOWLEDGEMENT

We are very grateful for the thoughtful comments provided by the late Professor Robert A. Surtees.

REFERENCES

1. Hauser WA, Annegers JF, Kurland LT. Incidence of epilepsy and unprovoked seizures in Rochester, Minnesota: 1935–1984. *Epilepsia* 1993; 34:453–468.
2. Camfield CS, Camfield PR, Gordon K, Wirrell E, Dooley JM. Incidence of epilepsy in childhood and adolescence: a population-based study in Nova Scotia from 1977 to 1985. *Epilepsia* 1996; 37:19–23.
3. Chevrie JJ, Aicardi J. Convulsive disorders in the first year of life: neurological and mental outcome and mortality. *Epilepsia* 1978; 19:67–74.
4. Chevrie JJ, Aicardi J. Convulsive disorders in the first year of life: persistence of epileptic seizures. *Epilepsia* 1979; 20:643–649.
5. Matsumoto A, Watanabe K, Sugiura M, Negoro T, Takaesu E, Iwase K. Long-term prognosis of convulsive disorders in the first year of life: mental and physical development and seizure persistence. *Epilepsia* 1983; 24:321–329.
6. Cavazzuti GB, Ferrari P, Lalla M. Follow-up study of 482 cases with convulsive disorders in the first year of life. *Dev Med Child Neurol* 1984; 26:425–437.
7. Czochanska J, Langner-Tyszka B, Losiowski Z, Schmidt-Sidor B. Children who develop epilepsy in the first year of life: a prospective study. *Dev Med Child Neurol* 1994; 36:345–350.
8. Battaglia D, Rando T, Deodato F, Bruccini G, Baglio G, Frisone MF *et al.* Epileptic disorders with onset in the first year of life: neurological and cognitive outcome. *Eur J Paediatr Neurol* 1999; 3:95–103.
9. Engel J Jr. A proposed diagnostic scheme for people with epileptic seizures and with epilepsy: report of the ILAE Task Force on Classification and Terminology. *Epilepsia* 2001; 42:796–803.
10. Engel J Jr. Report of the ILAE classification core group. *Epilepsia* 2006; 47:1558–1568.
11. Deonna T. Developmental consequences of epilepsy in infancy. In: Nehling A, Motte J, Moshe SL, Plouin P (eds) *Childhood Epilepsies and Brain Development.* London: John Libbey, 1999, pp. 113–122.
12. Holmes GL. Effects of seizures on brain development: lessons from the laboratory. *Pediatr Neurol* 2005; 33:1–11.
13. Neill JC, Liu Z, Sarkisian M, Tandon P, Yang Y, Stafstrom CE *et al.* Recurrent seizures in immature rats: effect on auditory and visual discrimination. *Brain Res Dev Brain Res* 1996; 95:283–292.

14. Sarisjulis N, Gamboni B, Plouin P, Kaminska A, Dulac O. Diagnosing idiopathic/cryptogenic epilepsy syndromes in infancy. *Arch Dis Child* 2000; 82:226–230.

15. Arzimanoglou A, Guerrini R, Aicardi J. Epilepsy in infants. In: Arzimanoglou A, Guerrini R, Aicardi J (eds) *Aicardi's Epilepsy in Children*. 3rd edn. Philadelphia: Lippincott Williams & Wilkins, 2004, pp. 210–219.

16. Dravet C, Catani C, Bureau M, Roger J. Partial epilepsies in infancy: a study of 40 cases. *Epilepsia* 1989; 30:807–812.

17. Saunders DE, Thompson C, Gunny R, Jones R, Cox T, Chong WK. Magnetic resonance imaging protocols for paediatric neuroradiology. *Pediatr Radiol* 2007; 37:789–797.

18. Wolf NI, Bast T, Surtees R. Epilepsy in inborn errors of metabolism. *Epileptic Disord* 2005; 7:67–81.

19. Clayton PT. B6-responsive disorders: a model of vitamin dependency. *J Inherit Metab Dis* 2006; 29:317–326.

20. Surtees R, Mills P, Clayton PT. Inborn errors affecting vitamin B6 metabolism. *Future Neurology* 2006; 1:615–620.

21. Mills PB, Struys E, Jakobs C, Plecko B, Baxter P, Baumgartner M *et al*. Mutations in antiquitin in individuals with pyridoxine-dependent seizures. *Nat Med* 2006; 12:307–309.

22. Plecko B, Stockler-Ipsiroglu S, Paschke E, Erwa W, Struys EA, Jakobs C. Pipecolic acid elevation in plasma and cerebrospinal fluid of two patients with pyridoxine-dependent epilepsy. *Ann Neurol* 2000; 48:121–125.

23. Baxter P. Pyridoxine-dependent and pyridoxine-responsive seizures. *Dev Med Child Neurol* 2001; 43:416–420.

24. Nabbout R, Soufflet C, Plouin P, Dulac O. Pyridoxine dependent epilepsy: a suggestive electroclinical pattern. *Arch Dis Child Fetal Neonatal Ed* 1999; 81:F125–F129.

25. Clayton PT, Surtees RA, DeVile C, Hyland K, Heales SJ. Neonatal epileptic encephalopathy. *Lancet* 2003; 361:1614.

26. Mills PB, Surtees RA, Champion MP, Beesley CE, Dalton N, Scambler PJ *et al*. Neonatal epileptic encephalopathy caused by mutations in the *PNPO* gene encoding pyridox(am)ine 5'-phosphate oxidase. *Hum Mol Genet* 2005; 14:1077–1086.

27. Hoffmann GF, Schmitt B, Windfur M, Wagner N, Strehl H, Franz AR *et al*. Pyridoxal 5'-phosphate may be curative in early-onset epileptic encephalopathy. *J Inherited Metab Dis* 2007; 30:96–99.

28. Wang HS, Kuo MF, Chou ML, Hung PC, Lin KL, Hsieh MY *et al*. Pyridoxal phosphate is better than pyridoxine for controlling idiopathic intractable epilepsy. *Arch Dis Child* 2005; 90:512–515.

29. Hyland K, Buist NR, Powell BR, Hoffman GF, Rating D, McGrath J *et al*. Folinic acid responsive seizures: a new syndrome? *J Inherit Metab Dis* 1995; 18:177–181.

30. Torres OA, Miller VS, Buist NM, Hyland K. Folinic acid-responsive neonatal seizures. *J Child Neurol* 1999; 14:529–532.

31. Hyland K, Arnold LA. Value of lumbar puncture in the diagnosis of infantile epilepsy and folinic acid-responsive seizures. *J Child Neurol* 2002; 17(Suppl 3):3S48–3S55.

32. Frye RE, Donner E, Golja A, Rooney CM. Folinic acid-responsive seizures presenting as breakthrough seizures in a 3-month-old boy. *J Child Neurol* 2003; 18:562–569.

33. Nicolai J, van Kranen-Mastenbroek VH, Wevers RA, Hurkx WA, Vles JS. Folinic acid-responsive seizures initially responsive to pyridoxine. *Pediatr Neurol* 2006; 34:164–167.

34. Hyland K. Folinic acid responsive seizures. In: Baxter P (ed.) *Vitamin Responsive Conditions in Paediatric Neurology*. London: Mac Keith Press, 2001, pp. 53–54.

35. Chiron C. Management of epilepsy in infants. In: Shorvon SD, Fish D, Perucca E, Dodson WE (eds) *The Treatment of Epilepsy*. Oxford: Blackwell Science, 2004, pp. 180–189.

36. Schwabe MJ, Dobyns WB, Burke B, Armstrong DL. Valproate-induced liver failure in one of two siblings with Alpers disease. *Pediatr Neurol* 1997; 16:337–343.

37. Dreifuss FE, Langer DH, Moline KA, Maxwell JE. Valproic acid hepatic fatalities. II. US experience since 1984. *Neurology* 1989; 39:201–207.

38. Hancock E, Osborne J, Milner P. Treatment of infantile spasms. *Cochrane Database Syst Rev* 2003; CD001770.

39. Mackay MT, Weiss SK, ms-Webber T, Ashwal S, Stephens D, Ballaban-Gill K *et al*. Practice parameter: medical treatment of infantile spasms: report of the American Academy of Neurology and the Child Neurology Society. *Neurology* 2004; 62:1668–1681.

40. Wang W, Murphy B, Dow KE, David AR, Fraser DD. Systemic adrenocorticotropic hormone administration down-regulates the expression of corticotropin-releasing hormone (CRH) and CRH-binding protein in infant rat hippocampus. *Pediatr Res* 2004; 55:604–610.

41. Rogawski MA, Reddy DS. Neurosteroids and infantile spasms: the deoxycorticosterone hypothesis. *Int Rev Neurobiol* 2002; 49:199–219.

42. Brunson KL, vishai-Eliner S, Baram TZ. ACTH treatment of infantile spasms: mechanisms of its effects in modulation of neuronal excitability. *Int Rev Neurobiol* 2002; 49:185–197.

43. Hrachovy RM, Frost JD, Glaze GD. High-dose, long duration versus low-dose, short duration corticotrophin therapy for infantile spasms. *J Pediatr* 1994; 124:803–806.

44. Yanagaki S, Oguni H, Hayashi K, Imai K, Funatuka M, Tanaka T et al. A comparative study of high-dose and low-dose ACTH therapy for West syndrome. *Brain Dev* 1999; 21:461–467.

45. Riikonen R. The latest on infantile spasms. *Curr Opin Neurol* 2005; 18:91–95.

46. Dulac O, Tuxhorn I. Infantile spasms and West syndrome. In: Roger J, Bureau M, Dravet C, Genton P, Tassinari C A, Wolf P (eds) *Epileptic Syndromes in Infancy, Childhood and Adolescence*. Montrouge, France: John Libbey Eurotext, 2005, pp. 53–72.

47. Hamano S, Yamashita S, Tanaka M, Yoshinari S, Minamitani M, Eto Y. Therapeutic efficacy and adverse effects of adrenocorticotropic hormone therapy in West syndrome: differences in dosage of adrenocorticotropic hormone, onset of age, and cause. *J Pediatr* 2006; 148:485–488.

48. Ito M, Aiba H, Hashimoto K, Kuroki S, Tomiwa K, Okuno T et al. Low-dose ACTH therapy for West syndrome: initial effects and long-term outcome. *Neurology* 2002; 58:110–114.

49. Oguni H, Yanagaki S, Hayashi K, Imai K, Funatsuka M, Kishi T et al. Extremely low-dose ACTH step-up protocol for West syndrome: maximum therapeutic effect with minimal side-effects. *Brain Dev* 2006; 28:8–13.

50. Lin HC, Young C, Wang PJ, Lee WT, Shen YZ. ACTH therapy for Taiwanese children with West syndrome – efficacy and impact on long-term prognosis. *Brain Dev* 2006; 28:196–201.

51. Chiron C, Dumas C, Jambaque I, Mumford J, Dulac O. Randomized trial comparing vigabatrin and hydrocortisone in infantile spasms due to tuberous sclerosis. *Epilepsy Res* 1997; 26:389–395.

52. Nicolson A, Leach JP, Chadwick DW, Smith DF. The legacy of vigabatrin in a regional epilepsy clinic. *J Neurol Neurosurg Psychiatry* 2002; 73:327–329.

53. Gross-Tsur V, Ben-Zeev B, Shalev RS. Malignant migrating partial seizures in infancy. *Pediatr Neurol* 2004; 31:287–290.

54. Russell-Eggitt IM, Mackey DA, Taylor DS, Timms C, Walker JW. Vigabatrin-associated visual field defects in children. *Eye* 2000; 14:334–339.

55. Malmgren K, Ben-Menachem E, Frisen L. Vigabatrin visual toxicity: evolution and dose dependence. *Epilepsia* 2001; 42:609–615.

56. Best JL, Acheson JF. The natural history of vigabatrin associated visual field defects in patients electing to continue their medication. *Eye* 2005; 19:41–44.

57. Spencer EL, Harding GF. Examining visual field defects in the paediatric population exposed to vigabatrin. *Doc Ophthalmol* 2003; 107:281–287.

58. Harding GF, Spencer EL, Wild JM, Conway M, Bohn RL. Field-specific visual-evoked potentials: identifying field defects in vigabatrin-treated children. *Neurology* 2002; 58:1261–1265.

59. Lux AL, Edwards SW, Hancock E, Johnson AL, Kennedy CR, Newton RW et al. The United Kingdom Infantile Spasms Study comparing vigabatrin with prednisolone or tetracosactide at 14 days: a multicentre, randomised controlled trial. *Lancet* 2004; 364:1773–1778.

60. Lux AL, Edwards SW, Hancock E, Johnson AL, Kennedy CR, Newton RW et al. The United Kingdom Infantile Spasms Study (UKISS) comparing hormone treatment with vigabatrin on developmental and epilepsy outcomes to age 14 months: a multicentre randomised trial. *Lancet Neurol* 2005; 4:712–717.

61. Dreifuss F, Farwell J, Holmes G, Joseph C, Lockman L, Madsen JA et al. Infantile spasms. Comparative trial of nitrazepam and corticotropin. *Arch Neurol* 1986; 43:1107–1110.

62. Hosain SA, Merchant S, Solomon GE, Chutorian A. Topiramate for the treatment of infantile spasms. *J Child Neurol* 2006; 21:17–19.

63. Mikaeloff Y, de Saint-Martin A, Mancini J, Peudenier S, Pedespan JM, Vallee L et al. Topiramate: efficacy and tolerability in children according to epilepsy syndromes. *Epilepsy Res* 2003; 53:225–232.

64. Zou LP, Ding CH, Fang F, Sin NC, Mix E. Prospective study of first-choice topiramate therapy in newly diagnosed infantile spasms. *Clin Neuropharmacol* 2006; 29:343–349.

65. Philippi H, Boor R, Reitter B. Topiramate and metabolic acidosis in infants and toddlers. *Epilepsia* 2002; 43:744–747.

66. Suzuki Y. Zonisamide in West syndrome. *Brain Dev* 2001; 23:658–661.
67. Yanai S, Hanai T, Narazaki O. Treatment of infantile spasms with zonisamide. *Brain Dev* 1999; 21:157–161.
68. Suzuki Y, Imai K, Toribe Y, Ueda H, Yanagihara K, Shimono K *et al*. Long-term response to zonisamide in patients with West syndrome. *Neurology* 2002; 58:1556–1559.
69. Lotze TE, Wilfong AA. Zonisamide treatment for symptomatic infantile spasms. *Neurology* 2004; 62:296–298.
70. Ohtsuka Y, Ogino T, Asano T, Hattori J, Ohta H, Oka E. Long-term follow-up of vitamin B(6)-responsive West syndrome. *Pediatr Neurol* 2000; 23:202–206.
71. Debus OM, Kurlemann G. Sulthiame in the primary therapy of West syndrome: a randomized double-blind placebo-controlled add-on trial on baseline pyridoxine medication. *Epilepsia* 2004; 45:103–108.
72. Kivity S, Lerman P, Ariel R, Danziger Y, Mimouni M, Shinnar S. Long-term cognitive outcomes of a cohort of children with cryptogenic infantile spasms treated with high-dose adrenocorticotropic hormone. *Epilepsia* 2004; 45:255–262.
73. Riikonen R. Long-term outcome of patients with West syndrome. *Brain Dev* 2001; 23:683–687.
74. Eisermann MM, DeLaRaillere A, Dellatolas G, Tozzi E, Nabbout R, Dulac O *et al*. Infantile spasms in Down syndrome – effects of delayed anticonvulsive treatment. *Epilepsy Res* 2003; 55:21–27.
75. Rener-Primec Z, Stare J, Neubauer D. The risk of lower mental outcome in infantile spasms increases after three weeks of hypsarrhythmia duration. *Epilepsia* 2006; 47:2202–2205.
76. Dravet C, Bureau M, Oguni H, Fukuyama Y, Cokar O. Severe myoclonic epilepsy in infancy: Dravet syndrome. *Adv Neurol* 2005; 95:71–102.
77. Harkin LA, McMahon JM, Iona X, Dibbens L, Pelekanos JT, Zuberi SM *et al*. The spectrum of *SCN1A*-related infantile epileptic encephalopathies. *Brain* 2007; 130:843–852.
78. Nabbout R, Gennaro E, Dalla BB, Dulac O, Madia F, Bertini E *et al*. Spectrum of *SCN1A* mutations in severe myoclonic epilepsy of infancy. *Neurology* 2003; 60:1961–1967.
79. Fukuma G, Oguni H, Shirasaka Y, Watanabe K, Miyajima T, Yasumoto S *et al*. Mutations of neuronal voltage-gated Na$^+$ channel alpha 1 subunit gene *SCN1A* in core severe myoclonic epilepsy in infancy (SMEI) and in borderline SMEI (SMEB) *Epilepsia* 2004; 45:140–148.
80. Fujiwara T, Sugawara T, Mazaki-Miyazaki E, Takahashi Y, Fukushima K, Watanabe M *et al*. Mutations of sodium channel alpha subunit type 1 (*SCN1A*) in intractable childhood epilepsies with frequent generalized tonic–clonic seizures. *Brain* 2003; 126:531–546.
81. Hurst DL. Epidemiology of severe myoclonic epilepsy of infancy. *Epilepsia* 1990; 31:397–400.
82. Guerrini R, Dravet C, Genton P, Belmonte A, Kaminska A, Dulac O. Lamotrigine and seizure aggravation in severe myoclonic epilepsy. *Epilepsia* 1998; 39:508–512.
83. Ohtsuka Y, Ohmori I, Ogino T, Ouchida M, Shimizu K, Oka E. Paroxysmal movement disorders in severe myoclonic epilepsy in infancy. *Brain Dev* 2003; 25:401–405.
84. Saito Y, Oguni H, Awaya Y, Hayashi K, Osawa M. Phenytoin-induced choreoathetosis in patients with severe myoclonic epilepsy in infancy. *Neuropediatrics* 2001; 32:231–235.
85. Chiron C, Marchand MC, Tran A, Rey E, d'Athis P, Vincent J *et al*. Stiripentol in severe myoclonic epilepsy in infancy: a randomised placebo-controlled syndrome-dedicated trial. STICLO study group. *Lancet* 2000; 11:1638–1642.
86. Thanh TN, Chiron C, Dellatolas G, Rey E, Pons G, Vincent J *et al*. [Long-term efficacy and tolerance of stiripentol in severe myoclonic epilepsy in infancy (Dravet syndrome)]. *Arch Pediatr* 2002; 11:1120–1127.
87. Trojnar MK, Wojtal K, Trojnar MP, Czuczwar SJ. Stiripentol. A novel antiepileptic drug. *Pharmacol Rep* 2005; 57:154–160.
88. Quilichini PP, Chiron C, Ben-Ari Y, Gozlan H. Stiripentol, a putative antiepileptic drug, enhances the duration of opening of GABA-A receptor channels. *Epilepsia* 2006; 47:704–716.
89. Coppola G, Capovilla G, Montagnini A, Romeo A, Spano M, Tortorella G *et al*. Topiramate as add-on drug in severe myoclonic epilepsy in infancy: an Italian multicenter open trial. *Epilepsy Res* 2002; 49:45–48.
90. Nieto-Barrera M, Candau R, Nieto-Jimenez M, Correa A, del Portal LR. Topiramate in the treatment of severe myoclonic epilepsy in infancy. *Seizure* 2000; 9:590–594.
91. Grosso S, Galimberti D, Farnetani MA, Cioni M, Mostardini R, Vivarelli R *et al*. Efficacy and safety of topiramate in infants according to epilepsy syndromes. *Seizure* 2005; 14:183–189.
92. Kanazawa O. Refractory grand mal seizures with onset during infancy including severe myoclonic epilepsy in infancy. *Brain Dev* 2001; 23:749–756.

93. Oguni H, Hayashi K, Oguni M, Mukahira A, Uehara T, Fukuyama Y *et al*. Treatment of severe myoclonic epilepsy in infants with bromide and its borderline variant. *Epilepsia* 1994; 35:1140–1145.

94. Sankar R, Wheless JW, Dravet C, Guerrini R, Medina MT, Bureau M *et al*. Treatment of myoclonic epilepsies in infancy and early childhood. *Adv Neurol* 2005; 95:289–298.

95. Ohtahara S, Yamatogi Y. Epileptic encephalopathies in early infancy with suppression–burst. *J Clin Neurophysiol* 2003; 20:398–407.

96. Djukic A, Lado FA, Shinnar S, Moshe SL. Are early myoclonic encephalopathy (EME) and the Ohtahara syndrome (EIEE) independent of each other? *Epilepsy Res* 2006; 70S:S68–S76.

97. Yamatogi Y, Ohtahara S. Early-infantile epileptic encephalopathy with suppression–bursts, Ohtahara syndrome; its overview referring to our 16 cases. *Brain Dev* 2002; 24:13–23.

98. Ohno M, Shimotsuji Y, Abe J, Shimada M, Tamiya H. Zonisamide treatment of early infantile epileptic encephalopathy. *Pediatr Neurol* 2000; 23:341–344.

99. Ozawa H, Kawada Y, Noma S, Sugai K. Oral high-dose phenobarbital therapy for early infantile epileptic encephalopathy. *Pediatr Neurol* 2002; 26:222–224.

100. Lortie A, Plouin P, Chiron C, Delalande O, Dulac O. Characteristics of epilepsy in focal cortical dysplasia in infancy. *Epilepsy Res* 2002; 51:133–145.

101. Dulac O. Epileptic encephalopathy. *Epilepsia* 2001; 42(Suppl 3):23–26.

102. Coppola G, Plouin P, Chiron C, Robain O, Dulac O. Migrating partial seizures in infancy: a malignant disorder with developmental arrest. *Epilepsia* 1995; 36:1017–1024.

103. Dulac O. Malignant migrating partial seizures in infancy. In: Roger J, Bureau M, Dravet C, Genton P, Tassinari C A, Wolf P (eds) *Epileptic Syndromes in Infancy, Childhood and Adolescence*. 4th edn. Montrouge, France: John Libbey Eurotext, 2005, pp. 73–76.

104. Hmaimess G, Kadhim H, Nassogne MC, Bonnier C, van Rijckeveorsel K. Levetiracetam in a neonate with malignant migrating partial seizures. *Pediatr Neurol* 2006; 34:55–59.

105. Okuda K, Yasuhara A, Kamei A, Araki A, Kitamura N, Kobayashi Y. Successful control with bromide of two patients with malignant migrating partial seizures in infancy. *Brain Dev* 2000; 22:56–59.

106. Freeman JM, Vining EPG, Pillas DJ. The efficacy of the ketogenic diet – 1998: a prospective evaluation of intervention in 150 children. *Pediatrics* 1998; 102:1358–1363.

107. Schwartz RH, Eaton J, Bower BD, Aynsley-Green A. Ketogenic diets in the treatment of epilepsy: short-term clinical effects. *Dev Med Child Neurol* 1989; 31:145–151.

108. Nordli D, Kuroda MM, Carroll J, Koenigsberger DY, Hirsch LJ, Bruner HJ *et al*. Experience with the ketogenic diet in infants. *Pediatrics* 2002; 108:129–133.

109. Kossoff EH, Pyzik PL, McGrogan JR, Vining EP, Freeman JM. Efficacy of the ketogenic diet for infantile spasms. *Pediatrics* 2002; 109:780–783.

110. Furth SL, Casey JC, Pyzik PL, Neu AM, Docimo SG, Vining EP *et al*. Risk factors for urolithiasis in children on the ketogenic diet. *Pediatr Nephrol* 2000; 15:125–128.

111. Vining EP, Pyzik PL, McGrogan JR, Hladky H, Anand AJ, Kriegler S *et al*. Growth of children on the ketogenic diet. *Dev Med Child Neurol* 2002; 44:796–802.

112. Wyllie E, Comair Y, Kotagal P, Raja S, Ruggieri PM. Epilepsy surgery in infants. *Epilepsia* 1996; 37:625–637.

113. Duchowny M, Jayakar P, Resnick T, Harvey AS, Alvarez L, Dean P *et al*. Epilepsy surgery in the first three years of life. *Epilepsia* 1998; 39:737–743.

114. Chugani HT, Shewmon DA, Shields WD, Sankar R, Comair Y, Vinters HV *et al*. Surgery for intractable infantile spasms: neuroimaging perspectives. *Epilepsia* 1993; 34:764–771.

115. Asarnow RF, LoPresti C, Guthrie D, Elliott T, Cynn V, Shields WD *et al*. Developmental outcomes in children receiving resection surgery for medically intractable infantile spasms. *Dev Med Child Neurol* 1997; 39:430–440.

116. Jonas R, Asarnow RF, LoPresti C, Yudovin S, Koh S, Wu JY *et al*. Surgery for symptomatic infant-onset epileptic encephalopathy with and without infantile spasms. *Neurology* 2005; 64:746–750.

117. Kung J, Scott R, Harkness W, Nicolaides P, Neville BG, Cross JH. Outcome of epilepsy surgery in children under three years of age. *Dev Med Child Neurol* 2005; 47:25.

118. Bittar RG, Rosenfeld JV, Klug GL, Hopkins IJ, Harvey AS. Resective surgery in infants and young children with intractable epilepsy. *J Clin Neurosci* 2002; 9:142–146.

119. Wyllie E, Comair YG, Kotagal P, Raja S, Ruggieri P. Epilepsy surgery in infants. *Epilepsia* 1996; 37:625–637.

120. Devlin AM, Cross JH, Harkness W, Chong WK, Harding B, Vargha-Khadem F *et al*. Clinical outcomes of hemispherectomy for epilepsy in childhood and adolescence. *Brain* 2003; 126:556–566.

121. Plouin P, Anderson VE. Benign familail and non familial neonatal seizures. In: Roger J, Bureau M, Dravet C, Genton P, Tassinari CA, Wolf P (eds) *Epileptic Syndromes in Infancy, Childhood and Adolescence*. 4th edn. Montrouge, France: John Libbey Eurotext, 2005, pp. 3–15.

122. Berkovic SF, Heron SE, Giordano L, Marini C, Guerrini R, Kaplan RE *et al*. Benign familial neonatal-infantile seizures: characterization of a new sodium channelopathy. *Ann Neurol* 2004; 55:550–557.

123. Vigevano F. Benign familial infantile seizures. *Brain Dev* 2005; 27:172–177.

124. Specchio N, Vigevano F. The spectrum of benign infantile seizures. *Epilepsy Res* 2006; 70(Suppl 1):S156–S167.

125. Okumura A, Watanabe K, Negoro T. Benign partial epilepsy in infancy long-term outcome and marginal syndromes. *Epilepsy Res* 2006; 70(Suppl 1):S168–S173.

126. Weber YG, Berger A, Bebek N, Maier S, Karafyllakes S, Meyer N *et al*. Benign familial infantile convulsions: linkage to chromosome 16p12-q12 in 14 families. *Epilepsia* 2004; 45:601–609.

127. Vanmolkot KR, Kors EE, Hottenga JJ, Terwindt GM, Haan J, Hoefnagels WA *et al*. Novel mutations in the Na⁺, K⁺-ATPase pump gene ATP1A2 associated with familial hemiplegic migraine and benign familial infantile convulsions. *Ann Neurol* 2003; 54:360–366.

128. Dravet C, Bureau M. Benign myoclonic epilepsy in infancy. *Adv Neurol* 2005; 95:127–137.

129. Auvin S, Pandit F, De BJ, Badinand N, Isnard H, Motte J *et al*. Benign myoclonic epilepsy in infants: electroclinical features and long-term follow-up of 34 patients. *Epilepsia* 2006; 47:387–393.

130. Herlenius E, Heron SE, Grinton BE, Keay D, Scheffer IE, Mulley JC *et al*. SCN2A mutations and benign familial neonatal-infantile seizures: the phenotypic spectrum. *Epilepsia* 2007; 48:1138–1142.

131. Aicardi J, Ohtahara S. Severe neonatal epilepsies with suppression–burst pattern. In: Roger J, Bureau M, Dravet C, Genton P, Tassinari C A, Wolf P (eds) *Epileptic Syndromes in Infancy, Childhood and Adolescence*. 4th edn. John Libbey Eurotext, 2005, pp. 39–50.

132. Ohtahara S, Yamatogi Y. Ohtahara syndrome: with special reference to its developmental aspects for differentiating from early myoclonic encephalopathy. *Epilepsy Res* 2006; 70(Suppl 1):S58–S67.

133. Fujiwara T. Clinical spectrum of mutations in *SCN1A* gene: severe myoclonic epilepsy in infancy and related epilepsies. *Epilepsy Res* 2006; 70(Suppl 1):S223–S230.

134. Kato M, Das S, Petras K, Sawaishi Y, Dobyns WB. Polyalanine expansion of ARX associated with cryptogenic West syndrome. *Neurology* 2003; 61:267–276.

135. Guerrini R, Moro F, Kato M, Barkovich AJ, Shiihara T, McShane MA *et al*. Expansion of the first PolyA tract of ARX causes infantile spasms and status dystonicus. *Neurology* 2007; 69:427–433.

136. Archer HL, Evans J, Edwards S, Colley J, Newbury-Ecob R, O'Callaghan F *et al*. CDKL5 mutations cause infantile spasms, early onset seizures, and severe mental retardation in female patients. *J Med Genet* 2006; 43:729–734.

137. Ferrari G, Lamantea E, Donati A, Filosto M, Briem E, Carrara F *et al*. Infantile hepatocerebral syndromes associated with mutations in the mitochondrial DNA polymerase-gammaA. *Brain* 2005; 128:723–731.

138. Horvath R, Hudson G, Ferrari G, Futterer N, Ahola S, Lamantea E *et al*. Phenotypic spectrum associated with mutations of the mitochondrial polymerase gamma gene. *Brain* 2006; 129:1674–1684.

139. de Koning TJ, Klomp LW. Serine-deficiency syndromes. *Curr Opin Neurol* 2004; 2:197–204.

140. Klepper J. Leiendecker B. GLUT1 deficiency syndrome. 2007 update. *Dev Med Child Neurol* 2007; 49:707–716.

141. Shih EV, Stöckler-Ipsiroglu S. Disorders of ornithine and creatine metabolism. In: Fernandes J, Saudubray J-M, van den Berghe G (eds) *Inborn Metabolic Disease*. 3rd edn. Dordrecht: Springer, 2000, pp. 233–240.

5

Treatment of the child or adolescent with newly diagnosed epilepsy

Renée A. Shellhaas, Dennis J. Dlugos

INTRODUCTION

Paediatric epilepsy is amazingly diverse. In some children, basic diagnosis, seizure classification and treatment are straightforward. Other patients have difficult-to-diagnose seizures, complicated seizure classification and a variable response to treatment. Some seizures are subclinical, others are barely noticeable, and occasionally they are life threatening. Many children with epilepsy have no associated disabilities, but all children with epilepsy are at increased risk for learning and behavioural difficulties. In many patients, even those with well-controlled seizures, epilepsy is only one element of a complex neurodevelopmental problem.

In children, epilepsy is typically defined as *a tendency toward recurrent seizures, with a history of at least two unprovoked seizures*. The first task when confronting a child with suspected seizures is to confirm that the episodes of concern are epileptic seizures, as there are many other conditions in children that may mimic seizures (see Chapter 6). The second task is to ensure that the seizures are unprovoked. Unprovoked seizures occur without an immediate trigger, such as fever, acute metabolic disturbance, acute head trauma or acute central nervous system (CNS) infection. Seizures associated with an immediate precipitant are provoked seizures. Since many children with a single unprovoked seizure will not have recurrent seizures [1], it is important to limit the diagnosis of paediatric epilepsy to those children who have had at least two unprovoked seizures. This is distinctly different from adults, in whom even a single seizure may have a significant impact on employment and driving.

TAKING A HISTORY IN A PATIENT WITH SEIZURES AND EPILEPSY

Treatment of newly diagnosed epilepsy begins with accurate diagnosis and appropriate seizure classification (Figure 5.1). A detailed history is essential, complemented by electroencephalography testing and neuroimaging in many cases. Elements of the history,

Renée A. Shellhaas, MD, Division of Pediatric Neurology, C. S. Mott Children's Hospital, University of Michigan, Ann Arbor, Michigan, USA

Dennis J. Dlugos, MD, MSCE, Associate Professor, Division of Neurology, The Children's Hospital of Philadelphia, University of Pennsylvania School of Medicine, Philadelphia, Pennsylvania, USA

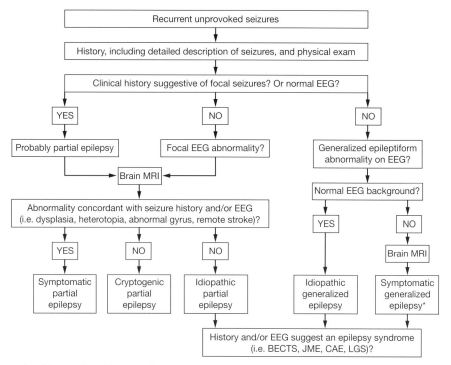

* Consider genetic and/or metabolic work-up, depending on clinical features.

Figure 5.1 Algorithm for classification of seizures and epilepsy syndromes [51].

if obtained correctly, will vastly facilitate classification. The following systematic approach is helpful (see Chapter 6):

(i)   Confirm by history that the episodes of concern are unprovoked. Common provoking factors include fever, metabolic derangements (e.g. hypoglycaemia, hyponatraemia, hypernatraemia, hypocalcaemia, hypomagnesaemia), CNS infection and acute head trauma.

(ii) Describe the clinical features of the episode from the beginning (aura) to the end (post-ictal state). Look for signs of focal onset, including any type of aura, focal twitching, tonic posturing or focal sensory phenomena such as dysaesthesias, visual symptoms or auditory symptoms. As the spell progresses, note any motor manifestations, such as focal–clonic shaking, tonic stiffening or loss of muscle tone. Assess the degree of responsiveness during the episode. Note the duration of the spell. Describe clinical manifestations during any post-ictal state, such as transient focal weakness.

(iii) If the episode is non-convulsive (i.e. staring, behavioural arrest and unresponsiveness), try to distinguish between focal seizures with altered awareness (complex partial seizures) and generalized non-convulsive seizures (absence seizures). Focal seizures with altered awareness often have a post-ictal state, while generalized non-convulsive seizures do not. Also, focal seizures with altered awareness typically are longer and occur less frequently than generalized non-convulsive seizures.

(iv) Note any possible precipitating factors, such as sleep deprivation, flashing lights, medications or illicit drug use. Note anything predictable about the timing of the episodes: do they always occur during sleep or within a few minutes of awakening? Since the unpredictability of seizures is frustrating and anxiety provoking, the identification of a reliable trigger can be very helpful to the patient.

(v) Establish the frequency of seizures and their impact on physical health (injuries and hospitalizations) and psychosocial well-being (embarrassment of seizures in school, anxiety over the next seizure and stress on the family).

DETERMINING AETIOLOGY

Once it is clear that the episodes are unprovoked seizures, a stepwise search for aetiology begins (see Figure 5.1).

EMERGENT OR URGENT EVALUATION OF A CHILD WITH A FIRST UNPROVOKED SEIZURE

Anxiety following a child's first unprovoked seizure often leads to extensive diagnostic testing in the emergency department, even if the child has returned to baseline. Usually, few diagnostic tests are needed following a first unprovoked seizure. A practice parameter from the American Academy of Neurology and the Child Neurology Society addresses these situations [2]. In the emergency department, a toxicology screen is reasonable. Measuring electrolytes and glucose levels is not required if the seizure has stopped and the child has returned to baseline and is not dehydrated. Except in selected cases, neuroimaging is not helpful in the emergency department [3, 4]. A hospital-based study in Boston made the following recommendations, based on 500 children presenting to the emergency department with a first-time seizure: emergent imaging with head computed tomography (CT) scan should be undertaken in children with a known bleeding or clotting disorder, a known history of malignancy, human immunodeficiency virus (HIV) infection or closed head injury, as well as in patients aged less than 33 months with a focal seizure [4].

In most cases, an electroencephalogram (EEG) is not needed in the emergency department, but should be obtained within 1 week after a first unprovoked seizure. Because some paroxysmal spells in children may be difficult to diagnose based on history alone, an abnormal EEG may help support the diagnosis of a seizure. However, a normal EEG in no way excludes the diagnosis of a seizure. An interictal EEG may also help to distinguish between focal-onset and generalized-onset seizures, which affects medication selection if the child goes on to develop epilepsy.

In addition, the interictal EEG provides valuable information regarding the risk of seizure recurrence. In a long-term, prospective cohort study in the Bronx, normal children with normal EEGs after a single unprovoked seizure had seizure recurrence rates of 28% and 32% at 2 and 5 years, while normal children with abnormal EEGs had seizure recurrence rates of 52% and 59% at 2 and 5 years. Not surprisingly, children with developmental disabilities and an abnormal EEG have an even higher risk of recurrent seizures [1].

EVALUATION OF THE CHILD WITH TWO OR MORE UNPROVOKED SEIZURES

In children with two or more unprovoked seizures (newly diagnosed epilepsy), appropriate diagnostic testing and treatment decisions depend on basic epilepsy classification (see Figure 5.1). At a minimum, the distinction between partial and generalized epilepsy should be made. A detailed history (see above) and neurological examination, combined with routine EEG, are usually sufficient for basic seizure classification. More detailed syndrome classification can often be made, which can be helpful for management decisions.

Electroencephalogram

If details of the seizure semiology are unavailable or are unclear, then EEG assumes an even more important role in seizure classification. An EEG with focal abnormalities, such as focal slowing or focal sharp waves, suggests a diagnosis of partial epilepsy. A normal routine EEG is more consistent with partial epilepsy (or non-epileptic events) than with generalized epilepsy. While the EEG may be normal in partial epilepsy, children with generalized epilepsy typically display generalized epileptiform abnormalities on their initial routine EEGs. If history, examination and routine EEG do not clarify whether the epilepsy is partial or generalized, additional EEG studies recording sleep and arousal from sleep may be helpful [5].

Magnetic Resonance Imaging

A magnetic resonance imaging (MRI) scan of the brain is usually required in the evaluation of children with symptomatic or cryptogenic partial epilepsy and symptomatic generalized epilepsy. In these patients, abnormalities on neuroimaging can direct further work-up (such as evaluation for a prothrombotic condition in a child with a stroke, genetic testing in the case of lissencephaly, or metabolic testing for a child with typical patterns on MRI). MRI is also typically required in the evaluation of children whose epilepsy begins before the age of 2 years, or whose seizures do not respond to appropriate therapy [6].

In contrast, neuroimaging is not required in children with idiopathic focal (e.g. benign epilepsy with centrotemporal spikes [BECTS]) or idiopathic generalized epilepsy syndromes (childhood absence epilepsy [CAE], juvenile myoclonic epilepsy [JME]). Note that in epilepsy syndrome classification, the term 'idiopathic' does not imply unknown cause. Rather, the patient with idiopathic epilepsy has no external cause or no cause beyond something inherently present in the individual [7]. Therefore, epilepsy with a genetic basis is usually considered idiopathic.

DECISION OF WHETHER TO TREAT THE NEWLY DIAGNOSED PATIENT

The decision to initiate anti-epileptic drugs (AEDs) depends on the balance between the risk of the AED and the risk of seizures (both the risk of seizure occurrence and the risk posed by the seizure itself – a simple partial seizure may be less worrisome than a generalized tonic–clonic convulsion). When treatment is begun, the goal is 'no seizures and no side-effects'. In those patients with epilepsy in whom AED treatment is not initiated, the goal is 'a life unaffected by seizures'.

Often initiation of treatment is motivated by fear – fear of injury or death, fear of brain damage and fear of social consequences. While these can be legitimate concerns, they do not constitute absolute requirements for anti-convulsant medication. Initiation of AEDs in children is often a more complex decision than it is in adults, for whom the loss of driving privileges, for example, has significant consequences and leads to a clear decision to begin AEDs. Not all children with newly diagnosed epilepsy require AED treatment at the time of presentation, although many do.

An intelligent decision to treat, or not to treat, a child's newly diagnosed epilepsy begins with syndrome classification (see Figure 5.1). Children may have relatively benign, self-limited epilepsy syndromes (e.g. BECTS) for which treatment may be entirely optional. On the other hand, few would disagree that an infant with newly diagnosed infantile spasms requires medical intervention. As in the treatment of most disorders, each patient's situation must be evaluated individually.

In most cases, initiation of an appropriate AED will not alter the natural history of the patient's epilepsy [1, 8]. However, suppression of seizures may have a significant effect on the patient's quality of life, as well as that of their parents [9].

SPECIFIC AEDs FOR SPECIFIC SEIZURE TYPES AND EPILEPSY SYNDROMES

AEDs can be broadly grouped into three categories: narrow spectrum, broad spectrum, and syndrome-specific (Table 5.1). In general, partial epilepsies may be treated with either narrow- or broad-spectrum AEDs. However, broad-spectrum AEDs are usually required for generalized or mixed epilepsy syndromes. Beyond the spectrum of action, selection of an AED also depends on the medicine's formulation – is the child able to swallow liquid, sprinkles or pills (Table 5.2)? Special consideration of the child's other medical conditions, such as obesity, migraine, mood disorder or any complex chronic illness, is also important. Certain AEDs will have clear advantages and disadvantages, depending on the patient's situation (Table 5.3). Dosing guidelines are found in Tables 5.4 and 5.5.

TREATMENT OF PARTIAL EPILEPSY

Symptomatic or Cryptogenic Partial Epilepsy

Initial treatment of partial epilepsy is typically with a 'narrow-spectrum' AED, but some broad-spectrum AEDs can also be used (see Table 5.1). The strongest evidence supports oxcarbazepine (OXC) as initial monotherapy [10]. Among the traditional AEDs, there is evidence to support the use of valproate (VPA), carbamazepine (CBZ), phenobarbital (PB) and phenytoin (PHT). However, these AEDs may have more side-effects than some of the newer medications. Clobazam (CLB) [11], levetiracetam (LVT), lamotrigine (LTG) and topiramate (TPM) [10] can also be used in the initial treatment of childhood partial epilepsy. The patient's seizure frequency, seizure severity, co-morbid conditions, ability to swallow the dosing formulation and insurance status/prescription plan all influence the choice of AED.

Idiopathic Partial Epilepsy

There is a paucity of research evaluating treatment regimens for these syndromes. Gabapentin (GBP) and sulthiame have both been shown to be more effective than placebo for treatment of BECTS [10]. In addition, AEDs which are effective for partial-onset seizures, in general can be considered as first-line therapies for BECTS. Many patients with idiopathic partial epilepsy, especially those with BECTS, do not require AEDs. For those who request treatment, single

Table 5.1 First-line anti-epileptic drugs (AEDs) by spectrum of action

Partial epilepsy (with or without second generalization): 'narrow-spectrum AEDs'	Partial and generalized epilepsy: 'broad-spectrum AEDs'	Full spectrum not yet defined	Syndrome-specific use
Carbamazepine (CBZ)	Clobazam (CLB)	Zonisamide (ZNS)	Ethosuximide (ETX) – childhood absence epilepsy
Gabapentin (GBP)	Lamotrigine (LTG)		Adrenocorticotropic hormone (ACTH) – infantile spasms
Oxcarbazepine (OXC)	Levetiracetam (LVT)		Vigabatrin (VGB) – infantile spasms in patients with tuberous sclerosis
Phenobarbital (PHB)	Topiramate (TPM)		
Phenytoin (PHT)	Valproate (VPA)		
Pregabalin (PGB)			

Table 5.2 Food and Drug Administration-approved indications for anti-epileptic drugs in patients under 16 years of age (as of September 2006)

Drug	Monotherapy indication in children	Adjunctive therapy indication in children	Paediatric-friendly formulation
Phenobarbital	Generalized and partial epilepsy		Suspension 20 mg/5 ml Chewable tablets 50 mg
Phenytoin (Dilantin)	GTCs and complex partial seizures		Suspension 125 mg/5 ml Chewable tablets 100 mg
Carbamazepine (Tegretol, Tegretol XR, Carbatrol)	Complex partial seizures, GTCs, mixed seizure patterns		Suspension 100 mg/5 ml Extended release sprinkle capsule 100 mg, 200 mg, 300 mg
Valproate (Depakote, Depakene)	Complex partial seizures in patients 10 years and older; simple and complex absence seizures		Sprinkle capsule 125 mg Suspension 250 mg/5 ml
Clobazam (Frisium)	No	No	No
Gabapentin (Neurontin)	No	Partial seizures in patients 3 years and over	Suspension 250 mg/5 ml
Lamotrigine (Lamictal)	Primary GTCs in patients 2 years and older	Partial seizures and generalized seizures in LGS in patients 2 years and older	Chewable tablet 2 mg, 5 mg, 25 mg
Levetiracetam (Keppra)	No	Partial seizures in patients 4 years and older; myoclonic seizures in JME patients 12 years and older	Suspension 500 mg/5 ml
Oxcarbazepine (Trileptal)	Partial seizures in patients 4 years and older	Partial seizures in patients 4 years and older	Suspension 300 mg/5 ml
Pregabalin (Lyrica)	No	No	No
Topiramate (Topamax)	Partial onset or primary GTCs in patients 10 years and older	Partial seizures, primary GTCs and generalized seizures in LGS in patients 2 years and over	Sprinkle capsule 15 mg, 25 mg
Vigabatrin (Sabril)	No	No	500-mg powder sachet
Zonisamide (Zonegran)	No	No	No

GTC, generalized tonic–clonic; JME, juvenile myoclonic epilepsy; LGS, Lennox–Gastaut syndrome.

Table 5.3 Advantages and disadvantages of anti-epileptic drugs [51, 52]

Drug	Advantages	Disadvantages
Carbamazepine (Tegretol, Tegretol XR, Carbatrol)	Possible mood stabilization Sustained-release formulation Readily available blood levels	Idiosyncratic leukopenia and aplastic anaemia Hepatic enzyme inducer May aggravate generalized epilepsies No i.v. formulation Rash and hypersensitivity reactions Not approved for use in the US
Clobazam (Frisium)	Broad spectrum of action Fewer cognitive side-effects than other benzodiazepines	
Gabapentin (Neurontin)	Well tolerated Rapid escalation if needed Effective against neuropathic pain	Limited spectrum of activity Three-times-per-day dosing Weight gain No i.v. formulation
Lamotrigine (Lamictal)	Favourable CNS profile Twice-daily dosing Broad spectrum Possible mood stabilization	Slow titration Interaction with VPA (VPA increases LTG levels) Rash and hypersensitivity reactions May exacerbate myoclonic epilepsy No i.v. formulation
Levetiracetam (Keppra)	Well tolerated Twice-daily dosing Rapid titration if needed No drug interactions i.v. formulation	Data lacking on use in monotherapy May exacerbate behavioural problems
Oxcarbazepine (Trileptal)	Twice-daily dosing Possible mood stabilization Well tolerated	Limited spectrum Hyponatraemia Rash and hypersensitivity reactions May exacerbate generalized epilepsy No i.v. formulation
Phenobarbital	i.v. formulation Can quickly load and bolus Long half-life Readily available blood levels	Hyperactivity in younger children Cognitive concerns Hepatic enzyme inducer Rash and hypersensitivity reactions

Continued overleaf

Table 5.3 Continued

Drug	Advantages	Disadvantages
Phenytoin (Dilantin)	i.v. formulation Can quickly load and bolus Long half-life Readily available blood levels	Cosmetic side-effects (gingival hypertrophy) Hepatic enzyme inducer Unpredictable pharmacokinetics at higher dosages Difficult to maintain therapeutic levels using oral dosing in infants Rash and hypersensitivity reactions
Pregabalin (Lyrica)	Twice-daily dosing Effective against neuropathic pain	No paediatric-friendly formulation Not FDA-approved for children
Topiramate (Topamax)	Twice-daily dosing Weight loss Migraine prevention	Adverse cognitive effects Weight loss Metabolic acidosis Renal stones, hypohidrosis Rare acute angle closure glaucoma No i.v. formulation
Valproate (Depakote, Depakene)	i.v. formulation Can quickly load and bolus Broad spectrum Possible mood stabilization Migraine prevention Extended-release formulation Readily available blood levels	Idiosyncratic reactions (pancreatitis, hepatic failure especially in children under 2 years old with polypharmacy) Dose-related thrombocytopenia Weight gain Tremor, hair loss Links to polycystic ovarian syndrome Teratogenicity, especially when combined with other AEDs High protein binding Hepatic enzyme inhibitor
Vigabatrin (Sabril)	Good efficacy in infants with tuberous sclerosis and infantile spasms	Retinal toxicity Not approved for use in the US Data lacking on use in children and generalized epilepsies Possible CNS adverse effects
Zonisamide (Zonegran)	Once- or twice-daily dosing Weight loss	Weight loss Metabolic acidosis Renal stones, hypohidrosis No i.v. formulation

CNS, central nervous system; FDA, Food and Drug Administration; i.v., intravenous; LTG, lamotrigine; VPA, valproate.

Table 5.4 Site of clearance, effect on hepatic enzymes and paediatric dosing ranges [51, 53, 54, 55]

Anti-epileptic drug	Site of clearance	Hepatic induction or inhibition	Initial dose (mg/kg/day)	Range of maintenance dose ()*(mg/kg/day)	Reference range for serum level (mg/l)
Carbamazepine (Tegretol, Tegretol XR, Carbatrol)	>95% hepatic	Inducer	5–10	15–40	4–12[†]
Clobazam (Frisium)	Hepatic		<2 years: 0.5–1	Maximum 40 mg/day	Not available
Gabapentin (Neurontin)	100% renal	None	2–16 years: 5 mg/day 1 month to 3 years: 30–40 3–12 years: 10–20	30–100	2–12
Lamotrigine (Lamictal)	90% hepatic	None	Monotherapy: 0.5 for 2 weeks, then 1 for 2 weeks, then increase by 1 every 1–2 weeks	With VPA: 1–5	4–20
			Added to valproate: 0.15 for 2 weeks, then 0.3 for 2 weeks then increase by 0.3 every 1–2 weeks Added to enzyme-inducing AED: with inducer – 0.6 for 2 weeks, then 1.2 for 2 weeks, then increase by 1.2 every 1–2 weeks	Monotherapy or with inducer: 5–20	
Levetiracetam (Keppra)	66% renal	None	10–20	30–90	5–40
Oxcarbazepine (Trileptal)	45% renal 45% hepatic	Induces OCPs at doses >1200 mg/day; specific inhibitor of CYP 2C19	8–10	30–50	12–30
Phenobarbital	75% hepatic 25% renal	Inducer	Neonates: 2–5 Children: 3–7	Neonates: 2–5 Children: 3–7	15–40[†]

Continued overleaf

Table 5.4 Continued

Anti-epileptic drug	Site of clearance	Hepatic induction or inhibition	Initial dose (mg/kg/day)	Range of maintenance dose ()* (mg/kg/day)	Reference range for serum level (mg/l)
Phenytoin (Dilantin)	>90% hepatic	Inducer	4–5	4–8	10–20† Free level: 0.5–3
Pregabalin (Lyrica)	100% renal	None	Adult: 150 mg/day	Adult maximum: 600 mg/day	Not available
Topiramate (Topamax)	30–50% hepatic 50–70% renal	Induces OCPs at doses >200mg/day; specific inhibitor of CYP 2C19	1–3	2–15 (higher for infantile spasms)	4–10
Valproate (Depakote, Depakene)	>95% hepatic	Inhibitor	15	15–60	50–130†
Vigabatrin (Sabril)	Renal	Reduces carbamazepine, phenobarbital, phenytoin levels	40	50–150	Not available
Zonisamide (Zonegran)	>90% hepatic	None	2–4	2–10 (higher for infantile spasms)	15–40

* For some patients, the usual maintenance dose may not be sufficient. AED dosing should be titrated individually for each patient according to efficacy and tolerability. †Indicates AED levels which are typically available with rapid turn-around. The others may not be available and/or may take days to receive results.

AED, anti-epileptic drug; OCP, oral contraceptive.

Table 5.5 Doses of anti-epileptic drugs used for control of acute recurrent or prolonged seizures

Age	Rectal diazepam*	Intranasal or buccal midazolam†
2–5 years	0.5 mg/kg/dose	0.5 mg/kg/dose
6–11 years	0.3 mg/kg/dose	0.5 mg/kg/dose
12 years and older	0.2 mg/kg/dose	0.5 mg/kg/dose
Maximum dose	20 mg	10 mg

*Doses of rectal diazepam should be rounded to the nearest 2.5 mg, to comply with available dosing formats for Diastat (10-mg or 20-mg syringe, programmed to specified dose by the pharmacist). †Midazolam is available as 5 mg/ml, supplied in 1-ml or 2-ml vials. The care-giver must draw required dose into syringe and administer in buccal mucosa or attach atomizer for intranasal administration.

nocturnal doses of an appropriate AED (e.g. GBP) may be sufficient. Although the approach is not evidence based and is not typically recommended, some children with BECTS choose to take AEDs on an intermittent basis, such as when going away to camp or sleeping at a friend's home [12].

TREATMENT OF GENERALIZED EPILEPSY

Idiopathic Generalized Epilepsy

Childhood Absence Epilepsy

There is evidence to support the use of VPA, ethosuximide (ETX), and LTG as initial monotherapy for CAE [10]. No evidence currently suggests that any of these has superior efficacy or effectiveness. There is, however, an ongoing multicentre trial, supported by the United States National Institutes of Health, to address this question.

Juvenile Myoclonic Epilepsy

Ideally, the goal in treating JME is to eliminate all seizure types. When this is not possible, targeting the most disabling seizure type, while avoiding obvious triggers (sleep deprivation and alcohol) is reasonable. While VPA has traditionally been used as the first-line AED in JME, there are no controlled trials to support this. In fact, no controlled trials have studied any AED as initial monotherapy for patients with JME. There is evidence from case series and open-label trials to support the use of VPA, LTG, LVT, TPM and zonisamide (ZNS) [10]. However, LTG has also been reported to exacerbate myoclonic seizures in JME. Therefore, in a patient for whom the myoclonus is the primary concern, with infrequent convulsions, LTG may not be the AED of choice [10].

Additional consideration should be given to the fact that JME patients typically require lifelong AED therapy. For adolescent females, concerns regarding teratogenicity may argue against VPA as a first-line agent [13]. Interactions with oral contraceptives should also be considered (see Table 5.4).

Primary Generalized Epilepsy with Tonic–Clonic Seizures Alone

There are few data to support evidence-based selection of AEDs for primary generalized tonic–clonic seizures alone. The available choices are the same as those discussed for JME: VPA, LTG, LVT, TPM and ZNS.

TREATMENT OF SYMPTOMATIC GENERALIZED EPILEPSY

Lennox–Gastaut Syndrome (LGS)

The classic triad of LGS is frequent seizures with multiple seizure types, interictal slow spike–wave and delayed mental development. The Food and Drug Administration (FDA) has approved felbamate (FBM), LTG and TPM for use in the treatment of LGS. TPM was shown to decrease drop attacks and convulsions when compared with placebo (33% of TPM patients had greater than 50% reduction in seizures, compared with 8% of placebo) [14]. Of patients treated with LTG vs. placebo, 33% vs. 16% had greater than 50% seizure reduction [15]. Patients treated with FBM had a 34% decrease in seizures, compared with a 16% decrease in placebo-treated patients [16].

Other AEDs often used in treatment of LGS, without data from controlled trials, include: VPA, vigabatrin (VGB), ZNS, PB, benzodiazepines and adrenocorticotropic hormone (ACTH) or prednisolone. Additional options include the ketogenic diet, vagus nerve stimulator or corpus callosotomy.

As with other epilepsy syndromes with multiple seizure types, targeting the most disabling seizures is important. In patients with LGS, tonic seizures cause injuries and are often the most disabling. Simple interventions, such as providing a helmet with face protection, can also be helpful.

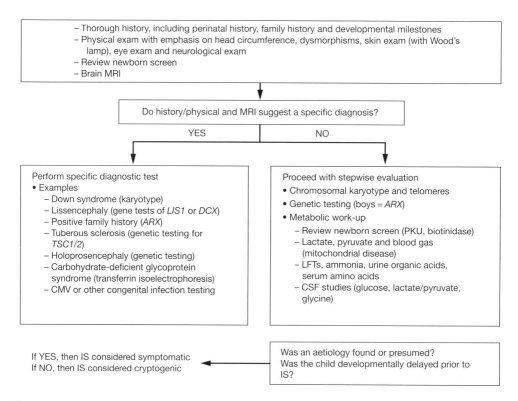

Figure 5.2 Evaluation of a child with infantile spasms. CMV, cytomegalovirus; CSF, cerebrospinal fluid; IS infantile spasm; LFT, liver function test; MRI, magnetic resonance imaging; PKU, phenylketonuria.

TREATMENT OF EPILEPTIC ENCEPHALOPATHIES

Infantile Spasms

West syndrome is the triad of infantile spasms (ISs), profoundly abnormal *interictal* EEG (hypsarrhythmia), and developmental arrest or regression. This is one of the classic catastrophic epilepsies of childhood. The prognosis and treatment of a child with IS often depends on the underlying aetiology of the disorder. For many infants, an extensive diagnostic work-up is required (Figure 5.2).

While prompt treatment of IS is typically viewed as important, there are remarkably few data available to support the various treatment choices. A recent practice parameter by the American Academy of Pediatrics and the Child Neurology Society concluded that ACTH is 'probably effective' for the short-term treatment of infantile spasms and resolution of hypsarrhythmia, but there is insufficient evidence to recommend optimal ACTH dosage or duration of treatment [17]. High-dose ACTH (150 units/m^2 daily) may have a slightly higher response rate than low-dose regimens, but there are increased side-effects with the increased steroid dose. Recent work has suggested that doses as low as 0.2–1.0 units/kg/day can be effective and have fewer serious side-effects [18].

In most current protocols, infants are started on a relatively low-dose ACTH regimen and monitored for response. If, by 2 weeks of treatment, the ISs resolve and the EEG improves, ACTH is tapered over approximately 4 weeks. If the seizures have not improved and side-effects are tolerable, the dose can be increased in an attempt to control the ISs. Ranitidine, or a similar agent, is used to avoid gastritis. Regular monitoring of blood pressure and routine stool guaiac testing may prevent serious adverse events. Some epilepsy centres also recommend co-trimazole as prophylaxis against *Pneumocystis carinii* pneumonia. Parents should be counselled that irritability is a common, but reversible, side-effect from this treatment regimen.

For patients who do not respond to ACTH, there are other options. VGB can be effective in doses of 25–150 mg/kg/day [19, 20]. However, VGB may take longer to produce a positive effect than ACTH [21], and the duration of IS and hypsarrhythmia may have implications for developmental outcome, especially in patients with cryptogenic IS.

Several studies have shown that patients whose ISs are caused by tuberous sclerosis have particularly good responses to VGB [22, 23]. For these patients, VGB is considered the most appropriate first-line therapy, despite risks of irreversible peripheral vision loss [24, 25]. VGB is not approved by the FDA for use in the United States.

Other second- or third-line AED choices for IS include VPA, pyridoxine, TPM, ZNS and LTG. In many cases, infants with newly diagnosed IS should be given a trial of 100-mg intravenous pyridoxine while an EEG is being recorded, to rule out pyridoxine dependency. High-dose pyridoxine has also been used as an ongoing treatment for IS, sometimes combined with low-dose ACTH. TPM and ZNS have shown efficacy in small case series of IS [26, 27].

ABORTIVE THERAPY IN NEWLY DIAGNOSED PATIENTS

The option of prescribing an abortive medication, such as rectal diazepam (see Table 5.5), may be a good one for the primary care physician who is caring for a child with a first unprovoked seizure or newly diagnosed epilepsy who must wait for several weeks prior to consultation with a neurologist. This may circumvent unnecessary prescription of a daily AED for a child who might not need such treatment. Additionally, it will avoid the situation in which an inappropriate medication is selected, which could exacerbate seizures in a patient with generalized epilepsy.

DISCONTINUING AEDs

About half of all children with epilepsy will eventually outgrow their disorder. For patients who are seizure free for a period of time (usually 2 years), a trial-off of AED is almost always reasonable. In this scenario, approximately 70% of children are successfully weaned from AEDs. Risk factors for recurrence of seizures after weaning AEDs include: (i) onset of epilepsy during adolescence; (ii) epileptiform discharges on EEG; and (iii) symptomatic (vs. idiopathic) epilepsy syndrome [28]. While none of these risk factors is an absolute contraindication for weaning AEDs, the patient and family must be made aware that the chances of success are reduced. Regardless, the risk of developing intractable epilepsy after withdrawing an AED in an appropriate clinical context is very low [29].

There is concern that rapid withdrawal of AEDs may precipitate status epilepticus. Therefore, slow tapering of AEDs is recommended. Generally, a taper of 6 weeks is appropriate for the child who is seizure free and is on monotherapy. There appears to be little or no advantage to using a longer taper [29, 30].

As mentioned above, typical patients with JME require lifelong AED treatment because of recurrent convulsions when AED tapers are attempted. Usually, by the time they achieve a period of seizure freedom, these patients are of driving age and prefer to continue the AED rather than give up their driving privileges.

Adults with a history of childhood-onset epilepsy are less likely than controls to obtain a driver's licence [31, 32]. Because driving is so important for social functioning, if at all possible we recommend a trial off of AEDs prior to the age of obtaining a licence. Doing this at age 12–14 years allows an adequate trial-off of AEDs, as well as enough time to regain seizure control should the wean be unsuccessful. Requirements of seizure freedom vary between states and countries, but most specify 6 months' to 2 years' remission prior to granting licences.

It is important that patients and care-givers have a plan of action in the case of recurrent seizures as AEDs are tapered and discontinued. They should know their specific epilepsy syndrome diagnosis and seizure type(s), AED dose at which the child was seizure free and whom to call in the case of a seizure. Plans should be clear regarding the need for emergency medical services in the case of recurrent seizures (care-giver knowledge of cardiopulmonary resuscitation [CPR] and a prescription for an emergency abortive medication are important). In addition, patients and care-givers should pay attention to any cognitive or behavioural changes that may occur when the child is off AEDs, as this could alter future treatment plans in the case of relapse.

ACADEMIC DIFFICULTIES AND PSYCHIATRIC CO-MORBIDITIES

Children with epilepsy, even those without other neurological impairment and with good seizure control, are at higher risk than their healthy peers for adverse psychosocial outcomes. In one study, 58% of all children with newly diagnosed epilepsy required special education services at some point in the first 5 years after diagnosis, compared with 13–14% of children in the general population [33]. Children with remote symptomatic epilepsy had the highest rates of special education services (88%), but even among children with idiopathic or cryptogenic epilepsy the rate was significantly higher than the general population (48%). These data have been reproduced in other study populations [34].

SYNDROMES ASSOCIATED WITH LEARNING DIFFERENCES

Studies of children with BECTS – a 'benign' epilepsy syndrome – have shown significant learning differences when compared with normal controls, with reduced auditory–verbal memory and learning, as well as poorer executive skills despite average intelligence [35, 36]. Another study of children with various epilepsy syndromes identified important deficits in reading compared with healthy controls, again despite normal intelligence and normal brain MRI [37]. Finally, a study of children with idiopathic epilepsy and normal-range intelligence quotient (IQ) had significantly lower academic achievement, IQ, memory and behaviour scores than their sibling controls [38].

Clearly, all seizure types can disrupt normal learning. Seizure control is the first step in optimizing achievement in children with epilepsy. While AEDs can contribute to learning difficulties, studies have shown that learning problems often pre-date initiation of AEDs and continue even after AEDs are tapered [38]. Despite the relatively good prognosis for seizure control in idiopathic childhood epilepsies, patients with these syndromes should be monitored for academic under-achievement in order to allow timely access to appropriate school supports. In addition, children with symptomatic epilepsy syndromes, more than 80% of whom require special education, must be evaluated early in their schooling to allow for optimal placement and resources [34]. Finally, in children with epilepsy there is an association between neuropsychological deficits and living in a disorganized unsupportive home environment [39], suggesting that family interventions may also be important.

BEHAVIOUR PROBLEMS

Parents of children with epilepsy report behaviour problems more often than parents of normal, healthy children [35, 38, 40, 41]. In addition, there is a very high rate of attention deficit hyperactivity disorder (ADHD) among children with epilepsy. In one recent rigorous study, 38% of children and adolescents with epilepsy had probable ADHD [42]. While there is concern that stimulants can lower a patient's seizure threshold, methylphenidate does appear to be safe and efficacious in children with the dual diagnoses of ADHD and epilepsy [43, 44]. Atomoxetine, a non-stimulant medication used to treat ADHD, is an alternative for children who cannot tolerate stimulants because of seizure exacerbation or other side-effects, but who need treatment for ADHD.

PSYCHIATRIC ISSUES

In addition to ADHD, psychiatric disorders such as depression are quite prevalent in children with epilepsy. Mental health disorders are too often overlooked. Patients with chronic disease, especially epilepsy, are more likely to experience depression, suicidal ideation and suicide attempts than patients who are otherwise healthy. Unfortunately, patients with epilepsy may have greater difficulty accessing the appropriate treatment for mental health disease. In one recent study, 61% of epilepsy patients qualified for *Diagnostic and Statistical Manual of Mental Disorders*, 4th edition (DSM-IV) diagnoses, but only half of those had ever received specific mental health care [45].

At the time of diagnosis of epilepsy, patients, parents and physicians tend to focus exclusively on seizure control. However, important issues such as school performance, anxiety, depression and other mental health problems must not be overlooked. Early on, physicians must ask questions about behaviour, mood, affect, aggression, anxiety, psychosis, obsessions and compulsions. Identification of psychiatric co-morbidity in its early stages, and appropriate referral to psychologists and psychiatrists, represent key interventions and may ultimately impact significantly on the patient's life [46].

ANTICIPATORY GUIDANCE: SAFETY PRECAUTIONS

Children with epilepsy are at risk for seizure-induced accidents and injuries. At the time of diagnosis, families should be reminded of several basic safety guidelines. It is practical to suggest that care-givers of children with epilepsy should be instructed in basic cardiopulmonary resuscitation. In order to minimize the risk of drowning, people with epilepsy should not bathe or swim alone. When swimming, the child should be supervised by an adult who is capable of assisting in the event of an emergency. Many clinicians recommend using a lifejacket when these patients swim in lakes or in the ocean.

On the whole, children with epilepsy participate in fewer organized sports and exercise less than their siblings without epilepsy [47]. However, there are few data, if any, to support such significant restrictions. Rather, it seems intuitive that allowing children with epilepsy to participate as fully as possible in normal childhood physical activities will have physical and psychological benefits. Reasonable precautions are appropriate. Use of a proper bicycle helmet should be mandatory for all children, but must be particularly enforced for children with epilepsy given their higher risk for bicycle accidents [48]. Restrictions on climbing to excessive heights should probably be suggested, to avoid serious injuries in case of a seizure [49]. However, there is no evidence to support restrictions on participation in contact sports [50].

CONCLUSIONS

Selection of appropriate medical therapy and diagnostic work-up for children with epilepsy begins with basic seizure and epilepsy syndrome classification. While the majority of children with epilepsy will eventually achieve remission of their seizures, behavioural, educational and social co-morbidities are often longlasting. Achieving seizure freedom and avoiding AED side-effects when possible are important initial goals. However, treatment of paediatric epilepsy extends beyond 'no seizures and no side-effects.' Consideration of mental health and social factors, such as school achievement and participation in sports and recreational activities, are also essential features in the comprehensive care of children and adolescents with epilepsy.

REFERENCES

1. Shinnar S, Berg AT, Moshe SL, O'Dell C, Alemany M, Newstein D et al. The risk of seizure recurrence after a first unprovoked afebrile seizure in childhood: an extended follow-up. *Pediatrics* 1996; 98:216–225.
2. Hirtz D, Ashwal S, Berg A, Bettis D, Camfield C, Camfield P et al. Practice parameter: evaluating a first nonfebrile seizure in children: report of the quality standards subcommittee of the American Academy of Neurology, The Child Neurology Society, and The American Epilepsy Society. *Neurology* 2000; 55:616–623.
3. Freeman JM. Less testing is needed in the emergency room after a first afebrile seizure. *Pediatrics* 2003; 111:194–196.
4. Sharma S, Riviello JJ, Harper MB, Baskin MN. The role of emergent neuroimaging in children with new-onset afebrile seizures. *Pediatrics* 2003; 111:1–5.
5. Panayiotopoulos CP. Idiopathic generalized epilepsies. In: Panayiotopoulos CP. *A Clinical Guide to Epileptic Syndromes and their Treatment*. Chipping Norton: Blandon Medical Publishing, 2002.
6. Epilepsy in adults and children: full guideline. UK National Institute for Health and Clinical Excellence guideline, 2004.
7. Proposal for revised classification of epilepsies and epileptic syndromes. Commission on Classification and Terminology of the International League Against Epilepsy. *Epilepsia* 1989; 30:389–399.
8. Marson A, Jocoby A, Kim L, Gamble C, Chadwick D; the Medical Research Council MESS Study Group. Immediate versus deferred antiepileptic drug treatment for early epilepsy and single seizures: a randomised controlled trial. *Lancet* 2005; 365:2007–2013.
9. Cottrell L, Kahn A. Impact of childhood epilepsy on maternal sleep and socioemotional functioning. *Clin Pediatr* 2005; 44:613–616.
10. Glauser T, Ben-Menachem E, Bourgeois B, Cnaan A, Chadwick D, Guerreiro C et al. ILAE treatment guidelines: evidence-based analysis of antiepileptic drug efficacy and effectiveness as initial monotherapy for epileptic seizures and syndromes. *Epilepsia* 2006; 47:1094–1120.
11. Canadian Study Group for Childhood Epilepsy. Clobazam has equivalent efficacy to carbamazepine and phenytoin as monotherapy for childhood epilepsy. *Epilepsia* 1998; 39:952–959.

12. Camfield P, Camfield C. Epileptic syndromes in childhood: clinical features, outcomes, and treatment. *Epilepsia* 2002; 43(Suppl 3):27–32.

13. Meador KJ, Baker GA, Finnell RH, Kalayjian LA, Liporace JD, Loring DW *et al*. In utero antiepileptic drug exposure: fetal death and malformations. *Neurology* 2006; 67:407–412.

14. Sachdeo RS, Glauser TA, Ritter F, Reife R, Lim P, Pledger G *et al*. A double-blind, randomized trial of topiramate in Lennox–Gastaut syndrome. *Neurology* 1999; 59:1882–1887.

15. Motte J, Trevathan E, Arvidsson JFV, Barrera MN, Mullens EL, Manasco P *et al*. Lamotrigine for generalized seizures associated with the Lennox–Gastaut syndrome. *New Eng J Med* 1997; 337:1807–1812.

16. The Felbamate Study Group in Lennox–Gastaut Syndrome. Efficacy of felbamate in childhood epileptic encephalopathy (Lennox–Gastaut syndrome). *New Eng J Med* 1993; 328:29–33.

17. Mackay MT, Weiss SK, Adams-Webber T, Ashwal S, Stephens D, Ballaban-Gill K *et al*. Practice parameter: medical treatment of infantile spasms. *Neurology* 2004; 62:1668–1681.

18. Oguni H, Yanagaki S, Hayashi K, Imai K, Funatsuka M, Kishi T *et al*. Extremely low-dose ACTH step-up protocol for West syndrome: maximum therapeutic effect with minimal side-effects. *Brain Dev* 2006; 28:8–13.

19. Appleton RE, Peters ACB, Mumford JP, Shaw DE. Randomised placebo-controlled study of vigabatrin as first-line treatment of infantile spasms. *Epilepsia* 1999; 40:1627–1633.

20. Mitchell WG, Shah NS. Vigabatrin for infantile spasms. *Pediatr Neurol* 2002; 27:161–164.

21. Lux AL, Edwards SW, Hancock E, Johnson AL, Kennedy CR, Newton RW *et al*. The United Kingdom Infantile Spasms Study (UKISS) comparing hormone treatment with vigabatrin on developmental and epilepsy outcomes to age 14 months: a multicentre randomized trial. *Lancet Neurology* 2005; 4:712–717.

22. Aicardi J, Mumford JP, Dumas C, Wood S; Sabril IS Investigator and Peer Review Groups. Vigabatrin as initial therapy for infantile spasms: a European retrospective survey. *Epilepsia* 1996; 37:638–642.

23. Elterman RD, Shields WD, Mansfield KA, Nakagawa J. Randomized trial of vigabatrin in patients with infantile spasms. *Neurology* 2001; 57:1416–1421.

24. Ascaso FJ, Lopez MJ, Mauri JA, Cristobal JA. Visual field defects in pediatric patients on vigabatrin monotherapy. *Doc Ophthalmol* 2003; 107:127–130.

25. McDonagh J, Stephen LJ, Dolan FM, Parks S, Dutton GN, Kelly K *et al*. Peripheral retinal dysfunction in patients taking vigabatrin. *Neurology* 2003; 61:1690–1694.

26. Hosain SA, Merchant S, Solomon GE, Chutorian A. Topiramate for the treatment of infantile spasms. *J Child Neurol* 2006; 21:17–19.

27. Yanagaki S, Oguni H, Yoshii K, Hayashi K, Imai K, Funatsuka M *et al*. Zonisamide for West syndrome: a comparison of clinical responses among different titration rate. *Brain Dev* 2005; 27:286–290.

28. Berg AT, Shinnar S, Levy SR, Testa FM, Smith-Rapaport S, Beckerman B *et al*. Two-year remission and subsequent relapse in children with newly diagnosed epilepsy. *Epilepsia* 2001; 42:1553–1562. (Erratum appears in *Epilepsia* 2002; 43:207–208.)

29. Camfield P, Camfield C. The frequency of intractable seizures after stopping AEDs in seizure-free children with epilepsy. *Neurology* 2005; 64:973–975.

30. Tennison M, Greenwood R, Lewis D, Thorn M. Discontinuing antiepileptic drugs in children with epilepsy. A comparison of a six-week and a nine-month taper period. *New Eng J Med* 1994; 330:1407–1410.

31. Sillanpää M, Shinnar S. Obtaining a driver's license and seizure relapse in patients with childhood-onset epilepsy. *Neurology* 2005; 64:680–686.

32. Wakamoto H, Nagao H, Masatoshi H, Morimoto T. Long-term medical, education, and social prognoses of childhood-onset epilepsy: a population-based study in a rural district of Japan. *Brain Dev* 2000; 22:246–255.

33. Berg AT, Smith SN, Frobish D, Levy SR, Testa FM, Beckerman B *et al*. Special education needs of children with newly diagnosed epilepsy. *Dev Med Child Neurol* 2005; 47:749–753.

34. Wodrich DL, Kaplan AM, Deering WM. Children with epilepsy in school: special service usage and assessment practices. *Psychology in the Schools* 2006; 43:169–181.

35. Croona C, Khilgren M, Lundberg S, Eeg-Olofsson O, Eeg-Olofsson KE. Neuropsychological findings in children with benign childhood epilepsy with centrotemporal spikes. *Dev Med Child Neurol* 1999; 41:813–818.

36. Giordani B, Caveney AF, Laughrin D, Huffman JL, Berent S, Sharma U *et al*. Cognition and behavior in children with benign epilepsy with centrotemporal spikes (BECTS). *Epilepsy Res* 2006; 70:89–94.

37. Vanasse CM, Beland R, Carmant L, Lassonde M. Impact of childhood epilepsy on reading and phonological processing abilities. *Epilepsy Behav* 2005; 7:288–296.

38. Bailet LL, Turk William R. The impact of childhood epilepsy on neurocognitive and behavioral performance: a prospective longitudinal study. *Epilepsia* 2000; 41:426–431.
39. Fastenau PS, Shen J, Dunn DW, Perkins SM, Hermann BP, Austin JK. Neuropsychological predictors of academic underachievement in pediatric epilepsy: moderating roles of demographic, seizure, and psychosocial variables. *Epilepsia* 2004; 45:1261–1272.
40. Høie B, Sommerfelt K, Waaler PE, Alsaker FD, Skeidsvoll H, Mykletun A. Psychosocial problems and seizure-related factors in children with epilepsy. *Dev Med Child Neurol* 2006; 48:213–219.
41. Wirrell EC, Camfield CS, Camfield PR, Dooley JM, Gordon KE, Smith B. Long-term psychosocial outcome in typical absence epilepsy: sometimes a wolf in sheep's clothing. *Arch Pediatr Adolesc Med* 1997; 151:152–158.
42. Dunn DW, Austin JK, Harezlak J, Ambrosius WT. ADHD and epilepsy in childhood. *Dev Med Child Neurol* 2003; 45:50–54.
43. Gross-Tsur V, Manor O, van der Meere J, Joseph A, Shalev RS. Epilepsy and attention deficit hyperactivity disorder: is methylphenidate safe and effective? *J Pediatr* 1997; 130:40–44.
44. Gucuyener K, Erdemoglu AK, Senol S, Serdaroglu A, Soysal S, Kockar AI. Use of methylphenidate for attention-deficit hyperactivity disorder in patients with epilepsy or electroencephalographic abnormalities. *J Child Neurol* 2003; 18:109–112.
45. Ott D, Siddarth P, Gurbani S, Koh S, Tournay A, Shields WD *et al.* Behavioral disorders in pediatric epilepsy: unmet psychiatric need. *Epilepsia* 2003; 44:591–597.
46. Baker G. Depression and suicide in adolescents with epilepsy. *Neurology* 2006; 66(Suppl 6):S5–S12.
47. Wong J, Wirrell EC. Physical activity in children/teens with epilepsy compared with that in their siblings without epilepsy. *Epilepsia* 2006; 47:631–639.
48. Wirrell EC, Camfield PR, Camfield CS, Dooley JM, Gordon KE. Accidental injury is a serious risk in children with typical absence epilepsy. *Arch Neurol* 1996; 53:929–932.
49. Kirsch R, Wirrell E. Do cognitively normal children with epilepsy have a higher rate of injury than their nonepileptic peers? *J Child Neurol* 2001; 16:100–104.
50. Dubow JS, Kelly JP. *Epilepsy in sports and recreation. Sports Med* 2003; 33:499–516.
51. Sullivan JE, Dlugos DJ. Antiepileptic drug monotherapy: pediatric concerns. *Semin Pediatr Neurol* 2005; 12:88–96.
52. Sander JW. The use of antiepileptic drugs – principles and practice. *Epilepsia* 2004; 45(Suppl 6):28–34.
53. French JA, Gidal BE. Antiepileptic drug interactions. *Epilepsia* 2000; 41(Suppl 8):S30–S36.
54. Perucca E, Dulac O, Shorvon S, Tomson T. Harnessing the clinical potential of antiepileptic drug therapy: dosage optimisation. *CNS Drugs* 2001; 15:609–621.
55. Levy HR, Mattson RH, Meldrum BS, Perucca E (eds). *Antiepileptic Drugs*. 5th edn. Philadelphia: Lippincott Williams & Wilkins, 2002.

6

Treatment of the child or adolescent with treatment-resistant epilepsy

Blaise F. D. Bourgeois

INTRODUCTION

Although children and adolescents may have well-known easily treatable epilepsy syndromes such as childhood or juvenile absence epilepsy or benign rolandic epilepsy, available evidence indicates that they are not less likely to suffer from treatment-resistant epilepsy than adults. Four main groups of aetiologies that are specific to the paediatric age range are responsible for the great majority of refractory epilepsies in this age group: (i) congenital or genetically determined structural abnormalities of the brain, such as migrational disorders, dysplasias, tuberous sclerosis or Aicardi syndrome; (ii) pre- or perinatally acquired brain insults (vascular or hypoxic–ischaemic); (iii) inborn metabolic or neurodegenerative disorders such as neuronal ceroid lipofuscinosis or glucose transporter defect; and (iv) severe cryptogenic or genetic epilepsy syndromes such as West syndrome, Lennox–Gastaut syndrome, severe myoclonic epilepsy of infancy (Dravet syndrome), Rett syndrome, ring chromosome 20 or acquired epileptic aphasia (Landau–Kleffner syndrome). This greater diversity of aetiologies responsible for treatment-resistant epilepsies in the paediatric population has two major consequences: a more elaborate diagnostic evaluation and a broader spectrum of applied therapeutic measures. This chapter will review these multiple diagnostic considerations, and the sequence of appropriate therapeutic options as a function of the aetiology or type of epilepsy in the difficult-to-control epilepsies of infancy, childhood or adolescence.

RE-ASSESSING THE DIAGNOSIS OF EPILEPSY

In any paediatric patient whose seizures seem to elude control by medication, one has to consider the possibility that the clinical events do not represent seizures. Since the interictal electroencephalogram (EEG) can be normal in patients with genuine epileptic seizures, it is not uncommon to have to diagnose epilepsy on the basis of clinical events alone. This obviously carries the risk of arriving at a diagnosis of epilepsy in a child that has non-epileptic paroxysmal events. The widespread availability of long-term video-electroencephalography monitoring and ambulatory electroencephalography has dramatically improved our ability to distinguish between non-epileptic and epileptic events. The spectrum of clinical events that may be mistaken for seizures is much broader in infants and children. Table 6.1 summarizes many conditions that can at times be mistaken for seizures.

Blaise F. D. Bourgeois, MD, Professor in Neurology, Harvard Medical School; Director, Division of Epilepsy and Clinical Neurophysiology, Children's Hospital Boston, Boston, Massachusetts, USA

Table 6.1 Paroxysmal clinical events that can be mistaken for seizures

Unusual movements	Tics, including Tourette's syndrome
	Benign sleep myoclonus
	Benign non-epileptic infantile spasms
	Non-epileptic head drops
	Startle response, hyperekplexia
	Paroxysmal torticollis
	Paroxysmal dyskinesias
	Episodic ataxias
	Gratification, self-stimulation and infantile masturbation
	Eye movements: benign paroxysmal vertigo, nystagmus, alternating hemiplegia
Loss of tone or consciousness	Syncopes: neurocardiogenic, orthostatic
	Narcolepsy/cataplexy
	Attention deficit/daydreaming
	Acute/alternating hemiplegia
	Migraine
Respiratory disorders	Apnoea
	Breath-holding spells
	Hyperventilation/panic attacks
Behaviour disorders and sleep disorders	Head banging (iactatio capitis)
	Night terrors, sleep walking, nightmares
	Rage attacks
	Narcolepsy/cataplexy
Psychiatric and mental disorders	Fugues, panic attacks
	Hallucinations
	Autism
	Pseudoseizures
	Munchhausen by proxy
Perceptual disturbances	Dizziness, vertigo
Episodic features of specific disorders	Hypoglycaemia, hypocalcaemia
	Periodic paralysis
	Hyperthyroidism
	Cardiac arrhythmias, long Q–T syndrome, tetralogy spells
	Hydrocephalic spells
	Gastroesophageal reflux/Sandifer syndrome, rumination
	Acute intoxications
	Cerebrovascular events

TICS

Among non-epileptic paroxysmal movements, tics can be mistaken for myoclonic seizures, and some infants can have clusters of movements that resemble spasms or head drops.

PAROXYSMAL DYSTONIAS

The paroxysmal dyskinesias can be mistaken for frontal lobe seizures, and the kinesigenic form usually responds well to medications such as carbamazepine and may indeed be in the borderland between a movement disorder and an epileptic disorder.

INFANTILE MASTURBATION

In a paediatric monitoring unit, it is not uncommon to see infants or young children who are treated for seizures and turn out to have a paroxysmal behavioural pattern referred to as gratification, or self-stimulation or infantile masturbation. Although the term infantile masturbation is used in the medical literature, there is of course no masturbation, but the movements have a sexually suggestive component.

ALTERNATING HEMIPLEGIAS

In alternating hemiplegia of childhood, the first symptoms may consist of erratic eye movements mistaken for seizures, and the episodes of transient hemiplegia may be mistaken for a Todd's paresis.

SYNCOPE

Patients with syncopes are often thought to have epileptic falls. One should keep in mind that most epileptic falls are seen in the context of certain syndromes that include cognitive impairment, such as Lennox–Gastaut syndrome.

DAYDREAMING

'Staring off', or daydreaming, is commonly considered by parents or teachers to represent absence seizures. This may especially be a problem in patients who have epileptic seizures that are actually controlled by medication.

MIGRAINE

Migraine, especially classic migraine, can cause transient neurological deficits that can be mistaken for seizures. Seizures may also be mistaken for migraine, since ictal vomiting and post-ictal headaches are indeed features of some seizures.

BREATH-HOLDING SPELLS

Breath-holding spells often resemble seizures and may have a convulsive component. The history of a triggering event with most events (pain, frustration, startle) is the single most reliable feature in establishing the diagnosis of breath-holding spells.

PARASOMNIAS

Parasomnias and sleep disorders are easily mistaken for seizures, especially frontal lobe seizures that often occur during nocturnal sleep.

PSYCHOGENIC NON-EPILEPTIC SEIZURES

Psychogenic non-epileptic seizures (pseudoseizures) do occur in adolescents and even in older children. Documenting their non-epileptic nature may take several months, or even remain an elusive goal, especially in patients who have a combination of epileptic and non-epileptic seizures. 'Munchhausen by proxy' is more specific to the paediatric age range, and its diagnosis may also represent a very arduous process.

MEDICAL DISORDERS

Finally, disorders that are not neurological or psychiatric may be associated with paroxysmal clinical events mimicking seizures, such as hypoglycaemia, hypocalcaemia, cardiac arrhythmias and tetralogy of Fallot. In infants, because of associated tonic posturing, rumination and gastroesophageal reflux (Sandifer syndrome) are often considered in the differential diagnosis of tonic seizures.

ESTABLISHING THE AETIOLOGY AND EPILEPSY DIAGNOSIS

In treatment-resistant patients in whom the diagnosis of epileptic seizures has been confirmed, the next step is to confirm the diagnosis of the seizure type, the epilepsy syndrome and the aetiology, if applicable. This is important to re-address during the course of treatment if seizure control is not achieved. Both the diagnosis of the seizure type or epilepsy syndrome and the underlying aetiology may have a significant impact on treatment decisions, and if patients have been incorrectly classified in the past, they may be receiving inappropriate treatments, resulting in apparent resistance to therapy.

TREATING BASED ON SEIZURE TYPE AND SYNDROME

Choices of medications in the treatment of epilepsy are always based on the seizure type, and often on the syndrome diagnosis (see Chapter 5). Anti-epileptic drugs (AEDs) that are effective specifically against partial seizures may not be effective against several types of generalized seizures, and may actually aggravate generalized epilepsies. A drug like ethosuximide is effective almost exclusively against absence seizures and not against generalized tonic–clonic seizures, and its use in monotherapy would be inappropriate in patients with juvenile absence epilepsy since it is known that more than one-half of these patients will at some point experience generalized tonic–clonic seizures. Partial seizures in benign epilepsy of childhood with centrotemporal spikes (rolandic epilepsy) may not respond best to the same medications as partial seizures that are cryptogenic or caused by a focal brain abnormality. Increasingly, randomized medication trials are now carried out in patients with a specific syndrome, such as felbamate, lamotrigine, topiramate and rufinamide in Lennox–Gastaut syndrome [1–4], sulthiame or gabapentin in benign epilepsy of childhood with centrotemporal spikes [5, 6], stiripentol in severe myoclonic epilepsy of infancy (Dravet syndrome) [7], vigabatrin in tuberous sclerosis or levetiracetam in juvenile myoclonic epilepsy [8].

TREATING BASED ON AETIOLOGY

Finally, knowledge of the underlying aetiology may affect the treatment in different ways. In patients with severe brain malformations such as hemimegalencephaly, or in patients diagnosed with Rasmussen's encephalitis, a decision is often made to operate rather than to continue attempts at medical therapy, based more on that diagnosis than on meticulously establishing criteria for medical intractability. Severe and medically refractory seizures occur in patients with a metabolic defect called glucose transporter defect [9]. These patients have impaired transport of glucose across the blood–brain barrier and their cerebrospinal fluid glucose level is one-third or less of the simultaneous value in plasma. These patients have been found to respond to the ketogenic diet much more readily than to anti-epileptic medications, and establishing this diagnosis is therefore crucial for optimal therapy. Pyridoxine dependency also causes medically intractable seizures, with atypical onset up to the age of 2 years [10]. No treatment will match the efficacy of daily doses of oral pyridoxine, and this diagnosis should not be missed.

Table 6.2 lists several diagnostic tests and consultations that can be considered in the evaluation of a paediatric or adolescent patient with epilepsy, either at the time of diagnosis or, particularly, if the seizures are resistant to treatment. Obviously, not all of these tests are indicated in the evaluation of every patient, nor is this list exhaustive of all tests that can be considered.

Table 6.2 Diagnostic tests to be considered in the evaluation of a paediatric or adolescent patient with epilepsy

Blood	Routine blood chemistries, electrolytes (anion gap), liver enzymes, ammonium
	Amino acids, lactate, pyruvate
	Pyridoxine trial with EEG recording
	Biotinidase
	Carnitine (total + free), acylcarnitines (short, middle, long chain)
	Transferrin isoelectric focusing (carbohydrate-deficient glycoprotein syndrome)
	Phytanic acid, urine and pyrimidine panel
	Lysosomal enzymes, peroxisomal enzymes panel (very low-chain fatty acids)
	Chromosomes: routine karyotype (e.g. ring chromosome 20); FISH analysis, molecular testing: fragile X chromosome, *ARX/CDKL5*, Prader–Willi syndrome, Angelman syndrome, Rett syndrome (*MECP2*), signature chip
Urine	Amino acids, organic acids
	Acylglycine, orotic acid, sulfites (molybdenium co-factor deficiency)
	Galactosyl/lactosyl sulfatide
Cerebrospinal fluid	Protein, glucose (simultaneous serum glucose), cells
	Lactate, pyruvate, amino acids
	Neurotransmitter metabolites, folinic acid dependency
	Tetrahydrobiopterin and neopterin
Neuroimaging	MR imaging, MR spectroscopy, MR angiogram, PET scan, SPECT scan
Electrophysiology	EEG, ambulatory EEG, long-term video-EEG monitoring, evoked potentials, electroretinogram
Consultations	Genetics and metabolism, ophthalmology, cardiology
Biopsies	Skin: microscopy, fibroblast culture (peroxisomal and lysosomal enzymes), chromosomes, electron microscopy (e.g. neuronal ceroid lipofuscinosis)
	Muscle: histology, biochemistry, mitochondrial disorder (electron transport chain abnormality)

EEG, electroencephalogram; FISH, fluorescent *in situ* hybridization; MR, magnetic resonance; PET, positron emission tomography; SPECT, single photon emission computed tomography.

PHARMACOKINETIC ISSUES IN CHILDREN

In paediatric patients who fail to respond to medications that are considered appropriate for their epilepsy diagnosis, it is important to determine that the dose is appropriate. Dosage requirements, in mg/kg/day, can be deceptively high, especially in infants. It has been shown that the clearance of AEDs, which determines the dose in mg/kg/day to achieve a certain steady-state plasma level, can be 2–3 times higher in infants compared with values in adults. This means that a level achieved with 10 mg/kg/day in an adult patient will only be achieved at a dose of 20–30 mg/kg/day in an infant.

DRUGS OF FIRST CHOICE AND SECOND CHOICE, AND THIRD-LINE ANTI-EPILEPTIC DRUGS IN CHILDREN

It should be ascertained in every child with medically refractory seizures that the drugs of first choice have been tried. For a discussion of drug choices related to seizure type and syndrome, see Chapter 5.

In the daily practice of treating patients with seizures, one cannot avoid the process of selecting the next drug if the current drug is failing, even if satisfactory scientific evidence to support the choice is lacking. Accordingly, Table 6.3 provides data on which drugs have class I, II or III evidence for effectiveness, and Table 6.4 summarizes, for various seizure types and syndromes, drugs that can be considered in patients who have remained refractory to first- and second-choice drugs. It should be emphasized that the choices listed in this table are a compromise, and that they are not based on scientific evidence and will always be open to debate. Also, over time, these treatment paradigms may suddenly or gradually change based on new information. Beyond the available knowledge regarding the spectrum of efficacy of various AEDs, safety and tolerability considerations as well as comfort factor are the main criteria used in the development of Table 6.4.

RESCUE THERAPIES

It is not uncommon for children with treatment-resistant epilepsy to have prolonged seizures, frequent seizures or clusters of multiple seizures over a period of minutes or hours (acute repetitive seizures). One important goal in the management of these patients is to prevent frequent visits to the emergency room by using so-called rescue therapies. By far the most widely used of these rescue therapies is the administration of different preparations of rectal diazepam (about 0.3 mg/kg), which can be quite effective and has represented a significant improvement in the management of children with severe intractable epilepsy. However, the administration of buccal and especially intranasal midazolam (0.2 mg/kg) is increasingly advocated because it seems to have a more rapid onset of action, it does not significantly affect respiration and oxygen saturation, it is easy to administer, and it is socially more acceptable [11–13]. In the hospital setting, intravenous lorazepam is preferable in the management of acute repetitive seizures.

THE KETOGENIC DIET

After a decline in use, the ketogenic diet has made a strong comeback since the early 1990s. It is now considered to be one of the standard medical therapies in children with epilepsy. It is not considered to be a treatment of first choice for any type of seizure or epilepsy syndrome, except for a few specific conditions that are particularly or exclusively responsive to the ketogenic diet, such as glucose transporter type I defect, pyruvate dehydrogenase complex deficiency, ketotic hypoglycaemia, and Rett syndrome. The main contraindications to the ketogenic diet are disorders of β-oxidation, acute intermittent porphyria, inability to comply (patient and/or parents). The ketogenic diet can be quite effective in patients who have failed to respond to medications, and in a variety of different seizure types. In a review of 11 studies, the retention rate on the ketogenic diet was about 50% at 1 year [14]. The seizure reduction was greater than 50% in 56% of the patients, greater than 90% in 32%, and 16% of the patients became seizure free. In a retrospective analysis of 134 children with a mean age of 7.5 years, 100 patients had generalized seizures and 34 had focal seizures [15]. The responder rate (patients with >50% seizure reduction) at 3 months, 6 months and 1 year for focal seizures was 27%, 30% and 24% respectively, and for generalized seizures the responder rate was 46%, 46% and 42% respectively. The difference in response between those with focal seizures and those with generalized seizures was not statistically significant. Three patients

Table 6.3 Evidence-based analysis of anti-epileptic drug efficacy and effectiveness as initial mono-therapy for epileptic seizures and syndromes (Glauser). Summary of studies and level of evidence for each seizure type and epilepsy syndrome

Seizure type or epilepsy syndrome	Class I	Class II	Class III	Level of efficacy and effectiveness (alphabetical)
Children with partial-onset seizures	1	0	17	Level A: OXC Level B: None Level C: CBZ, PB, PHT, TPM, VPA
Children with generalized-onset tonic–clonic seizures	0	0	14	Level A: None Level B: None Level C: CBZ, PB, PHT, TPM, VPA
Children with absence seizures	0	0	6	Level A: None Level B: None Level C: ESM, LTG, VPA
Rolandic epilepsy	0	0	2	Level A: None Level B: None Level C: CBZ, VPA
Juvenile myoclonic epilepsy	0	0	0	Level A: None Level B: None Level C: None

CBZ, carbamazepine; ESM, ethosuximide; LTG, lamotrigine; OXC, oxcarbazepine; PB, phenobarbital; PHT, phenytoin; TPM, topiramate; VPA, valproate.

Table 6.4 Choice of anti-epileptic drugs in children by seizure type and syndrome

Seizure type or syndrome	First choice	Second choice	Consider
Partial seizures with/without secondary generalization	OXC, LVT	LTG, GBP, VPA, TPM, ZNS	PB, PHT, PGB
Generalized tonic–clonic	VPA, LTG, TPM	LVT, CBZ, OXC, PHT	PB, ZNS
Childhood absence	ESM, VPA	LTG	MSM, LVT, ZNS, TPM, AAA
Juvenile absence	VPA	LTG	ESM, MSM, LVT, ZNS, TPM, AAA
Juvenile myoclonic epilepsy	VPA	LTG, LVT, TPM	PRM, CZP, ZNS
Infantile spasms	ACTH, VGB	VPA, TPM	BDZ, pyridoxine, LTG, ZNS, LVT, KGD
Lennox–Gastaut syndrome	VPA	TPM, LTG	KGD, FBM, BDZ, LVT, ZNS, PB, steroids
Benign rolandic epilepsy	GBP, sulthiame	VPA, LVT	LTG, OXC, BDZ, ESM, steroids, immunoglobulins

AAA, acetazolamide; ACTH, adrenocorticotropic hormone; BDZ, benzodiazepine; CBZ, carbamazepine; CZP, clonazepam; ESM, ethosuximide; FBM, felbamate; GBP, gabapentin; KGD, ketogenic diet; LTG, lamotrigine; LVT, levetiracetam; MSM, methsuximide; OXC, oxcarbazepine; PB, phenobarbital; PHT, phenytoin; PRM, primidone; TPM, topiramate; VGB, vigabatrin; VPA, valproate; ZNS, zonisamide.

with acquired epileptic aphasia (Landau–Kleffener syndrome) refractory to traditional treatment were treated with the ketogenic diet and experienced a lasting improvement of language, behaviour and seizures for 12, 24 and 26 months respectively [16]. Like any other medical treatment, the ketogenic diet may have several side-effects, including constipation, renal stones (5–10%), acidosis, elevated serum lipids, growth inhibition (especially under the age of 2 years), anorexia, lethargy, impaired neutrophil function, recurrent infections, vitamin deficiency and gastroesophageal reflux. In one series, 5 out of 52 children developed serious adverse events: severe hypoproteinaemia (two patients, one also lipaemia and haemolytic anaemia); Fanconi's renal tubular acidosis (one patient); and marked elevation of liver enzymes (two patients, AST 283/8,580; ALT 120/10,080) [17]. Other side-effects included significant bruising or bleeding (16 out of 51: 31.4%), hypocalcaemia, pancreatitis (fatal), optic nerve neuropathy and prolonged Q–T interval. Arguments in favour of using the ketogenic diet are that it can be effective when AEDs have failed, it is not a 'drug', it allows a more active role by the parents, and there are no cognitive effects and no allergic reactions. Arguments against the ketogenic diet are that the term 'diet' misleads parents into thinking that it will be very simple and harmless, it is often unpalatable and restrictive, and it is time-consuming. Also, it requires easy access to an experienced centre, there are no blinded-controlled studies, like AEDs it has side-effects and the parents may take a failure personally.

MONOTHERAPY VS. COMBINATION THERAPY

In the child whose seizures are resistant to treatment, the question almost invariably arises as to whether combination therapy might be superior to sequential monotherapies. The rationale for polytherapy is based on the assumption that AEDs interact synergistically and that multiple drugs can provide more seizure protection together than one drug alone. However, combining drugs can produce more side-effects than administering one drug alone. More recently, the concept of monotherapy and sequential monotherapy has gained wide acceptance. A number of studies with careful observations demonstrated that the severity or number of side-effects often diminished following a reduction in the number of AEDs, in most cases without appreciable loss in seizure control. They also indicated that the beneficial effect of adding a second drug after the failure of a first drug was modest [18]. This led to the practice of 'high-dose monotherapy' [19]. A recent return to careful introduction of drug combinations in treatment-resistant patients is based mainly on two factors: (i) the realization that about one-third of patients still remained refractory even to high-dose monotherapy and (ii) the release of several newer AEDs after 1993 with fewer or no pharmacokinetic interactions.

There have been very few clinical studies of AED combinations based on systematic comparisons between the effect of two drugs administered both in monotherapy and their effect in combination. Comparing the effect of adding a second drug with the result of monotherapy with the first drug is not sufficient to demonstrate the superiority of the combination. Success with add-on therapy should be considered as success of alternative therapy until proven otherwise. AED combinations that were shown to be possibly superior to monotherapy in appropriate clinical trials included lamotrigine and valproate [20, 21], carbamazepine with vigabatrin [22], as well as valproate and ethosuximide [23].

The temptation to combine AEDs will not subside as long as single-drug therapy fails to render patients seizure free. However, the benefit of any given drug combination must be well documented in every patient if the combination is to be maintained, taking into account the known disadvantages of combination therapy. It is best to choose a drug combination by selecting the safest drugs known to be effective against the child's seizure type or epilepsy syndrome, or two drugs that have both shown some efficacy in a given patient. Whether a polytherapy regimen is rational cannot be predicted and must be demonstrated for every patient according to the following definition: when the patient does better in terms of seizure control vs. side-effects while taking drugs A and B together (at any dose) than the patient had done on drug A alone and on drug B alone at their respective optimal doses [18]. However, it can be appropriate under certain circumstances to maintain a drug combination even when the above definition is not met. There may be an instance when a patient responds partially to a first drug and subsequently experiences further seizure reduction after addition of the second drug. Another patient may become seizure free after addition of a second drug, although there had been no apparent response to the first drug. Understandably, the patient and the physician may be reluctant to make any change in such cases. Overall, however, the need to reduce over-treatment of patients with epilepsy may be at least as common in clinical practice as the need to find an appropriate drug combination [24].

SEIZURE AGGRAVATION

Whether at the time of initiation of anti-epileptic therapy, or in the patient whose seizures have not yet yielded to therapy, it is always important to keep in mind that AEDs may paradoxically worsen seizure frequency or induce new seizure types [25]. This is more common in the epilepsies of childhood than in adult patients, and more common with generalized epilepsies than with focal epilepsies. Many AEDs have been shown to occasionally be the cause of seizure exacerbation. The mechanisms by which AEDs aggravate seizures have not been established with any degree of certainty, and several hypotheses have been proposed. In general, those AEDs that can exacerbate epilepsy are more likely to have only one mechanism of action, which is mostly an increase in γ-aminobutyric acid-mediated transmission or inhibition of voltage-gated sodium channels [25].

Absence seizures may be exacerbated by carbamazepine, phenytoin and vigabatrin, and to a lesser extent by oxcarbazepine, gabapentin, tiagabine or even by valproate [26]. Myoclonic seizures in general, and those occurring in juvenile myoclonic epilepsy in particular, can be aggravated by carbamazepine and phenytoin, and to a lesser extent by oxcarbazepine, gabapentin and vigabatrin. A seizure increase in patients with Lennox–Gastaut syndrome or myoclonic astatic epilepsy (Doose syndrome) can be caused by carbamazepine, phenytoin, vigabatrin and certain benzodiazepines, as well as by oxcarbazepine, lamotrigine and gabapentin. Exacerbation of severe myoclonic epilepsy of infancy has been reported with lamotrigine, carbamazepine and vigabatrin. Aggravation of benign rolandic epilepsy has been associated with carbamazepine, lamotrigine and even valproate [27]. Finally, it has also been shown that phenytoin can aggravate the course of the Baltic type of progressive myoclonic epilepsy (Unverricht–Lundborg disease). Whenever there is seizure worsening or new seizures appear after the introduction of any AED, the possibility of drug-induced seizure aggravation should be considered, and the accuracy of the seizure or epilepsy diagnosis should be critically reassessed.

CO-MORBIDITY

Children with treatment-resistant epilepsy are more likely to be affected by co-existing disorders, also called co-morbidity [28]. These co-morbidities can fall into four main groups: they may be due to the same underlying cause as the epilepsy itself (e.g. mental retardation due to brain malformation, or cardiac rhabdomyoma due to tuberous sclerosis), they can be a consequence of the clinical seizure activity (e.g. depression or social maladjustment), they may be related to the AED therapy (e.g. cognitive impairment or decreased bone mineralization) or they may be totally unrelated (e.g. asthma).

Co-morbidities that can cause epilepsy include:

- cortical dysplasias
- cerebral injury/damage

- inborn errors of metabolism
- neurodegenerative processes
- chromosomal disorders
- neoplasms
- infections.

Co-morbidities that can result from epilepsy (other than ictal or post-ictal events) include:

- learning disorders/cognitive impairment
- behavioural dysfunction
- social maladjustment
- sleep disturbances
- results of repeated injuries.

Co-morbidities that are possibly related to the same underlying disorder include:

- cerebral palsy
- autism
- mental retardation/intellectual disabilities
- behavioural disorders
- depression/anxiety migraine
- personality disorders
- liver disease, renal disease, heart disease and non-central nervous system (CNS) tumours.

Unrelated disorders include:

- asthma
- diabetes
- infectious diseases
- liver disease, renal disease, heart disease, and non-CNS tumours.

Among children with epilepsy, learning disabilities or attention-deficit disorder (mostly without hyperactivity) can be found in as many as 50%, mental retardation is present in 35–40%, and various behavioural disturbances such as depression, anxiety, neurotic behaviour, anti-social behaviours and aggression can be seen in about 20–50% of the patients. These are very high percentages, and identifying these co-morbidities as well as coordinating their proper management, if necessary with appropriate referrals, is an integral part of the care of a child with chronic uncontrolled epilepsy.

One important aspect of the co-morbidities in children with epilepsy is the fact that they can influence the choice of AEDs, as well as monitoring of the side-effects and drug levels. AED therapy must be tailored, based on the possible impact of the co-morbidities (pharmacokinetics, drug–drug interactions with the drugs used for the treatment of the co-morbid conditions) or the possible effects on the co-morbidities (worsened short- and long-term adverse events of the AEDs, drug–drug interactions with the drugs used for the treatment of the co-morbid conditions). A number of drugs used commonly in paediatric patients with co-morbidities (both short-term and long-term) can potentially interact with AEDs and the choice of AEDs may be influenced by the fact that they are or will be administered. These drugs include psychostimulants, psychotropics, erythromycin, clarithromycin, isoniazid, propoxyphene, theophylline, chemotherapeutic agents, anti-coagulants, cyclosporine, steroids and digoxin (see Chapter 13). Some drugs used for the treatment of co-morbidities, such as psychostimulants and psychotropic drugs, are considered to have a potential for lowering the seizure threshold. Finally, among children with treatment-resistant epilepsy, side-effects of therapies – such as behavioural changes in an autistic child, cognitive changes in a child with mental retardation, ataxia in a physically handicapped child and decreased bone mineral density in a wheelchair-bound patient – may be less recognizable.

COGNITIVE SIDE-EFFECTS

All AEDs have the potential for causing cognitive impairment, and some have been identified more often than others [29, 30]. Ascertaining that a certain drug is actually causing cognitive problems in a given child may at times be easy because of an obvious temporal relationship with the introduction of the drug, but it is more often quite difficult. The reason is that cognitive impairment is common in children with epilepsy. Those with treatment-resistant epilepsy are particularly vulnerable because they are more likely to take a greater number of drugs for longer periods of time. The causes are multiple and they include the underlying brain pathology, the epilepsy itself, ongoing electrographic epileptiform activity and psychosocial problems, in addition to drug effect. Therefore, it may at times be virtually impossible to separate the various causes of the cognitive problems that a patient is experiencing at a given time, and the literature on this issue is often ambiguous or contradictory. Children should be monitored closely for changes in cognitive function when an AED is added or removed. Although phenobarbital, benzodiazepines and topiramate have been most consistently identified as a cause of cognitive impairment in published studies, it is important to keep in mind that there is no AED that has never been implicated.

PSYCHOSOCIAL NEEDS

The comprehensive care of a child with treatment-resistant epilepsy goes well beyond therapeutic measures aimed at reducing seizures. The primary goal of this care is not merely seizure control, but rather the child's and the family's overall quality of life. The need to recognize and properly manage co-morbidities, especially those that involve cognitive and psychiatric issues, has been addressed earlier. However, other important issues that need to be addressed include the impact of the child's epilepsy on parents and siblings, the impact of the diagnosis of epilepsy on the parents' attitude towards the child, and helping the child and the parents to deal with the stigma of epilepsy [31]. A child with severe uncontrolled epilepsy can put a substantial strain on the family dynamics. Referral to a social worker is at times warranted. The parents often need help to obtain optimal accommodations within the school system. Teachers as well as parents tend to lower their expectations when a child carries a diagnosis of epilepsy, which can be unnecessarily detrimental to the child. Although certain restrictions are necessary in many patients, in particular in relation to water safety and climbing, those restrictions should not be excessive and unwarranted. Inversely, children with epilepsy should also be expected to live up to all the expectations that are appropriate for their individual condition, and they should not be overprotected. Finally, the parents should be offered help to gain access to support groups, or to other families with affected children, assuming that all parties involved consent to it.

THE CONCEPT OF MEDICAL INTRACTABILITY

Although many more medical therapies are currently available for the treatment of epilepsy in children, there has been no evidence that the proportion of patients whose seizures remain refractory to medical treatment has decreased. Other therapies are now widely available, in particular resective epilepsy surgery and vagus nerve stimulation. It is therefore important to determine in every patient at which point the benefit vs. risk ratio of an alternative therapy, specifically epilepsy surgery, exceeds the benefit vs. risk ratio of any additional medical treatment, such as another AED or the ketogenic diet. The availability of epilepsy surgery has created the need to define medical intractability. Defining medical intractability and declaring a patient medically intractable serves no useful therapeutic purpose unless it is done in the context of defining the optimal point in time when a patient should be evaluated for the possibility of epilepsy surgery (see Chapter 2).

Epilepsy was formerly considered medically refractory when most available AEDs had been tried alone and in various combinations. However, with the number of currently available drugs, this would now be unrealistic. The definition of medical intractability has to be based on the type and number of the drugs that have failed despite adequate trials. After each drug failure, the statistical probability of seizure control by the next drug becomes lower, but is never zero. No single step in treatment defines medical intractability and the certainty that the patient will remain refractory to medications can only be approached in an asymptomatic manner. Intractability could be defined as a probability of seizure control of ≤5% [32]. Although until recently there was no generally accepted definition of intractability, such a concept has evolved markedly during the past decade. Various studies in adults and children have addressed the question of the likelihood of seizure control as patients with epilepsy go through sequential therapeutic steps [33–37]. Overall, the results of these studies are in strong agreement and the concept that has emerged is that patients whose seizures have failed to come under control despite adequate trials at good therapeutic doses with two or three appropriate medications have a less than 10% probability of experiencing seizure control with any additional AED. It is now widely accepted that those patients should be evaluated for the possibility of epilepsy surgery. If they are not good candidates for surgery, they should be considered for vagus nerve stimulator implantation. There is now extensive experience with epilepsy surgery and with vagus nerve stimulation in the paediatric age range, and results are as good as in adult patients [38, 39]. In assessing medical intractability for the purpose of surgical consideration in any given patient, it is important to keep in mind that the likelihood of ultimate success with medical therapy varies widely in function of the underlying aetiology of the epilepsy. This has been well demonstrated by long-term follow-up in a large group of patients who were treated medically (Table 6.5) [40]. When determining the optimal timing of evaluation for surgery in any patient, it is important to weigh the likelihood of surgical success against the likelihood of medical control. According to Table 6.5, a patient with hippocampal sclerosis would be a good example of low probability of medical success with high probability of surgical success. Such a patient should certainly be considered for surgery sooner than a patient with cryptogenic partial epilepsy.

Table 6.5 Proportion of patients achieving long-term seizure control on medication as a function of the underlying aetiology [40]

Aetiology of epilepsy	Percentage controlled (>1 year seizure free)
Idiopathic generalized epilepsy	82
Cryptogenic partial epilepsy	45
Symptomatic partial epilepsy	35
Extra-temporal partial epilepsy	36
Head injury	30
Dysgenesis	24
Temporal lobe epilepsy (TLE)	20
TLE with hippocampal sclerosis (HS)	11
TLE without HS	31
Dual pathology (HS + neocortical dysplasia)	3

CONCLUSION

Treatment-resistant epilepsy affects about one-third of paediatric patients diagnosed with epilepsy. They differ from adult patients with treatment-resistant epilepsy in many ways. Several aetiologies of epilepsy are specific to the paediatric age range such as congenital or genetically determined structural abnormalities of the brain, pre- or perinatally acquired brain insults, inborn metabolic or neurodegenerative disorders, and severe cryptogenic or genetic epilepsy syndromes. Also, children not only can experience a greater variety of paroxysmal clinical events that may mimic epileptic seizures, but they can also present with a greater variety of different seizure types and epilepsy syndromes. Accordingly, paediatric patients are more likely to need a more elaborate diagnostic evaluation and a broader spectrum of applied therapeutic measures. Establishing appropriate treatment paradigms for the paediatric population is more challenging, not only because of the multitude of epilepsy syndromes, but also because there is a greater lack of randomized controlled trials and evidence-based guidelines in this age range. Seizure aggravation by anti-epileptic medications is more common in the paediatric epilepsy syndromes. Co-morbidities are common among children with uncontrolled epilepsies. Some are obvious, but others tend to be under-recognized, in particular attention deficit disorder and depression. Cognitive side-effects of AEDs may also be more difficult to recognize in children. Some of the psychosocial needs of children with epilepsy differ from those of adult patients. They centre predominantly on family dynamics, schooling, appropriate restrictions and parental expectations. Unfortunately, the introduction of many newer AEDs over the past 15 years has had no recognizable impact on the occurrence of treatment resistance among children with epilepsy. These treatment-resistant children need to be identified and considered for alternative therapies in a timely fashion.

REFERENCES

1. The Felbamate Study Group in Lennox–Gastaut syndrome. Efficacy of felbamate in childhood epileptic encephalopathy (Lennox–Gastaut syndrome). *N Engl J Med* 1993; 328:29–33.
2. Motte J, Trevathan E, Arvidsson JFV *et al*. Lamotrigine for generalized seizures associated with the Lennox–Gastaut syndrome. *N Engl J Med* 1997; 337:1807–1812.
3. Sachdeo RC, Glauser TA, Ritter F *et al*. A double-blind, randomized trial of topiramate in Lennox–Gastaut syndrome. *Neurology* 1999; 52:1882–1887.
4. Deeks ED, Scott LJ. Rufinamide. *CNS Drugs* 2006; 20:751–760.
5. Rating D, Wolf C, Bast T. Sulthiame as monotherapy in children with benign childhood epilepsy with centrotemporal spikes: a 6-month randomized, double-blind, placebo-controlled study. Sulthiame Study Group. *Epilepsia* 2000; 41:1284–1288.
6. Bourgeois BFD, Brown LW, Pellock JM *et al*. Gabapentin BECTS Study Group (945–94) Gabapentin (Neurontin) monotherapy in children with benign childhood epilepsy with centrotemporal spikes (BECTS): a 36-week, double-blind, placebo-controlled study. *Epilepsia* 1998; 39(Suppl 6):163.
7. Chiron C, Marchand MC, Tran A *et al*. Stiripentol in severe myoclonic epilepsy in infancy: a randomized placebo-controlled syndrome-dedicated trial. STICLO study group. *Lancet* 2000; 356:1638–1642.
8. Specchio LM, Gambardella A, Giallonardo AT *et al*. Open label, long-term, pragmatic study on levetiracetam in the treatment of juvenile myoclonic epilepsy. *Epilepsy Res* 2006; 71:32–39.
9. De Vivo DC, Trifiletti RR, Jacobson RI *et al*. Defective glucose transport across the blood–brain barrier as a cause of persistent hypoglycorrhachia, seizures, and developmental delay. *N Engl J Med* 1991; 325:703–709.
10. Goutieres F, Aicardi J. Atypical presentations of pyridoxine-dependent seizures: a treatable cause of intractable epilepsy in infants. *Ann Neurol* 1985; 17:117–120.
11. Scott RC. Buccal midazolam as rescue therapy for acute seizures. *Lancet Neurol* 2005; 4:592–593.
12. Bhattacharyya M, Kalra V, Gulati S. Intranasal midazolam vs rectal diazepam in acute childhood seizures. *Pediatr Neurol* 2006; 34:355–359.
13. Kyrkou M, Harbord M, Kyrkou N *et al*. Community use of intranasal midazolam for managing prolonged seizures. *J Intellect Dev Disabil* 2006; 31:131–138.

14. Lefevre F, Aronson N. Ketogenic diet for the treatment of refractory epilepsy in children: a systematic review of efficacy. *Pediatrics* 2000; 105:E46.
15. Maydell BV, Wyllie E, Akhtar N *et al*. Efficacy of the ketogenic diet in focal versus generalized seizures. *Pediatr Neurol* 2001; 25:208–212.
16. Bergqvist AG, Chee CM, Lutchka LM, Brooks-Kayal AR. Treatment of acquired epileptic aphasia with the ketogenic diet. *J Child Neurol* 1999; 14:696–701.
17. Ballaban-Gil K, Callahan C, O'Dell C *et al*. Complications of the ketogenic diet. *Epilepsia* 1998; 39:744–748.
18. Bourgeois BFD. Combination drug therapy (monotherapy versus polytherapy). In: Pellock JM, Bourgeois BFD, Dodson WE, Nordli DR, Sankar R (eds) *Pediatric Epilepsy: Diagnosis and Therapy*. 3rd edition. New York: Demos, 2008, pp. 441–448.
19. Lesser RP, Pippinger CE, Lüders H *et al*. High-dose monotherapy in the treatment of intractable seizures. *Neurology* 1984; 34:707–711.
20. Brodie MJ, Yuen AW. Lamotrigine substitution study: evidence for synergism with sodium valproate? 105 Study Group. *Epilepsy Res* 1997; 26:423–432.
21. Pisani F, Oteri G, Russo MF *et al*. The efficacy of valproate–lamotrigine comedication in refractory complex partial seizures: evidence for a pharmacodynamic interaction. *Epilepsia* 1999; 40:1141–1146.
22. Tanganelli P, Regesta G. Vigabatrin vs. carbamazepine monotherapy in newly diagnosed focal epilepsy: a randomized response conditional cross-over study. *Epilepsy Res* 1996; 25:257–262.
23. Rowan AJ, Meijer JW, de Beer-Pawlikowski N *et al*. Valproate–ethosuximide combination therapy for refractory absence seizures. *Arch Neurol* 1983; 40:797–802.
24. Bourgeois BFD. Overtreatment in epilepsy – mechanisms and management: reducing overtreatment. *Epilepsy Res* 2002; 52:53–60.
25. Sazgar M, Bourgeois BFD. Aggravation of epilepsy by antiepileptic drugs. *Pediatr Neurol* 2005; 33:227–234.
26. Lerman-Sagie T, Watemberg N, Kramer U *et al*. Absence seizures aggravated by valproic acid. *Epilepsia* 2001; 42:941–943.
27. Prats JM, Garaizar C, Garcia-Nieto ML *et al*. Antiepileptic drugs and atypical evolution of idiopathic partial epilepsy. *Pediatr Neurol* 1998; 18:402–406.
28. Duchowny MS, Bourgeois BFD. Coexisting disorders in children with epilepsy. *Johns Hopkins – Advanced Studies in Medicine* 2003; 3:S680–S683.
29. Bourgeois BFD. Differential cognitive effects of antiepileptic drugs. *J Child Neurol* 2002; 17:2S28–2S33.
30. Bourgeois BFD. Determining the effects of antiepileptic drugs on cognitive function in pediatric patients with epilepsy. *J Child Neurol* 2004; 19(Suppl 1):S15–S24.
31. Dunn DW, Austin JK. Social aspects. In: Wallace SJ, Farrell K (eds) *Epilepsy in Children*. London: Arnold, 2004, pp. 463–473.
32. Bourgeois BFD. General concepts of medical intractability. In: Lüders H, Comair Y (eds) *Epilepsy Surgery*. 2nd edition. Philadelphia: Lippincott Williams & Wilkins, 2001, pp. 63–68.
33. Gilman JT, Duchowny M, Jayakar P *et al*. Medical intractability in children evaluated for epilepsy surgery. *Neurology* 1994; 44:1341–1343.
34. Hermanns G, Noachtar S, Tuxhorn I *et al*. Systematic testing of medical intractability for carbamazepine, phenytoin, and phenobarbital or primidone in monotherapy for patients considered for epilepsy surgery. *Epilepsia* 1996; 37:675–679.
35. Bourgeois BFD, Elkis LC. Efficacy of a second antiepileptic drug after failure of one drug in children with partial epilepsy. In: Tuxhorn I, Holthausen H, Boenigk HE (eds) *Pediatric Epilepsy Syndromes and their Surgical Treatment*. London: John Libbey, 1997, pp. 99–103.
36. Kwan P, Brodie MJ. Early identification of refractory epilepsy. *N Engl J Med* 2000; 342:314–319.
37. Dlugos DJ, Sammel MD, Strom BL *et al*. Response to first drug trial predicts outcome in childhood temporal lobe epilepsy. *Neurology* 2001; 57:2259–2264.
38. Gupta A, Wyllie E, Bingaman WE. Epilepsy surgery in infants and children. In: Wyllie E (ed) *The Treatment of Epilepsy: Principles and Practice*. 4th edition. Philadelphia: Lippincott Williams & Wilkins, 2006, pp. 1143–1157.
39. Wheless JW. Vagus nerve stimulation therapy. In: Wyllie E (ed.) *The Treatment of Epilepsy: Principles and Practice*. 4th edition. Philadelphia: Lippincott Williams & Wilkins, 2006, pp. 969–980.
40. Semah F, Picot MC, Adam C *et al*. Is the underlying cause of epilepsy a major prognostic factor for recurrence? *Neurology* 1998; 51:1256–1262.

Section III

Epilepsy in adulthood

7

Treatment of adults with newly diagnosed epilepsy

John Paul Leach, Rajiv Mohanraj

INTRODUCTION

Epilepsy can be defined as a tendency towards recurrent seizures unprovoked by systemic or neurological insult [1]. As described elsewhere, the diagnosis of epilepsy is made in patients who have suffered more than one seizure and an acute neurological or systemic precipitant has been excluded by physical examination and investigations. Once the diagnosis is made, the decision to initiate anti-epileptic drug (AED) treatment is based on the perceived risk of seizure recurrence. Clearly, the patient's attitudes and expectations play a major role in this process. In this chapter, we will attempt to address the issue of timing and choice of AED treatment, in the light of available evidence. In order to gain a reasonable sense of perspective on the benefits of treatment, we have to understand the natural history of single unprovoked seizures and the effects of treatment. In order to help plan treatment schedules, the relative benefits of individual drugs should be assessed as should the effects of specific combinations. We should look at these and see if they enlighten our choices in individual patients.

INCIDENCE OF UNPROVOKED SEIZURES AND EPILEPSY

Of the studies examining the incidence of unprovoked seizures, two population-based studies from Rochester, Minnesota and Iceland provide the most robust data. Over a 50-year period from 1935 [2] the age-adjusted incidence of unprovoked seizures was 61 per 100000 person-years. Highest incidence was seen in the first year of life and in persons older than 75 years. In the study performed in rural Iceland, the mean annual incidence of first unprovoked seizures was 56.8 per 100000 person-years [3].

Studies addressing the incidence of epilepsy are more numerous. In the Rochester and Iceland studies, the age-adjusted incidence of epilepsy was 44 and 47 per 100000 person-years respectively [2, 3]. The cumulative incidence of epilepsy up to 74 years of age was 3.1% [2]. A systematic review of all published incidence studies found the incidence in developing countries to be higher than in industrialized countries (median 68.7 vs. 43.4 per 100000 person-years) [4].

John Paul Leach, MD, FRCP, Consultant Neurologist and Neurophysiologist, Department of Neurology, Southern General Hospital; Epilepsy Unit, Western Infirmary, Glasgow, UK

Rajiv Mohanraj, PhD, MRCP, Consultant Neurologist, Hope Hospital, Manchester, UK

WHEN TO INITIATE AED TREATMENT

RISK OF SEIZURE RECURRENCE

The Rochester study referred to above also provides useful insights into the likelihood of seizure recurrence in patients presenting with the first unprovoked seizure. In a prospective study of 244 patients, Hauser and colleagues found that the cumulative risks of recurrence were 16% at 12 months, 21% at 24 months and 27% at 36 months after the initial seizure [5]. An extended follow-up study of the same cohort found recurrence rates of 14%, 29% and 34% at 1, 3 and 5 years following the first unprovoked seizure. There was a 2.5-fold increase in recurrence risk in those with a pre-existing neurological insult, especially if there was a history of status epilepticus, a prior acute symptomatic seizure, or Todd's paresis. Patients with generalized spike–wave abnormalities on electroencephalogram (EEG), or a family history of an affected sibling also have an increased risk of recurrence. Among various patient groups with different risk factor profiles, the recurrence risk at 5 years following a first seizure ranges from 23% to 80% [6].

A number of other studies have also examined the risk of recurrence after a first seizure in adults and children. Berg and Shinnar reviewed 17 such studies [7] and showed that variations in methodology markedly affect estimates of recurrence risk. Prospective studies recruiting patients presenting with the first-ever seizure had a pooled seizure recurrence rate of 40% by 2 years. Studies employing retrospective case ascertainment with prospective follow-up had a higher pooled seizure recurrence rate of 52%. This higher recurrence rate is presumably due to ascertainment bias, where patients experiencing a recurrent seizure are more likely to be recruited to retrospective studies.

Examining the factors predictive of seizure recurrence, Berg and Shinnar [7] found that the presence of a neurological abnormality increased the recurrence risk from 32% to 57%. Similarly, epileptiform electroencephalographic abnormalities increased the recurrence risk, from 27% to 58%. Patients with non-specific EEG changes had a recurrence risk of 37%. With a combination of these risk factors, more accurate estimates of risk can be made, with lowest risk (24%) in those with no antecedent neurological insult and a normal EEG. The risk of seizure recurrence was 48% in patients with antecedent neurological injury or an abnormal EEG, with a recurrence risk of around 65% in patients with both. The authors were unable to draw meaningful conclusions from analysis of other risk factors such as presence of partial seizures, history of neonatal or febrile seizures, age, gender, family history of epilepsy, history of other provoked seizures or status epilepticus and anti-convulsant treatment.

Once patients have suffered a second seizure, the risk of further seizures appears to increase considerably. Further follow-up of the Mayo clinic series showed that the overall rate of a second seizure was 33%, but among those with a second seizure, the risk of a third unprovoked seizure was 73%, and among those with a third unprovoked seizure, the risk of a fourth was 76% [8]. Most recurrences occurred within 1 year of the second or third seizure. The UK Medical Research Council study of the effect of early vs. delayed AED treatment in patients with single seizures and early epilepsy (the MESS study) also identified multiple seizures as a risk factor for recurrence [9]. A prognostic model based on individual patient data from MESS-stratified patients at low, medium or high risk of seizure recurrence is presented in Table 7.1. Increasing number of seizures prior to randomization, presence of a neurological disorder and an abnormal EEG were significant factors in the prognostic model. Thus, once unprovoked seizures recur, the risk of seizure recurrence does increase substantially, and patients should be offered AED treatment.

Table 7.1 Prognostic index of seizure recurrence in patients with single seizures and early epilepsy [24]

Starting value	Prognostic index
One seizure prior to presentation	0
Two or three seizures prior to presentation	1
Four or more seizures prior to presentation	2
Add if present	
Neurological disorder or deficit, learning disability or developmental delay	1
Abnormal electroencephalogram	1
Risk classification group for seizure recurrence	*Final score*
Low risk	0
Medium risk	1
High risk	2–4

IS AED TREATMENT INDICATED AFTER THE FIRST UNPROVOKED SEIZURE? THE FIRST TRIAL GROUP

Although studies of seizure recurrence have quantified the risk of and identified risk factors associated with further seizures, the impact of AED treatment on the natural history of early epilepsy remains to be clarified. None of the currently available AEDs have displayed convincing anti-epileptogenic properties, and are perhaps more accurately described as anti-seizure drugs. Whether a purely symptomatic effect of preventing seizures would alter the natural course of the epilepsy is a moot point. Sir William Gowers stated in his treatise 'Epilepsy and other chronic convulsive disorders' that 'The tendency of the disease is toward self-perpetuation; each attack facilitates the occurrence of the next by increasing the instability of the nerve elements' [10]. This came to be known as the 'seizures beget seizures' hypothesis. A century later, Reynolds and colleagues supported this view, stating 'Chronic epilepsy is very difficult to control and may best be prevented by more effective treatment at the onset of the disorder' [11]. Some animal experiments have been cited in support of this view, which show that repeated seizures cause mossy fibre sprouting and neuronal loss leading to excitatory recurrent circuits [12].

Neuropsychological studies showing cognitive decline over time in patients with uncontrolled seizures [13–15], and serial imaging studies demonstrating progressive loss of cerebral volume in certain subgroups of patients with epilepsy [16, 17] would appear to support the view that epilepsy is a progressive condition, at least in some patients. However, studies in drug-naive patients in developing countries, where AED treatment has not been readily available, paints a different picture. In their study of treatment outcomes in patients in Kenya, Feksi and colleagues found that even patients who had suffered over 100 generalized seizures had remission rates comparable with patients who were treated after a few seizures [18]. Moreover, epidemiological studies examining the incidence and prevalence of epilepsy have consistently found prevalence rates much lower than would be expected from cumulative incidence rates. This suggests that a significant proportion of epilepsy does enter remission spontaneously [19].

Such conflicting data from various sources regarding the natural history of epilepsy do not aid the clinician in deciding when best to initiate AED treatment in patients with seizures. If seizures do beget seizures, effective AED treatment early on in the course of the disorder may well result in better outcomes, specifically in fewer patients developing refractory epilepsy. The Italian FIRST seizure trial group study was the first prospective study to investigate the effects of AED treatment on prognosis for achieving 1 and 2 years of seizure freedom in patients presenting with the first-ever unprovoked seizure [20]. Patients aged over 2 years, seen within 7 days of a first unprovoked seizure, were recruited. A total of 419 patients were randomized to immediate AED treatment or to a group to be treated only in the event of recurrence of seizures. Over the first 2 years of follow-up, 24% of patients starting AED treatment suffered seizure recurrence compared with 42% of those who did not start AED treatment after the first seizure. Patients younger than 16 years, with secondarily generalized seizures, a history of remote aetiological factors, and epileptiform abnormalities on EEG were at a higher risk of relapse. The cumulative probability of seizure recurrence at 1 and 2 years of follow-up was 17% and 26% respectively for the immediate-treatment group compared to 37% and 45% respectively for the deferred-treatment group. Thus, the risk of seizure recurrence was approximately 50% lower in patients receiving immediate AED treatment after presentation with the first seizure (relative risk [RR] 0.5, 95% confidence interval [CI] 0.3–0.6) [21].

In the immediate-treatment group, 78% entered a 12-month seizure-free period within the first 3 months, compared with 63% of the deferred-treatment group [22]. By 2 years, this figure was 90% for the immediately-treated group, and 92% for the untreated group. The prognosis for entering a 2-year seizure-free period within the follow-up period of the study was 20% higher for the treated group, but the difference was not significant (RR 1.2, 95% CI 0.97–1.56). The authors reported that any differences between the cohorts in the likelihood of entering a 1- or 2-year period of seizure freedom had disappeared by 2 years of follow-up (Figure 7.1). This conclusion is borne out by longer follow-up of the cohorts. In a further publication in 2006, the authors reported that the probability of treated patients achieving a 2-year remission was 72% during the first 3 months of follow-up, 84% at 3 years and 85% at 10 years; the corresponding figures for untreated patients were 57%, 79% and 86% [23]. Thus, treatment with AEDs after the first unprovoked seizure decreased the likelihood of seizure recurrence in the short term, but did not affect the longer term prognosis in this study.

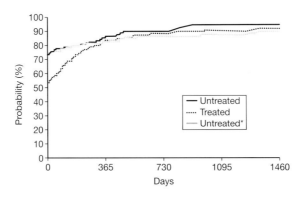

Figure 7.1 Cumulative time-dependent probability of initiating a period of 1-year seizure free according to whether an anti-epileptic drug was given after the first seizure [22]. *Considers as entry time the time of treatment initiation.

DOES EARLY TREATMENT IMPROVE OUTCOME IN EPILEPSY? THE MESS STUDY

While the FIRST trial data provide a clear basis for rational management of patients presenting with the first-ever unprovoked seizures, there remain several situations in which the indication for AED treatment is far from clear. These include patients who have suffered very infrequent seizures and those who have suffered only a single clinical seizure but are deemed to be at high risk of seizure recurrence because of the presence of risk factors. The MESS study, funded by the UK Medical Research Council, was designed as a pragmatic unblinded study to examine seizure recurrence and longer term outcomes with a policy of immediate vs. delayed AED treatment in patients with single seizures or early epilepsy, where the clinician and the patient were uncertain about starting treatment [24]. A total of 1443 patients were randomized equally to starting AED treatment immediately, and to delaying the start of AED treatment until the patient and physician agreed that treatment was necessary for any reason. The proportion of patients with only one seizure was 56% in either group, with 25% having suffered two seizures, and the remainder having suffered more than two seizures.

Over the whole study, 43% in the immediate-treatment group suffered a seizure recurrence, while the delayed-treatment group had a recurrence rate of 53%. At 2 years of follow-up, 32% of those starting treatment immediately had recurrence of seizures, compared with 39% in the deferred-treatment group. Time to first seizure was significantly shorter in patients in the deferred-treatment group. Time to second seizure also differed significantly between groups, but, instructively, there was no difference with respect to time to fifth seizure. Similarly, actuarial estimates for achieving 2 years of seizure freedom showed significant differences at 2 years (i.e. in the proportion of patients achieving immediate seizure control), with 64% in the immediate-treatment group and 52% in the deferred group achieving this outcome. The difference was more marked for patients with multiple seizures before randomization (57% vs. 39%). However, the difference in the proportion of patients in remission diminished with the passage of time, with the actuarial curves converging by 6 years from randomization for patients with a single seizure, and by 8 years for those with multiple seizures prior to randomization (Figure 7.2). This is reflected in the proportion of patients remaining seizure free between the first and third years, and third and fifth years

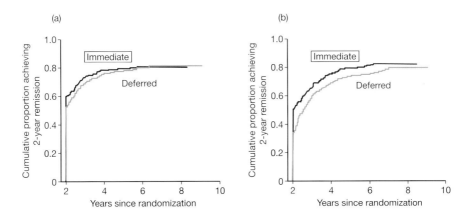

Figure 7.2 Time to achieving 2-year seizure freedom in patients with single seizures (a) and early epilepsy (b) randomized to immediate and deferred anti-epileptic drug treatment [24].

of follow-up. At 3 years, 74% of the immediate-treatment group and 71% of the deferred-treatment group had been seizure free for the preceding 2 years. At 5 years, 76% of the immediate-treatment and 77% of the deferred-treatment group had been seizure free for the preceding 2 years. The differences were not significant at either time point. Indeed, immediate treatment resulted in 17% more patients receiving anti-epileptic drugs 5 years into the study to achieve the same outcome as a policy of deferred treatment.

There were no significant differences in the scores for anxiety or depression between the patient groups, but patients assigned immediate treatment were more likely to express a preference for the alternative treatment policy than those who were randomized to deferred treatment, and those randomized to deferred treatment were more likely than those treated immediately to express uncertainty about their treatment preference. The only area where patients randomized to deferred treatment were disadvantaged was driving [25]. A total of 54 deaths were reported during follow-up, 31 in the immediate- and 23 in the deferred-treatment group; six were sudden unexplained deaths (four in the immediate group, two in the deferred group). Injuries ascribable to seizures and incidence of status epilepticus were also similar in the two groups.

Results from the MESS study indicate that in patients with single seizures and early epilepsy, the short-term risk of seizure recurrence is reduced by AED treatment, but the longer term prognosis is unaffected. The risks attached to seizure recurrence such as injuries, status epilepticus and sudden death were not altered by early treatment in this study. Given the long-term nature of AED therapy in most patients, a policy of deferring treatment until the patient and the physician are both certain of the need for treatment may be appropriate in patients presenting with infrequent seizures or single seizures with high risk of recurrence.

CHOICE OF AED

There are a large number of AEDs licensed for use worldwide, the majority having emerged since the late 1980s (see Figure 7.3). Only a few drugs, however, would be considered first-line monotherapies. Over several decades of use, a wealth of information has been gleaned about the efficacy and safety of these AEDs, which can help inform choice in patients with newly diagnosed epilepsy. Of the newer drugs, lamotrigine, oxcarbazepine and levetiracetam have gone on to acquire monotherapy licence. Such expansion in the choice of AEDs has been of benefit to patients with epilepsy, but has made the task of choosing the best drug for each patient more complicated.

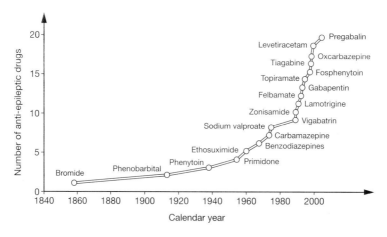

Figure 7.3 Timeline of anti-epileptic drug development.

COMPARING AEDs

Prospective Studies

Prospective randomized studies employing pragmatic dosing adjustments and follow-up periods long enough to measure clinically meaningful outcomes are required to assess the relative merits of AEDs in a 'real life' setting. The Veterans Affairs studies in the USA were the first attempt at determining the best initial treatment in newly diagnosed epilepsy in a randomized prospective manner. In a double-blind study comparing phenytoin, phenobarbital, primidone and carbamazepine in 622 adults with partial and secondary generalized seizures, Mattson and colleagues found that more treatment failures occurred with barbiturates than with phenytoin and carbamazepine, mainly on account of differences in side-effect profile [26]. There were no significant differences among the drugs in their efficacy in controlling generalized seizures, but carbamazepine was clearly superior to phenobarbital and primidone in controlling partial seizures. Further analysis of these data suggested that carbamazepine produced fewer adverse effects on concentration/attention and was superior to the other three drugs in the study with regard to cognitive adverse effects [27].

Heller *et al.* [28] compared treatment with phenobarbital, phenytoin, carbamazepine and sodium valproate in 243 adults with newly diagnosed generalized tonic–clonic seizures and partial seizures. No difference was found among the three drugs in the primary efficacy measure of 12-month seizure freedom, but phenobarbital had the highest withdrawal rates because of adverse effects.

A second Veterans Affairs study [29] compared carbamazepine with valproate in the treatment of complex partial and secondary generalized seizures in 480 patients. There was no difference between the drugs in controlling generalized tonic–clonic seizures, but carbamazepine was significantly superior in controlling complex partial seizures. A composite score reflecting efficacy and tolerability favoured carbamazepine and this was accordingly proposed as the drug of choice for partial seizures.

Systematic Reviews and Meta-Analyses

Randomized controlled trials (RCTs) of AEDs used as add-on therapy employ generally similar designs, and such data lend themselves readily to meta-analysis [30]. This enables comparison, albeit indirect, amongst new AEDs as add-on therapy. When assessing the relative merits of AEDs as monotherapy, meta-analysis of RCTs is far less informative. Many of the older AEDs did not undergo such rigorous RCTs before being used as monotherapy, and few data are available for comparison. Moreover, the number of monotherapy RCTs involving the newer AEDs are unlikely to increase dramatically. The success rates for current therapies and the danger of uncontrolled epilepsy mean that ethical considerations will preclude, or at least inhibit, placebo-controlled trials in newly diagnosed patients. Systematic reviews by the Cochrane collaboration of studies comparing phenobarbital with phenytoin [31] and carbamazepine [32] confirmed that phenobarbital was significantly more likely to be withdrawn than the other two drugs. Reviews comparing carbamazepine and phenytoin showed no significant differences in time to withdrawal or achievement of 6 or 12 months' seizure freedom [33]. Confidence intervals were, however, wide and important differences could not be discounted.

Tudur Smith and colleagues also reviewed studies comparing valproate with phenytoin in generalized and partial epilepsies respectively. Among 669 patients, no important differences were found, but only one of the studies counted absences and myoclonus separately (potentially confounding classification) and it was therefore not possible to draw any firm conclusions from this analysis [34]. Another review of 1265 patients from five trials comparing valproate and carbamazepine found some support for use of carbamazepine in patients with partial seizures but not for use of valproate in generalized seizures [35]. However, the age distribution of patients classified as having idiopathic generalized epilepsy (IGE) in these studies suggested that misclassification of epilepsy was a likely confounding factor.

COMPARISON OF NEW AND OLD AEDs

Randomized Controlled Studies of New AEDs

The largest study in epilepsy care has been the Standard and New Antiepileptic Drugs (SANAD) study, which was conceived as a pragmatic, prospective randomized study comparing efficacy and tolerability of standard treatment and new AEDs. Recruited patients were older than 4 years of age and were diagnosed as having epilepsy. Patients were recruited from a number of centres within the UK between December 1999 and August 2004, and were reviewed at 3, 6 and 12 months after randomization and at least annually thereafter. Primary outcome measures were time to treatment failure and time to 12-month seizure freedom. Time to 24-month seizure freedom, adverse effects, quality-of-life measures and cost effectiveness were secondary outcome measures.

The localization-related epilepsy arm of the study (Arm A) compared carbamazepine (the accepted 'gold standard' for partial epilepsies) with lamotrigine, gabapentin, topiramate and oxcarbazepine [36] in 1721 patients with newly diagnosed epilepsy. From 2001, oxcarbazepine was included as an additional comparator.

In the primary outcome measure of time to treatment failure, lamotrigine was significantly least likely to fail for any reason compared with carbamazepine, topiramate and gabapentin (Figure 7.4). The lower number of patients randomized to oxcarbazepine (the latecomer) meant that comparison of this drug with the others lacked sufficient statistical power to draw definite conclusions (except for comparison with gabapentin, where oxcarbazepine was superior). Lamotrigine was therefore the most effective AED for localization-related epilepsy overall. Treatment failure because of lack of efficacy was significantly more likely to occur with gabapentin than with any of the other drugs, while withdrawal due to intolerable adverse effects was most frequently observed with carbamazepine and topiramate. Intention-to-treat analysis of time to 12-month seizure freedom suggested that

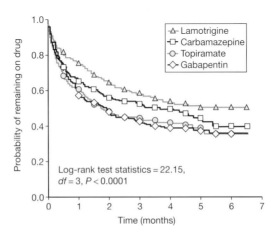

Figure 7.4 Time to treatment failure for any reason after initiation of AED treatment in patients randomized to lamotrigine, carbamazepine, topiramate or gabapentin [36].

patients randomized to carbamazepine achieved this end-point sooner, but this observation is misleading as many patients had switched to other drugs because of tolerability problems. Per-protocol analysis (including only patients remaining on the randomized drug) showed that 29% of patients receiving carbamazepine achieved seizure freedom at the end of the first year, compared with 25% on lamotrigine. There were no differences in the proportion of seizure-free patients at the end of the second year, while lamotrigine showed a non-significant superiority at 4, 5 and 6 years. The authors consider this to be sufficient to support non-inferiority of lamotrigine compared with carbamazepine for efficacy. In the analysis of time to first seizure, carbamazepine was significantly superior to all the other drugs in this arm of the study, as a result of the longer titration times for initiation of lamotrigine. The differences in initiation and titration may account for the superior early efficacy and worse adverse effect profile of carbamazepine compared with lamotrigine.

In the cost-effectiveness analysis, incremental costs per quality-adjusted life year (QALY) gained and per seizure avoided were examined by using quality of life (QoL) questionnaires. Such questionnaires are subject to responder bias, with patients who did not achieve seizure freedom less likely to complete the QoL questionnaires compared with those who did. Over the whole study period, lamotrigine proved the most cost effective, with each QALY gained at a cost of £11 851. When analysis was restricted to patients recruited after July 2001, oxcarbazepine was the most cost-effective option, with each incremental QALY costing only £6200, but the relevance of this is uncertain because the study did not support non-inferiority of oxcarbazepine compared with carbamazepine. Another measure, cost per seizure avoided, again favoured lamotrigine, with each £80 of additional expenditure resulting in one fewer seizure. After July 2001, oxcarbazepine was the most cost-effective option, as the additional expenditure required to avoid one seizure was £35.

Based on these results, the authors recommend that lamotrigine replace carbamazepine as the first-choice monotherapy for patients with localization-related epilepsy.

Arm B of the SANAD study compared valproate (the 'gold standard' treatment for IGEs) with lamotrigine and topiramate in the treatment of generalized and unclassified epilepsy [37]. Inclusion and exclusion criteria and outcome measures were the same as in Arm A. A total of 716 patients were randomized to the three drugs: 62.9% had an IGE syndrome, while 26.7% had unclassified epilepsy. The remainder comprised those with symptomatic or cryptogenic partial or a variety of other syndromes. Of the three drugs, valproate was significantly superior to lamotrigine and topiramate for the primary end-points of time to treatment failure and time to 12-month seizure freedom. Lamotrigine was least efficacious, and topiramate was worst tolerated. In the analysis restricted to patients with IGE, the superiority of valproate was even more striking, with topiramate being significantly better than lamotrigine. In the cost-effectiveness analysis of QALYs, topiramate appeared to be most cost effective (note potential responder bias above), while in terms of costs per seizure avoided, valproate was the cheapest and the most effective option.

Thus, robust conclusions can be drawn from this arm of the study in spite of low recruitment, which is due to greater than expected differences in the primary outcome measures between the three drugs. The authors recommend that valproate continue to be used as the drug of choice for patients with generalized and unclassified epilepsy. Subgroup analysis of individual epilepsy syndromes was not performed as the numbers would have been inadequate to reach definitive conclusions. Similarly, certain patient groups, such as women of childbearing age, were under-represented in the study because of concerns regarding the use of valproate in this group.

The SANAD study represents the first attempt to prospectively determine the best initial monotherapy for epilepsy since the advent of the newer AEDs. While the pragmatic nature of the study helped maintain a high rate of recruitment, it is important that certain limitations are borne in mind while interpreting the emerging data. The possibility of investigator bias is inescapable in unblinded studies, especially with self-fulfilling prophesies in recording adverse events. Furthermore, three new AEDs (levetiracetam, pregabalin and zonisamide) have been licensed in the UK since the initiation of the SANAD study, and the place of these drugs in newly diagnosed epilepsy is not addressed in SANAD. Further studies are required to address these issues.

Some important differences have been consistently observed, mainly in trials comparing lamotrigine with carbamazepine. Early RCTs comparing the two drugs as monotherapy in newly diagnosed patients showed that lamotrigine was less likely to be withdrawn, while producing comparable seizure freedom rates [38]. Gillham and colleagues [39] studied 260 patients with newly diagnosed epilepsy who were randomized to treatment with carbamazepine or lamotrigine, recording health-related QoL as the main outcome measure; in this study, lamotrigine was associated with better tolerability and QoL. A systematic review of 1384 participants from five RCTs showed lamotrigine to be significantly less likely to be withdrawn than carbamazepine [40]. Results for time to first seizure suggested that carbamazepine may be superior in terms of seizure control, but the short duration of trials did not allow measurement of important seizure outcomes such as time to 12-month remission.

Oxcarbazepine underwent a placebo-controlled monotherapy trial in the USA, and was also compared to phenytoin, valproate and carbamazepine as monotherapy [41–43]. These studies showed no significant differences in efficacy measures, although oxcarbazepine was better tolerated than phenytoin and carbamazepine, but not valproate. A meta-analysis of individual patient data found that oxcarbazepine was significantly less likely to be withdrawn than phenytoin, but no conclusions could be drawn regarding comparative clinical efficacy of the two drugs [44].

A recent RCT comparing levetiracetam with controlled-release carbamazepine using flexible dosing schedules found virtually identical 6-month remission rates [45]. There were no differences between the drugs in time to withdrawal or incidence of adverse effects.

Retrospective Outcome Studies

While non-randomized observational studies of treatment outcomes are subject to biases in recruitment and follow-up [46], such studies tend to reflect the use of AEDs in the real world, and can occasionally complement data from controlled studies. Mohanraj and Brodie analysed treatment-known outcomes in 780 adolescents and adults diagnosed with epilepsy over a 20-year period in a single clinic in Glasgow, UK [47]. Response to treatment was defined as attainment of 12-month seizure freedom. A total of 558 of the cohort had localization-related epilepsy, 103 had IGE and the remaining 119 had unclassified epilepsy. For purposes of treatment outcomes, unclassified epilepsies were considered along with IGEs.

Classification of epilepsy can help predict outcome: among localization-related epilepsy syndromes, lamotrigine (63% response rate) produced significantly better responder rates than any other AED ($P = 0.001$). This observation held true for cryptogenic seizures, while the numbers were insufficient to show significant differences amongst the various drugs in other localization-related epilepsy syndromes. In IGE and unclassified epilepsies, treatment with valproate produced the highest response rate (68%), significantly better than with carbamazepine (36%, $P = 0.006$), but not significantly better than lamotrigine (57%). When specific IGE syndromes were analysed, responder rates in juvenile myoclonic epilepsy were significantly higher with valproate (75%) than with lamotrigine (39%, $P = 0.014$).

In this analysis, significant differences in tolerability were only found in patients with IGE. Additionally, carbamazepine is known to worsen certain types of IGE syndromes and may cause seizure exacerbation [48] and is thus inappropriate as a first-line monotherapy agent for IGE patients [49].

RESPONSE TO INITIAL MONOTHERAPY IN NEWLY DIAGNOSED EPILEPSY

Receiving a diagnosis of epilepsy can have a devastating impact on patients. The ramifications are related not only to health, but also to social and economic implications. For the majority of adults, the onset of epilepsy leads to several lifestyle restrictions [50]. The unpredictable and uncontrollable nature of seizures can engender a potentially debilitating sense of 'loss of control'. Certain seizure sequelae such as incontinence can also be a source of embarrassment, further worsening restricted social activity and isolation. Loss of driving privileges is probably the most frequent cause for concern for adult patients and can have a significant impact on QoL for patients in the developed world. Furthermore, loss of employment in potentially hazardous occupations, such as operating machinery or working at heights, can have significant financial effects. Regaining a normal lifestyle requires a useful prediction of prognosis, and so, for a patient diagnosed with epilepsy, the most important question is often 'How likely are the seizures to stop?'

Studies examining response to AED treatment in newly diagnosed epilepsy generally paint an encouraging picture. A prospective study of 280 patients with newly diagnosed epilepsy found that the prospect of 12-month seizure freedom was 62% by 1 year after onset of treatment, 81% by 2 years, 92% by 3 years and 98% by 5 years. The UK National General Practice Survey of Epilepsy (NGPSE) reported a 3-year remission rate of 86% (95% CI 81–90) in a population-based cohort with definite epilepsy after 9 years of follow-up [51]. Other studies have reported less optimistic results. One population-based study from Sweden reported a 3-year remission rate of 64% after 10 years of follow-up [52], but much of the variability can be explained on the basis of recruitment bias and differences in referral patterns.

In the series of 780 newly diagnosed patients, 50% became seizure free on the first AED. Indeed, 31% never had another seizure after starting AED [53]. Overall, 56% of patients achieved remission with the first or second AED regimen, generally with a modest dose of AEDs. In the majority of cases, early response to treatment correlates with a good long-term prognosis. Patients who remained seizure free during the first 3 months of treatment achieved remission in 88% of cases, with the figure rising to 94% after 2 years of seizure freedom.

FACTORS DETERMINING RESPONSE TO TREATMENT

Several studies have shown that response to initial AED treatment is the most important indicator of prognosis [54–56]. In the Glasgow series, 387 of 780 patients failed to achieve seizure control with the initial AED treatment, 82 (11%) due to adverse effects and 305 (39%) due to lack of efficacy. A total of 103 patients (27%) of those failing the first drug subsequently achieved remission. Remission was significantly more likely if the reason for failure was lack of tolerability rather than lack of efficacy (47% vs. 21%, $P<0.001$). Thus, for patients failing initial monotherapy due to adverse effects, the subsequent chance of remission was similar to that in a drug-naive population, whereas failure due to lack of efficacy signified a worse outcome. Individuals not responding to two or three well-tolerated regimens had a greater than 90% or 95% chance respectively of remaining uncontrolled and could, therefore, be considered to have refractory epilepsy. These observations held good for both idiopathic and localization-related (focal) epilepsies [53].

Hitiris and colleagues [57] analysed factors influencing response to AED treatment in a cohort of patients with newly diagnosed epilepsy. Of 780 patients, 462 (59.6%) had achieved 12-month seizure freedom after commencing AED treatment. Pharmacoresistance, defined as failure to achieve 12-month seizure freedom, was associated with family history of epilepsy, prior febrile seizures, traumatic brain injury, intermittent recreational drug use and psychiatric co-morbidity. Depression alone accounted for 85% of the psychiatric diagnoses and was itself associated with lack of response to treatment (odds ratio [OR] 2.27; 95% confidence interval [CI] 1.38–3.73; $P = 0.001$). A multi-variable logistic regression

Table 7.2 Co-morbidities and AEDs useful in their treatment

Co-morbidity	Anti-epileptic drug
Depression	Pregabalin
Anxiety	Pregabalin
Neuropathic pain	Pregabalin
	Gabapentin
Obesity	Topiramate
Migraine	Topiramate
	Valproate

model demonstrated that family history of epilepsy, febrile seizures, traumatic brain injury, recreational drug use, psychiatric co-morbidity and more than 10 pre-treatment seizures all remained significantly associated with a poor prognosis.

Other studies have suggested that a large number of seizures before starting treatment was a poor prognostic indicator, raising the question of whether repeated seizures themselves can lead to refractory epilepsy [54, 58]. However, a detailed analysis of Shorvon and Reynolds' data suggests that this holds true only for patients with complex partial seizures [59]. It is likely that the prognosis is determined by the underlying epilepsy syndrome rather than purely by the number of seizures. It follows that the epileptogenic process responsible for a large number of complex partial seizures probably has a higher inherent tendency to pharmacoresistance.

Overall, the trial data are not strong enough to support the immediate choice of any single AED for all new patients with epilepsy. Given the relatively high response rates for newly diagnosed epilepsy, this would prove difficult. Since there is no unanimous winner, a number of factors have to be taken into consideration when prescribing. These are listed below.

Seizure Classification

As described above, the choice of drug will be heavily influenced by the epilepsy classification.

Concomitant Medication

Where the patient is already on medication, the choice of an enzyme-inducing AED may reduce their effectiveness. Such interactions could prove life threatening (e.g. with warfarin) or life changing (e.g. with oestrogen-containing contraceptives).

Side-effects

Where other medical conditions are present, the side-effect profile of some AEDs may prove problematic (e.g. valproate-induced weight gain in patients with diabetes or asthma).

Fertility

Where the patient may be considering pregnancy in the future, some AEDs may frustrate this desire by reducing fertility (e.g. valproate) or may be potentially be hazardous to the fetus. While much attention has rightly been placed on the risks of teratogenesis, it has become increasingly apparent that some drugs may have selective effects on childhood development; a story that will undoubtedly progress in time.

Side Benefits

Where co-morbidities are present, whether these are related to the seizure disorder (e.g. anxiety or depression) or unrelated (e.g. obesity, neuropathic pain or migraine) then some AEDs can prove helpful in their treatment. Many modern AEDs have sought and have had granted product licences for these other indications (Table 7.2).

SUMMARY AND CONCLUSIONS

It is usual for patients with newly diagnosed epilepsy to do well on treatment. While studies have struggled to show that the response rate will be significantly higher with the newer drugs, there is a consistent trend showing that these newer drugs are better tolerated than their older counterparts. Such improved tolerability is a boon to patients who have to take daily medications for a paroxysmal disorder, and it is likely that this improved tolerability will also prove beneficial in improving adherence. Since studies have not shown a clear winner in terms of response rates, the choice of initial monotherapy depends on several factors. In choosing the drug, some of the factors that may be considered are listed above. It is important that the choice of drug is made after discussion of the likely prognosis, potential benefits and drawbacks. Provision of this information will help the patient stick with the treatment and withstand temporary side-effects. Such motivation is the first step in improving patient compliance in the long term. In keeping with the findings of SANAD, many clinicians (in the UK at least) would use lamotrigine or carbamazepine for partial epilepsies and valproate where the epilepsy is idiopathic generalized or unclassified, especially in males. The provision of information about the condition is as important as inclusion in the process of choosing medication; both processes will help empower the patient and leave them more able to face the hurdles presented by this condition. Where medical resources are scarce, the help presented by specialist nurses may be vital. The increasing demand for informed support will prove difficult to ignore in the coming years.

REFERENCES

1. Blume WT, Luders HO, Mizrahi E, Tassinari C, van Emde Boas W, Engel J Jr. Glossary of descriptive terminology for ictal semiology: report of the ILAE task force on classification and terminology. *Epilepsia* 2001; 42:1212–1218.
2. Hauser WA, Annegers JF, Kurland LT. Incidence of epilepsy and unprovoked seizures in Rochester, Minnesota: 1935–1984. *Epilepsia* 1993; 34:453–468.
3. Olafsson E, Hauser WA, Ludvigsson P, Gudmundsson G. Incidence of epilepsy in rural Iceland: a population-based study. *Epilepsia* 1996; 37:951–955.
4. Kotsopoulos IA, van Merode T, Kessels FG, de Krom MC, Knottnerus JA. Systematic review and meta-analysis of incidence studies of epilepsy and unprovoked seizures. *Epilepsia* 2002; 43:1402–1409.
5. Hauser WA, Anderson VE, Loewenson RB, McRoberts SM. Seizure recurrence after a first unprovoked seizure. *N Engl J Med* 1982; 307:522–528.
6. Hauser WA, Rich SS, Annegers JF, Anderson VE. Seizure recurrence after a 1st unprovoked seizure: an extended follow-up. *Neurology* 1990; 40:1163–1170.
7. Berg AT, Shinnar S. The risk of seizure recurrence following a first unprovoked seizure: a quantitative review. *Neurology* 1991; 41:965–972.
8. Hauser WA, Rich SS, Lee JR, Annegers JF, Anderson VE. Risk of recurrent seizures after two unprovoked seizures. *N Engl J Med* 1998; 338:429–434.
9. Kim LG, Johnson TL, Marson AG, Chadwick DW; MRC MESS Study group. Prediction of risk of seizure recurrence after a single seizure and early epilepsy: further results from the MESS trial. *Lancet Neurol* 2006; 5:317–322.
10. Gowers WR. *Epilepsy and Other Chronic Disorders: Their Causes, Symptoms and Treatment*. London: William Wood & Co., 1885.
11. Reynolds EH, Elwes RD, Shorvon SD. Why does epilepsy become intractable? Prevention of chronic epilepsy. *Lancet* 1983; 2:952–954.

12. Dudek FE, Spitz M. Hypothetical mechanisms for the cellular and neurophysiologic basis of secondary epileptogenesis: proposed role of synaptic reorganization. *J Clin Neurophysiol* 1997; 14:90–101.

13. Jokeit H, Ebner A. Long term effects of refractory temporal lobe epilepsy on cognitive abilities: across sectional study. *J Neurol Neurosurg Psychiatry* 1999; 67:44–50.

14. Oyegbile TO, Dow C, Jones J, Bell B, Rutecki P, Sheth R *et al*. The nature and course of neuropsychological morbidity in chronic temporal lobe epilepsy. *Neurology* 2004; 62:1736–1742.

15. Marques CM, Caboclo LO, da Silva TI, Noffs MH, Carrete H Jr, Lin K *et al*. Cognitive decline in temporal lobe epilepsy due to unilateral hippocampal sclerosis. *Epilepsy Behav* 2007; 10:477–485.

16. Fuerst D, Shah J, Kupsky WJ, Johnson R, Shah A, Hayman-Abello B *et al*. Volumetric MRI, pathological, and neuropsychological progression in hippocampal sclerosis. *Neurology* 2001; 57:184–188.

17. Briellmann RS, Berkovic SF, Syngeniotis A, King MA, Jackson GD. Seizure-associated hippocampal volume loss: a longitudinal magnetic resonance study of temporal lobe epilepsy. *Ann Neurol* 2002; 51:641–644.

18. Feksi AT, Kaamugisha J, Sander JW, Gatiti S, Shorvon SD. Comprehensive primary health care antiepileptic drug treatment programme in rural and semi-urban Kenya. ICBERG (International Community-based Epilepsy Res Group). *Lancet* 1991; 337:406–409.

19. Kwan P, Sander JW. The natural history of epilepsy: an epidemiological view. *J Neurol Neurosurg Psychiatry* 2004; 75:1376–1381.

20. Beghi E, Musicco M, Viani F, Bordo B, Hauser WA, Nicolosi A. A randomized trial on the treatment of the first epileptic seizure. Scientific background, rationale, study design and protocol. First Seizure Trial Group (FIRST Group). *Ital J Neurol Sci* 1993; 14:295–301.

21. First Seizure Trial Group. Randomized clinical trial on the efficacy of antiepileptic drugs in reducing the risk of relapse after a first unprovoked tonic–clonic seizure. *Neurology* 1993; 43:478–483.

22. Musicco M, Beghi E, Solari A, Viani F. Treatment of first tonic–clonic seizure does not improve the prognosis of epilepsy. First Seizure Trial Group (FIRST Group). *Neurology* 1997; 49:991–998.

23. Leone MA, Solari A, Beghi E; FIRST Group. Treatment of the first tonic–clonic seizure does not affect long-term remission of epilepsy. *Neurology* 2006; 67:2227–2229.

24. Marson A, Jacoby A, Johnson A, Kim L, Gamble C, Chadwick D; Medical Research Council MESS Study Group. Immediate versus deferred antiepileptic drug treatment for early epilepsy and single seizures: a randomised controlled trial. *Lancet* 2005; 365:2007–2013.

25. Jacoby A, Gamble C, Doughty J, Marson A, Chadwick D; Medical Research Council MESS Study Group. Quality of life outcomes of immediate or delayed treatment of early epilepsy and single seizures. *Neurology* 2007; 68:1188–1196.

26. Mattson RH, Cramer JA, Collins JF, Smith DB, Delgado-Escueta AV, Browne TR *et al*. Comparison of carbamazepine, phenobarbital, phenytoin, and primidone in partial and secondarily generalized tonic–clonic seizures. *N Engl J Med* 1985; 313:145–151.

27. Smith DB, Mattson RH, Cramer JA, Collins JF, Novelly RA, Craft B. Results of a nationwide Veterans Administration Cooperative Study comparing the efficacy and toxicity of carbamazepine, phenobarbital, phenytoin, and primidone. *Epilepsia* 1987; 28(Suppl 3): S50–S58.

28. Heller AJ, Chesterman P, Elwes RD, Crawford P, Chadwick D, Johnson AL *et al*. Phenobarbital, phenytoin, carbamazepine, or sodium valproate for newly diagnosed adult epilepsy: a randomised comparative monotherapy trial. *J Neurol Neurosurg Psychiatry* 1995; 58:44–50.

29. Mattson RH, Cramer JA, Collins JF. A comparison of valproate with carbamazepine for the treatment of complex partial seizures and secondarily generalized tonic–clonic seizures in adults. The Department of Veterans Affairs Epilepsy Cooperative Study No. 264 Group. *N Engl J Med* 1992; 327:765–771.

30. Mohanraj R, Brodie MJ. Measuring the efficacy of antiepileptic drugs. *Seizure* 2003; 12:413–443.

31. Taylor S, Tudur Smith C, Williamson PR, Marson AG. Phenobarbital versus phenytoin monotherapy for partial onset seizures and generalized onset tonic–clonic seizures. *Cochrane Database Syst Rev* 2001; (4):CD002217.

32. Tudur Smith C, Marson AG, Williamson PR. Carbamazepine versus phenobarbital monotherapy for epilepsy. *Cochrane Database Syst Rev* 2003; (1):CD001904.

33. Tudur Smith C, Marson AG, Clough HE, Williamson PR. Carbamazepine versus phenytoin monotherapy for epilepsy. *Cochrane Database Syst Rev* 2002; (2):CD001911.

34. Tudur Smith C, Marson AG, Williamson PR. Phenytoin versus valproate monotherapy for partial onset seizures and generalized onset tonic–clonic seizures. *Cochrane Database Syst Rev* 2001; (4):CD001769.

35. Marson AG, Williamson PR, Clough H, Hutton JL, Chadwick DW; Epilepsy Monotherapy Trial Group. Carbamazepine versus valproate monotherapy for epilepsy: a meta-analysis. *Epilepsia* 2002; 43:505–513.

36. Marson AG, Al-Kharusi AM, Alwaidh M, Appleton R, Baker GA, Chadwick DW *et al.*; SANAD study group. The SANAD study of effectiveness of carbamazepine, gabapentin, lamotrigine, oxcarbazepine, or topiramate for treatment of partial epilepsy: an unblinded randomised controlled trial. *Lancet* 2007; 369:1000–1015.

37. Marson AG, Al-Kharusi AM, Alwaidh M, Appleton R, Baker GA, Chadwick DW *et al.*; SANAD study group. The SANAD study of effectiveness of valproate, lamotrigine, or topiramate for generalised and unclassifiable epilepsy: an unblinded randomised controlled trial. *Lancet* 2007; 369:1016–1026.

38. Brodie MJ, Richens A, Yuen AW. Double-blind comparison of lamotrigine and carbamazepine in newly diagnosed epilepsy. UK Lamotrigine/Carbamazepine Monotherapy Trial Group. *Lancet* 1995; 345:476–479. Erratum in: *Lancet* 1995; 345:662.

39. Gillham R, Kane K, Bryant-Comstock L, Brodie MJ. A double-blind comparison of lamotrigine and carbamazepine in newly diagnosed epilepsy with health-related quality of life as an outcome measure. *Seizure* 2000; 9:375–379.

40. Gamble C, Williamson PR, Chadwick DW, Marson AG. A meta-analysis of individual patient responses to lamotrigine or carbamazepine monotherapy. *Neurology* 2006; 66:1310–1317 (Review).

41. Bill PA, Vigonius U, Pohlmann H, Guerreiro CA, Kochen S, Saffer D *et al.* A double-blind controlled clinical trial of oxcarbazepine versus phenytoin in adults with previously untreated epilepsy. *Epilepsy Res* 1997; 27:195–204.

42. Christe W, Kramer G, Vigonius U, Pohlmann H, Steinhoff BJ, Brodie MJ *et al.* A double-blind controlled clinical trial: oxcarbazepine versus sodium valproate in adults with newly diagnosed epilepsy. *Epilepsy Res* 1997; 26:451–460.

43. Dam M, Ekberg R, Loyning Y, Waltimo O, Jakobsen K. A double-blind study comparing oxcarbazepine and carbamazepine in patients with newly diagnosed, previously untreated epilepsy. *Epilepsy Res* 1989; 3:70–76.

44. Muller M, Marson AG, Williamson PR. Oxcarbazepine versus phenytoin monotherapy for epilepsy. *Cochrane Database Syst Rev* 2006; (2):CD003615.

45. Brodie MJ, Perucca E, Ryvlin P, Ben-Menachem E, Meencke HJ; Levetiracetam Monotherapy Study Group. Comparison of levetiracetam and controlled-release carbamazepine in newly diagnosed epilepsy. *Neurology* 2007; 68:402–408.

46. Chadwick DW, Marson AG. Choosing a first drug treatment for epilepsy after SANAD: trials, systematic reviews, guidelines and treating patients. *Epilepsia* 2007; 48:1259–1263.

47. Mohanraj R, Brodie MJ. Pharmacological outcomes in newly diagnosed epilepsy. *Epilepsy Behav* 2005; 6:382–387.

48. Perucca E, Gram L, Avanzini G, Dulac O. Antiepileptic drugs as a cause of worsening seizures. *Epilepsia* 1998; 39:5–17.

49. Benbadis SR, Tatum WO 4th, Fieron M. Idiopathic generalised epilepsy and choice of antiepileptic drugs. *Neurology* 2003; 61:1793–1795.

50. Gilliam F, Kuzniecky R, Faught E, Black L, Carpenter G, Schrodt R. Patient-validated content of epilepsy-specific quality-of-life measurement. *Epilepsia* 1997; 38:233–236.

51. Cockerell OC, Johnson AL, Sander JW, Hart YM, Shorvon SD. Remission of epilepsy: results from the National General Practice Study of Epilepsy. *Lancet* 1995; 346:140–144.

52. Lindsten H, Stenlund H, Forsgren L. Remission of seizures in a population-based adult cohort with a newly diagnosed unprovoked epileptic seizure. *Epilepsia* 2001; 42:1025–1030.

53. Mohanraj R, Brodie MJ. Diagnosing refractory epilepsy: response to sequential treatment schedules. *Eur J Neurol* 2006; 13:277–282.

54. Sillanpää M, Jalava M, Kaleva O, Shinnar S. Long-term prognosis of seizures with onset in childhood. *N Engl J Med* 1998; 338:1715–1722.

55. Kwan P, Brodie MJ. Early identification of refractory epilepsy. *N Engl J Med* 2000; 342:314–319.

56. Dlugos DJ, Sammel MD, Strom BL, Farrar JT. Response to first drug trial predicts outcome in childhood temporal lobe epilepsy. *Neurology* 2001; 57:2259–2264.

57. Hitiris N, Mohanraj R, Norrie J, Sills GJ, Brodie MJ. Predictors of pharmacoresistant epilepsy. *Epilepsy Res* 2007; 75:192–196.

58. Shorvon SD, Reynolds EH. Early prognosis of epilepsy. *BMJ* 1982; 285:1699–1701.

59. Shinnar S, Berg AT. Does antiepileptic drug therapy prevent the development of 'chronic' epilepsy? *Epilepsia* 1996; 37:701–708.

8

Treatment of adults with treatment-resistant epilepsy

Patrick Kwan, Howan Leung

INTRODUCTION

In the clinical context, since anti-epileptic drugs (AEDs) are the mainstay of treatment, treatment-resistant epilepsy usually refers to resistance to AED therapy. Long-term outcome studies suggest that up to one-third of patients continue to have seizures despite appropriate drug treatment [1, 2]. This chapter reviews the treatment options that may be considered for adult patients who are considered to have drug-resistant epilepsy, and gives a brief overview on what other approaches might become available in future. Primarily, adult data will be reviewed, although paediatric evidence will also be highlighted where appropriate. Before the various treatment strategies are discussed, it is necessary to address the issues related to the definition of drug resistance that these strategies aim to tackle.

RULING OUT PSEUDORESISTANCE

'Pseudoresistance', in which seizures persist because the disorder has not been adequately or appropriately treated, must be excluded or corrected before AED treatment can be declared as having failed [3]. It may arise in a number of situations (Table 8.1), of which misdiagnosis of epilepsy is probably one of the most common. Conditions that frequently mimic epileptic seizures include vasovagal syncope, cardiac arrhythmias and metabolic disturbances [4]. Pseudoseizures or non-epileptic psychogenic seizures are estimated to account for 10% to 45% of patients with apparently refractory epilepsy [5]. Mistaking other conditions for epilepsy can lead to unnecessary and potentially harmful treatments and delays in initiating appropriate therapy.

Incorrect classification of syndrome or seizure type is another common cause of drug failure. This is because various AEDs have different profiles of activity. AEDs may be inappropriately chosen for a particular seizure type, resulting in increase in seizure frequency and/or severity, presumably due to adverse pharmacodynamic interactions between the mode of action of the specific drug and the pathogenetic mechanisms underlying the specific seizure type. The idiopathic generalized epilepsies seem to be more vulnerable to aggravation by

Patrick Kwan, MD, PhD, Division of Neurology, Department of Medicine and Therapeutics, The Chinese University of Hong Kong, Prince of Wales Hospital, Hong Kong, People's Republic of China

Howan Leung, MD, Division of Neurology, Department of Medicine and Therapeutics, The Chinese University of Hong Kong, Prince of Wales Hospital, Hong Kong, People's Republic of China

Table 8.1 Some reasons for 'pseudoresistance' to anti-epileptic drug therapy

Wrong diagnosis	Syncope, cardiac arrhythmia, etc.
	Malingering, pseudoseizures
	Underlying brain neoplasm
Wrong drug(s)	Inappropriate for seizure type
	Kinetic/dynamic interactions
Wrong dose	Too low (ignore target range)
	Side-effects preventing dose increase
Wrong lifestyle	Poor compliance with medication
	Inappropriate lifestyle (e.g. alcohol or drug abuse)

inappropriately chosen AEDs compared with focal epilepsies [6]. For instance, carbamazepine and oxcarbazepine are well documented to aggravate generalized seizures, including typical and atypical absence seizures, myoclonic and atonic seizures in a substantial proportion of patients [7, 8]. In a retrospective series, lamotrigine was reported to worsen seizure control in 80% of patients with severe myoclonic epilepsy in infancy, although the drug appears to be generally effective in other idiopathic generalized epilepsies [9].

In some circumstances, an AED fails to control seizures satisfactorily because it is not prescribed at optimal dosage. This may arise due to injudicious reliance on monitoring serum drug concentration, including a 'therapeutic range' that can be interpreted as dictating dosage adjustment without adequate clinical correlation. Instead, an individualized approach must be adopted when titrating an AED because wide interindividual variability exists in the dosages at which beneficial and toxic effects are observed as a result of genetic and environmental factors [10].

Other possible causes of 'pseudoresistance' are related to the patient's lifestyle or behaviour. As with other chronic medical conditions, imperfect adherence to the therapeutic regimen is one of the most common factors resulting in epilepsy treatment failure. Abuse of alcohol and recreational drugs can cause seizures as well as non-compliance to AED treatment. Sleep deprivation and stress are common precipitating factors for seizures. Therefore, social and lifestyle factors should be considered when evaluating the efficacy of pharmacological treatment.

RECOGNITION OF DRUG-RESISTANT EPILEPSY

Before the specific treatment strategies for drug-resistant epilepsy are discussed, it is important to first consider who should receive such treatment; that is, when is drug resistance recognized? Such consideration has practical implications, particularly given that some of the treatments for drug-resistant epilepsy may be associated with permanent complications, as in the case of surgery.

ELEMENTS OF DEFINITION

A unifying definition of drug resistance in epilepsy remains hotly debated [11]. The term is often used interchangeably with 'medical intractability', pharmacoresistance or refractory epilepsy. It should be emphasized that, by default, intractability is a relative concept rather than an absolute designation, which is influenced by the context in which it is intended to apply. Thus, the definition may vary in different settings, such as selection of patients for epilepsy surgery, recruitment in experimental drug trials, or identification for inclusion in epidemiological studies. As for the selection of candidates to receive treatment for AED-resistant epilepsy, a clinically relevant, pragmatic definition of drug resistance must take into account the potential success of the alternative treatment modalities under consideration. Interestingly, in spite of seemingly high variability in the definitions of medical intractability used by investigators in the medical literature, strong agreement was observed in some cases when applied to a cohort of children with newly diagnosed epilepsy [12] (Table 8.2). The essential elements of any definitions should include number of AEDs failed, frequency of seizures and duration of treatment [11].

NUMBER OF DRUGS FAILED

An implicit assumption in any definition of medical intractability is that remission will not, or is very unlikely to, be attained with further manipulation of AED treatment. Therefore, the most important element in defining medical drug resistance is the number of AEDs failed at optimal dosage. Any definition must be based on an assessment of the probability of subsequent remission after each drug failure, which requires an understanding of the relationship between outcome and course of AED treatment.

This issue has been specifically addressed in an ongoing, long-term study of patients with newly diagnosed epilepsy, conducted in Glasgow, UK, since 1982. In the first analysis reported in 2000, 525 unselected adolescent and adult patients (median age at onset, 26 years) were given a diagnosis of epilepsy, commenced on AED therapy, and followed for up to 16 years, with a median of 5 years [1]. Among the 470 patients who had never before received AED treatment, 64% entered terminal remission for at least 1 year. Forty-seven per cent of patients became and remained seizure free on their first drug, 13% on the second drug, but only 4% on the third drug or a combination of two drugs. Similar results were obtained in an updated analysis performed 5 years later [2]. These observations suggest that when two appropriately chosen AEDs have failed, the chance of success with a third agent is slim (Figure 8.1).

Table 8.2 Six selected definitions of drug resistance applied to a prospective cohort of 617 children with newly diagnosed epilepsy* [12]

	Criteria	
Study/Reference	Minimum AEDs failed	Seizures
Connecticut [81]	2	1 seizure per month for ≥18 months and ≤3 months seizure free during that time
Holland [82]	Not specified	At 6 months after diagnosis, failure to be ≥3 months seizure free
Philadelphia [83]	2	At 2 years after diagnosis, failure to be ≥6 months seizure free
Canada [84]	3	≥1 seizure every 2 months in last year of follow-up
Scotland [1]	2	<1 year seizure free at last follow-up
Surgery [16]	2	Not explicitly stated

*Observed and chance-adjusted agreement was measured using Kappa statistics, with possible values ranging from +1 (perfect agreement) via 0 (no agreement above that expected by chance) to −1 (complete disagreement). Kappa ranged from 0.39 to 0.79 (median 0.63). All were strongly associated with remission status as of last follow-up.

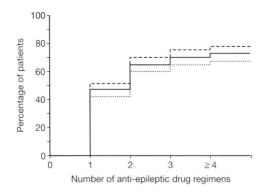

Figure 8.1 Probability of seizure freedom in patients with newly diagnosed epilepsy, according to the number of anti-epileptic drug regimens. Dotted lines represent 95% confidence intervals [73].

SEIZURE FREQUENCY

There is no universal agreement as to how frequent and over what period of time seizures must be occurring to constitute intractability. Seizure frequency used by different authors in defining intractability has ranged from one per month to one per year, in an almost arbitrary fashion (Table 8.2). However, studies including patients treated surgically [13] or medically [14] suggest that absolute seizure freedom is the only relevant outcome consistently associated with improvement in quality of life. In many countries, having even one seizure per year poses restrictions on driving. Therefore, the impact of seizure frequency on a patient's lifestyle should be taken into consideration when defining intractability pragmatically.

DURATION OF PERSISTENT SEIZURES AND TIME-DEPENDENT COURSE

Even when the criteria for number of drugs failed and seizure frequency are fulfilled, it is unclear how long recurrent seizures should persist before the patient's epilepsy can be declared drug resistant and alternative treatment considered. This question relates to the possibility of patients 'crossing' from one drug response status to the other over time. The critical issue for such a patient would be how much longer should he or she wait before the more specific treatment for refractory epilepsy is instituted.

In the updated analysis of the Glasgow database including 780 adult patients with newly diagnosed epilepsy, 504 (64.4%) patients became seizure free for at least 1 year. Although seizures relapsed in 105 (21%) of these initial responders, seizure control was regained in the majority (63 patients) [2]. It was reported that 276 (35.4%) of the entire cohort never obtained adequate control of seizures for any 1-year period during follow-up, suggesting a refractory course at the outset for such patients.

On an individual level, it is likely that the treatment outcome is highly dependent upon the underlying epilepsy syndromes, some of which might display a progressive or remitting–relapsing course [15]. In a retrospective survey of 333 patients who underwent resective surgery for medically refractory epilepsy (88% of whom had anterior temporal lobectomy), the average time to failure of two first-line AEDs was 9.1 years (median, 5 years). Of 284 patients from the cohort, 26% recalled a previous period of at least 1 year of seizure freedom since the onset of their epilepsy [16]. This suggests that for some patients with temporal lobe epilepsy, medical intractability may not declare itself in the early stages of the disorder.

Recent reports suggest that such a fluctuating or remitting–relapsing course might be particularly common in childhood-onset epilepsy. In a cohort of 613 children, more than half with delayed intractability (defined as more than 3 years after initial diagnosis) had previously been in remission for at least 1 year, and of the 83 children with intractable epilepsy initially, 13% were in remission when last contacted [17]. Another observational study with a smaller sample size described the outcome of 144 children with epilepsy onset in the 1960s over an average of 37 years [18]. Delayed remission was observed in 50% of children and relapse after initial remission in 33%. Unfortunately, the relationship with drug treatment was not detailed in the report. The extent to which such a remitting–relapsing course might be present in adult patients, who have different epilepsy syndromes and aetiologies from children, and the relationship between changes in seizure control status and in drug therapy, need to be determined by further prospective studies.

OPERATIONAL DEFINITION

A pragmatic, operational definition of drug resistance constituting the elements discussed above is needed in order to apply treatment rationally. Based on currently available data in adult patients, it would appear that defining medical intractability as a function of the number of AEDs failed represents a more consistent criterion than duration of illness, which is more arbitrary. Many authors have empirically used the failure of two or three AEDs as a cut-off for the definition of medical intractability (see Table 8.2). Data from the Glasgow studies lend further support to an operational definition of refractory epilepsy as failure of two appropriately chosen AEDs in adequate doses due to lack of efficacy.

TREATMENT OPTIONS

For adults with refractory epilepsy, current evidence supports the use of several treatment options, including epilepsy surgery, vagus nerve stimulation and 'rational' polytherapy.

EPILEPSY SURGERY

It is recommended that patients whose epilepsy remains uncontrolled despite treatment with two appropriately chosen AEDs, either singly or in combination, in adequate doses should be evaluated for the suitability of epilepsy surgery [11]. Aided by technical advances in neuroimaging and video-electroencephalography monitoring, improvements in technique, and a better understanding of the anatomical and pathophysiological basis of the epilepsies, resective surgery has become a highly effective and safe treatment modality for certain remediable syndromes, the prototype of which is mesial temporal lobe epilepsy. The effectiveness of epilepsy surgery for patients with surgically remediable syndromes refractory to AED treatment, in particular anterior temporal lobectomy for mesial temporal lobe epilepsy, has been documented in a number of uncontrolled studies [19, 20] and confirmed in a randomized controlled trial [21]. With a reported remission rate of 60% to 70% from centres across the world, mortality close to zero, and permanent neurologic morbidity <5%, anterior temporal lobectomy has made mesial temporal lobe epilepsy, an often medically intractable condition, highly surgically treatable in appropriately selected patients [22]. In addition, with advances in imaging technology, the range of surgically remediable syndromes is ever expanding. Details of pre-surgical evaluation and epilepsy surgery are discussed in Chapter 2.

VAGUS NERVE STIMULATION

Vagus nerve stimulation (VNS) was approved in 1997 by the US Food and Drug Administration as adjunctive treatment for refractory partial-onset seizures. The modern therapeutic use of vagus nerve stimulators was based on the concept that VNS induces electroencephalogram (EEG) desynchronization in animals [23]. In humans, about 80% of the nerve fibres consist of afferent fibres that terminate in the nucleus solitarius located in the dorsal medullary complex of the vagus [24]. The nucleus solitarius, in turn, transmits and modulates the anti-seizure effect of VNS by virtue of its extensive projections to a number of potential epileptogenic structures such as the insula, amygdala and hippocampus.

The VNS system consists of an implantable lithium-powered generator with a bipolar lead. The titanium-encased generator is implanted subcutaneously in the left infraclavicular fossa in a fashion resembling that of a cardiac pacemaker. Following exposure of the left vagus nerve via latero-cervical incision under general anaesthesia, the connecting lead, comprising three discrete platinum helical coils, is wrapped around the cervical section of the vagus nerve. The left vagus nerve is chosen as it carries (theoretically) fewer parasympathetic fibres that innervate the ventricles. The generator may deliver electrical pulses in programmable parameters, which can be adjusted using an external telemetry wand linked to a computer. In the long term, high-intensity stimulation is used: typically signal on-time 30s, signal off-time 5 minutes, pulse duration 500ms and frequency 30Hz. Output current can be stepped up at 0.25-mA intervals up to a maximum of 2.5mA.

Two seminal studies of VNS therapy were published in the mid 1990s. Both were multicentre, double-blind, randomized controlled trials. In the E03 study [25], 114 patients with complex partial or secondarily generalized seizures were recruited, whereas in the E05 study [26], 199 patients with simple partial, complex partial seizures or secondarily generalized seizures were evaluated. In these two trials, post-treatment seizure frequencies were compared with baseline values established during the 12 to 16 weeks before implantation. Patients were randomly assigned to either high (30Hz, 30s on, 5 minutes off, 500-μs pulse width) or low (1Hz, 30s on, 90–180 minutes off, 130-μs pulse width) stimulation. Low stimulation has minimal efficacy. For the high-stimulation groups in both studies, the mean percentage of seizure reduction was significantly higher in the E03 (24.5% vs. 6.1%) and E05 study (28% vs. 15%). By the end of 2 years, up to 8.3% of patients achieved seizure freedom. Subsequent long-term observational studies suggest that efficacy was maintained without development of habituation [27, 28].

The advantages of VNS include a relative lack of systemic or cognitive side-effects, absence of potential drug interaction and an automatic delivery which minimizes the problem of compliance. The disadvantages include a relatively high cost, moderate efficacy, requirement for battery renewal and the palliative nature of the intervention.

'RATIONAL' POLYTHERAPY

As previously discussed, drug resistance is a relative state rather than an absolute designation, and a proportion (albeit small) of such patients may still benefit from further drug manipulation. Whether AEDs can be combined 'rationally' to achieve 'synergism' has been under intense debate. With at least 15 AEDs available to treat partial seizures, 105 duotherapy combinations are possible. Such an overwhelming number of options makes 'rational' polytherapy not only of academic interest but a practical necessity. The goal is to achieve better seizure control with combinations that may produce supra-additive (synergistic) efficacy and/or infra-additive toxicity, while paying attention to any potential undesirable pharmacokinetic drug–drug interactions [29].

Pharmacomechanistic Approach to AED Combinations

Combining drugs with different mechanisms of action is a common strategy in the treatment of many medical disorders. Polytherapy is also used routinely in some neurological conditions, even at treatment initiation. Thus, in patients with Parkinson's disease, levodopa is combined with a dopa decarboxylase or catechol-o-methyltransferase inhibitor to reduce its systemic breakdown. Likewise, it is plausible to obtain a synergistic (supra-additive) effect in the drug treatment of epilepsy by combining agents with potentially complementary mechanisms of action (Table 8.3). It might even be argued that, since many AEDs possess multiple (and possibly undiscovered) modes of action [30, 31], mechanistic combinations already exist even when a single drug is used. Deckers and colleagues [32] comprehensively reviewed the available animal and human data and concluded that combinations involving a Na$^+$ channel blocker and a drug with γ-aminobutyric acid (GABA)-ergic properties appeared to be particularly beneficial. Observation from the Glasgow database tended to support the addition of an AED with multiple mechanisms of action [33]. However, selecting drug combinations based on their mode of action remains an untested hypothesis. In addition, while it is convenient to conceptualize and categorize the mechanisms of action of AEDs, it is important to bear in mind that our understanding of the pathogenesis of seizure generation and propagation and, indeed, how drugs modulate these processes in the individual patient, remains rudimentary. It is likely, too, that some AEDs possess as yet unrecognized modes of action. Thus, many possible AED combinations remain to be evaluated, and only a few have hinted at evidence of particular efficacy.

Table 8.3 Perceived mechanisms of action of anti-epileptic drugs [30, 31]

	↓ Na$^+$ channels	↓ Ca^{2+} channels*	↑ GABA transmission	↓ Glutamate transmission
Established anti-epileptic drugs				
Benzodiazepines			+ +	
Carbamazepine	+ +			
Ethosuximide		+ + (T-type)		
Phenobarbital	?		+ +	?
Phenytoin	+ +			
Valproate	?	? (T-type)	+	?
New anti-epileptic drugs				
Felbamate	+	?	+	+
Gabapentin	?	++ ($\alpha2\delta$)	+	
Lamotrigine	+ +	?		
Levetiracetam†		?	?	?
Oxcarbazepine	+ +			
Pregabalin		++ ($\alpha2\delta$)		
Tiagabine			+ +	
Topiramate	+	+	+	+
Vigabatrin			+ +	
Zonisamide	+	+ (T-type)		

+ +, primary action; +, probable action; ?, possible action.
*Unless otherwise stated, action on high voltage activated Ca^{2+} channels.
†Levetiracetam acts by binding to synaptic vesicle protein 2A (SV2A).
GABA, γ-aminobutyric acid.

Clinical evidence of synergistic combinations

The most scientifically valid approach to study such potential interactions is the isobolographic method (Figure 8.2), in which two AEDs are given in various dose proportions to identify the most effective regimen in terms of seizure control [34]. This approach has been successfully applied in animal studies [35], but presents logistic difficulties in the clinical trial setting because of the wide inter-individual variation in the pharmacokinetics and pharmacodynamics of different AEDs. The ideal way to test for synergism in the clinical setting has not been agreed upon [29].

There is a paucity of data on the comparative efficacy of different AED combinations in clinical practice. The only published head-to-head, double-blind, randomized trial conducted for such a purpose compared gabapentin and vigabatrin as the first add-on drug for partial seizures that had not been controlled by monotherapy [36]. Unfortunately, this study was terminated prematurely due to emerging concerns regarding vigabatrin-associated visual field defects. There was no significant difference in the improvement rate, proportion of seizure-free patients, or quality of life scores between the drug groups during the 8-week treatment period.

The best non-randomized controlled data in favour of true synergism exist with valproate and lamotrigine for partial-onset and generalized seizures [37, 38]. Brodie *et al.* [37] added lamotrigine in 345 patients with uncontrolled epilepsy receiving a single AED (valproate, carbamazepine or phenytoin). The addition of lamotrigine to valproate produced a significantly better response than adding it to carbamazepine or phenytoin despite similar lamotrigine concentrations (Figure 8.3). Pisani *et al.* [38] performed a well-designed, crossover study in 20 patients. Among the 13 patients who did not respond to the consecutive monotherapy with valproate and lamotrigine, four became seizure free and an additional four experienced >60% seizure reduction when both drugs were given in combination, despite lower doses and serum concentrations than during separate administration.

Other 'recommended' combinations are largely based on anecdotal reports or studies with small sample sizes. They include valproate with ethosuximide for absence seizures [39], phenobarbital and phenytoin for generalized tonic–clonic and partial seizures [40], carbamazepine and vigabatrin or valproate for partial seizures [41], vigabatrin and tiagabine for partial seizures [42] and lamotrigine with topiramate for a range of seizure types [43].

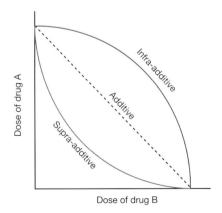

Figure 8.2 Hypothetical isobologram showing the doses of two drugs required to produce a specified effect (either efficacy or toxicity) where the drugs have additive, supra-additive (synergistic) or infra-additive (antagonistic) effects [29].

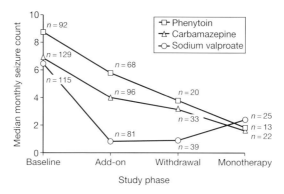

Figure 8.3 Median monthly seizure counts for patients receiving add-on lamotrigine to baseline treatment with phenytoin, carbamazepine or valproate. The study consisted of a 12-week 'baseline phase', followed by the 'add-on phase', when lamotrigine was introduced with baseline medication unchanged. Patients showing at least 50% reduction in seizure frequency compared with baseline entered the 12-week 'withdrawal phase' when the baseline anti-epileptic drug was tapered off. Patients who successfully completed the withdrawal phase entered the lamotrigine 'monotherapy phase' of 12 weeks' duration [37].

Avoiding Excessive Toxicity

In combining AEDs, supra-additivity in terms of adverse effects via pharmacodynamic interactions should be avoided, although this issue has not been well explored in clinical studies. There is some evidence that adverse pharmacodynamic interactions are more likely to occur when AEDs share similar mechanisms of action. For instance, excessive neurotoxic adverse effects have been reported in patients treated with carbamazepine or oxcarbazepine in combination with lamotrigine, all of which block voltage-gated Na^+ channels [37, 44, 45]. However, a similar adverse effect profile does not seem to occur when lamotrigine is combined with phenytoin, which also blocks voltage-gated Na^+ channels [37]. Attention should also be paid to the total drug load, which has been shown to be related to the incidence of dose-related adverse events [46].

Unfavourable Pharmacokinetic Interactions between Anti-Epileptic Drugs

In combining AEDs, it is beneficial to avoid complex pharmacokinetic interactions which may lead to reduced efficacy and/or increased toxicity. The older AEDs are notorious for their ability to produce pharmacokinetic interactions among themselves as well as with other medications via their effect on the hepatic cytochrome P450 (CYP) enzyme superfamily [47]. Phenobarbital, primidone, phenytoin and carbamazepine all induce CYP enzymes that accelerate the breakdown of CYP-metabolized AEDs as well as many commonly prescribed lipid-soluble drugs, including oral contraceptives, cytotoxics, cardiac anti-arrhythmics and warfarin. Valproate is a weak inhibitor of mono-oxygenase and conjugating enzymes, which can slow the clearance of other AEDs, such as phenytoin and lamotrigine [47]. In comparison, few of the newer AEDs interfere with CYP enzymes and they are generally less likely to affect the metabolism of other AEDs to a clinically significant extent (Table 8.4) [47]. In particular, gabapentin and pregabalin are excreted unchanged in the urine and have not been implicated in pharmacokinetic drug interactions [48, 49]. Levetiracetam is believed to partially undergo metabolism by enzymatic hydrolysis, primarily in the blood. There is recent evidence that its serum concentration may be modestly reduced by concomitant enzyme-inducing AEDs, although the clinical significance of this is unclear [50]. Oxcarbazepine has been reported to

Table 8.4 Pharmacokinetic interactions between anti-epileptic drugs

AED	Undergoes hepatic metabolism	Affects hepatic cytochrome P450 enzymes	Affects metabolism of other anti-epileptic drugs	Metabolism affected by other anti-epileptic drugs
Established anti-epileptic drugs				
Carbamazepine	Yes	Yes	Yes	Yes
Clobazam	Yes	No	No	Yes
Clonazepam	Yes	No	No	Yes
Ethosuximide	Yes	No	No	Yes
Phenobarbital	Yes	Yes	Yes	Yes
Phenytoin	Yes	Yes	Yes	Yes
Primidone	Yes	Yes	Yes	Yes
Valproate	Yes	Yes	Yes	Yes
Modern anti-epileptic drugs				
Felbamate	Yes	Yes	Yes	Yes
Gabapentin	No	No	No	No
Lamotrigine	Yes	No	No	Yes
Levetiracetam	No	No	No	Yes*
Oxcarbazepine	Yes	Yes	Yes*	Yes
Pregabalin	No	No	No	No
Tiagabine	Yes	No	No	Yes
Topiramate	Yes	Yes	Yes*	Yes
Vigabatrin	No	No	Yes*	No
Zonisamide	Yes	No	No	Yes

*Effect modest, see text.

reduce the serum concentrations of lamotrigine, topiramate and levetiracetam, and increase those of phenytoin [51]. Topiramate may slightly inhibit the metabolism of phenytoin and induce that of valproate [52]. Vigabatrin appears to decrease the blood concentration of phenytoin through an unidentified mechanism [47]. However, these interactions are modest and generally have limited clinical consequences [47].

TREATMENT STRATEGIES UNDER INVESTIGATION FOR DRUG-RESISTANT EPILEPSY

It should be apparent from the previous discussion that current strategies for the treatment of drug-resistant epilepsy have limited efficacy and are associated with risks of adverse effects/complications. To overcome treatment resistance, a number of innovative techniques are under investigation. Some of the approaches already in clinical development will be briefly reviewed [53]. Strategies currently in the pre-clinical stage of development, such as stem cell transplantation and gene therapy, will not be discussed.

NOVEL DRUG TARGETS/CHEMICAL STRUCTURES

The new generation of AEDs have not proved to produce significant improvement in seizure control for the majority of patients refractory to traditional agents. It has been suggested that this is due to the intrinsic limitations of AED development approaches resulting in new chemical entities having similar, often overlapping, mechanisms of action that afford similar spectra of action and efficacy to the established AEDs [54].

To address this limitation, compounds acting on new molecular targets are being developed [55]. For example, retigabine (RGB) exhibits a selective and potent M-current potassium channel opening effect at the KCNQ2/3 and KCNQ3/5 potassium channels, resulting in membrane stabilization [56]. Talampanel (TPL) is a potent non-competitive antagonist at a novel allosteric site of the α-amino-3-hydroxy-5-methyl-4-isoxazeoleproprionic acid (AMPA) subtype of glutamate receptors [57]. AMPA antagonists are thought to give rise to anti-convulsant activity by limiting neuronal hyperexcitability and by preventing glutamate-driven neuronal damage. Lacosamide, the R-enantiomer of 2-acetamido-N-benzyl-3-methoxypro-pionamide, is a new chemical compound developed for treatment of epilepsy and neuropathic pain. It belongs to a class of compounds referred to as 'functionalized amino acids', and its precise mechanism of action is presently unclear. A pivotal phase III trial evaluating oral lacosamide as adjunctive therapy in adults with uncontrolled partial seizures demonstrated statistically significant and clinically relevant improvements over placebo [58]. Application of lacosamide for regulatory approval has been filed. Other potential AEDs under advanced clinical development that act on more novel targets include ganaxolone (neuroactive steroid), NS1209 (competitive AMPA receptor antagonist) and rufinamide (triazole) [55].

CIRCUMVENTION OF EFFLUX DRUG TRANSPORTERS

Data supporting the potential role of cerebral efflux drug transporters in pharmacoresistance raises the possibility of improving AED efficacy by co-administration of transporter inhibitors/modulators [59]. Efflux drug transporters are transmembrane molecules present in blood–tissue barriers (including the blood–brain barrier) that function as active 'pumps' to drive the flux of their substrates against the concentration gradient, thereby reducing the accumulation of substrates inside the cell. The most studied drug transporter is P-glycoprotein, which has been shown to be over-expressed in epileptic brain tissues resected from patients with drug-resistant epilepsy. Tariquidar (XR9576), a potent, specific third-generation inhibitor of P-glycoprotein, has been demonstrated to enhance the anti-seizure effect of phenytoin, a weak P-glycoprotein substrate, in a rat model of temporal lobe epilepsy [60].

The idea of inhibiting P-glycoprotein to achieve higher brain concentration of substrate AEDs may be intuitively attractive. However, because of the influence of P-glycoprotein in key pharmacokinetic stages through its physiological expression in organs with excretory functions (e.g. gut enterocytes, renal tubular cells), any attempt to modulate its function in one step could have complex knock-on effects on others. In addition, given the presumed protective role of drug transporters in the blood–brain barrier (BBB) and other tissue barriers, any plan to modulate their function must take into consideration these potential associated hazards [53].

NEW DRUG DELIVERY SYSTEMS

Several modes of delivering AEDs directly to the brain are being investigated [61]. The theoretical advantages of such a drug delivery system include improved efficacy with higher local drug concentrations, and avoidance of systemic adverse effects and pharmacokinetic drug–drug interactions. Conantokin-G (CGX-1007), an N-methyl-D-aspartate (NMDA) receptor antagonist, is being developed as a novel AED to be delivered intrathecally via a subcutaneously implanted infusion pump to patients with epilepsy [62]. The safety of intrathecal administration of CGX-1007 was tested in animal studies, and clinical studies are under way.

Another novel drug delivery system is to implant AED-containing polymers onto the seizure focus in the brain, thereby bypassing the BBB. This may allow the use of compounds that have anti-convulsant properties *in vitro* but that cannot be administered systemically either because of poor BBB penetration or because of significant systemic toxicity. Patients with epileptogenic lesions not amenable to resection, such as owing to the risk of damaging eloquent cortex, could have the polymers placed in the vicinity of the seizure focus. Advances in neurosurgical techniques have made possible the implantation of polymers of 2–3 mm in diameter into the brain stereotactically via cannulae, without resorting to craniotomy. Implantation of adenosine-releasing and GABA-releasing polymers into rat models of epilepsy reduced or attenuated seizures [63, 64]. Controlled-release polymers containing chemotherapy placed in the tumour bed during debulking operation have already been tested clinically in patients with high-grade gliomas [65]. The safety and efficacy of AED-releasing polymers for seizure control in humans remain to be tested.

ELECTRICAL BRAIN STIMULATION

Following the success of treatment for movement disorders, deep brain stimulation (DBS) is under active investigation as a non-pharmacological therapeutic modality for patients with medically intractable epilepsy who are not eligible for resective surgical procedures [66]. A variety of anatomical structures may be targeted, including deep brain structures [67, 68]. Interest in the stimulation of subcortical structures stems from the recognition of widespread non-specific anterior and intralaminar nuclear connections to many other parts of brain and the progressive recruitment of substantia nigra, subthalamic nucleus and midline thalamic nuclei in animal models of epilepsy [66]. Furthermore, automated seizure detection can be incorporated into an electrical brain stimulator to form a closed-loop system so that electrical stimulation is delivered to the epileptogenic zone when onset of ictal activity is detected [69, 70]. Recent understanding in seizure dynamics also helps decipher the collective action of large neuronal assemblies and can potentially help advance protocols for closed-loop brain stimulation. For example, it was shown that the correlation structure of seizure at onset was usually decreased, rather than 'hypersynchronous', and towards the end of seizure, the correlation increased again [71]. Several large-scale randomized clinical trials of DBS for intractable partial or secondarily generalized seizures targeting various brain structures with or without a seizure detection system are under way [72].

DIETARY MODIFICATION

In a paediatric population, the ketogenic diet is a recognized therapy for refractory epilepsy. It mimics the effects of starvation, with provision of high fat, low to moderate protein and very low carbohydrate diet. However, evidence to support its use in adult patients is very limited. One recent case series reported the use of the Atkins diet, which is akin to the ketogenic diet, with restriction of carbohydrates but not overall calories or proteins, in six patients aged between 7 and 52 years with refractory epilepsy [73]. Although three of the patients attained good seizure reduction, it was difficult to conclude whether or not the Atkins diet can be recommended as therapy for adult refractory epilepsy patients. In this cohort, only one of three adult patients (aged ≥18 years) maintained adherence to the diet, ketosis on urine testing and good seizure response to the therapy. By comparison, two of three paediatric patients (aged <18 years) attained good seizure response. The authors of the report raised questions about the level of restrictions on calories and protein imposed by a ketogenic diet. They recommended a maximum of 10 g of carbohydrate per day at the induction phase of the ketogenic diet.

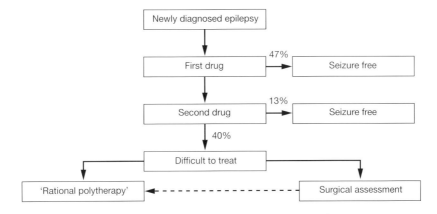

Figure 8.4 Practical treatment approach for epilepsy [75].

PRACTICAL TREATMENT APPROACH

A 'staged' approach is recommended for the treatment of epilepsy [74] (Figure 8.4). This means that monotherapy should be initiated for the newly diagnosed patients, the majority of whom will become seizure free with a single AED, often at modest or moderate dosage [1, 75]. A drug should be chosen with a spectrum of activity and side-effect and interaction profiles that has the potential to produce seizure freedom without intolerable toxicity or long-term sequelae for that individual. The choice should ideally be matched to the patient's seizure type(s) and/or epilepsy syndrome, age, gender, weight, psychiatric history, other disease states, concomitant medication and lifestyle [76].

If the first AED produces an idiosyncratic reaction, side-effects at low or moderate dosage, or fails to improve seizure control, an alternative should be substituted. If the drug is well tolerated, the dose can be increased towards the limit of tolerability aiming for complete seizure freedom. If there is no impact on the patient's seizures, it should be substituted. However, if seizure control has been greatly improved but complete freedom proves elusive, we feel that another AED can be added in [29]. Before combination therapy is instituted, the possibility of 'pseudo-failure' or 'pseudo-resistance' must be considered since the majority of newly diagnosed patients (60–70%) will respond to monotherapy.

If the patient becomes seizure free after the addition of a second agent without added toxicity, it would be reasonable to continue prescribing both drugs. Combination therapy should also be considered after failure of two monotherapy attempts, since the chance of success with a third choice is slim. It should be stated, however, that further evidence is needed to support this strategy. The dose of the original AED can often be reduced, particularly if the patient has or develops side-effects, to reduce potential drug load. If seizures are not fully controlled on the first two drugs as monotherapy or the initial choice and first combination, evaluation for epilepsy surgery should be considered early, particularly if a potentially operable structural abnormality, such as mesial temporal sclerosis, has been identified [77]. VNS can be considered if the patient is deemed an unsuitable candidate for surgery after thorough evaluation at an experienced epilepsy surgery centre.

The choice of agent to add as second or third drug is often influenced by the existing monotherapy. Based on current – albeit limited – data, it is reasonable to attempt with combinations that have potential complementary modes of action. Broad-spectrum drugs such as valproate, lamotrigine, topiramate, levetiracetam and zonisamide may be preferred over those with a more limited clinical range such as oxcarbazepine, tiagabine or pregabalin, particularly in patients with more than one seizure type [29]. If the patient is established on an enzyme-inducer (e.g. carbamazepine, phenytoin or phenobarbital), the addition of an AED carrying a low risk of clinically relevant pharmacokinetic interactions (e.g. topiramate, levetiracetam, zonisamide, pregabalin) may be a desirable option [47].

If a two-drug regimen is particularly well tolerated and substantially reduces seizure frequency and/or severity, triple therapy can be attempted by adding a small dose of a third AED with different pharmacological properties. Again, in order to avoid excessive drug load, reducing the dose of one or more AEDs will help accommodate its introduction. Third-line agents, including tiagabine, clobazam and acetazolamide, can be tried. Adjunctive piracetam can be used in patients with refractory myoclonic seizures. Vigabatrin and felbamate remain drugs of last resort because of their propensity to produce visual field defects [78] and aplastic anaemia and hepatotoxicity [79] respectively. Some patients will do well on duotherapy. A few more will become seizure free on three AEDs, but treatment with four or more is unlikely to be successful [80].

CONCLUSION

Despite appropriate AED treatment, up to one-third of epilepsy patients have uncontrolled seizures. A consensus is being reached, at least for adult patients, that, for operational purposes, medical refractoriness can be suspected when two appropriately chosen, well-tolerated, first-line AEDs or one monotherapy and one combination have failed due to lack of efficacy [74]. Clinical approaches that may be considered in such situations include the early use of 'rational polytherapy', selection of patients for epilepsy surgery and VNS. The biological mechanisms underlying medical intractability remain unclear but a number of novel strategies to overcome drug resistance are under investigation. It is hoped that these exciting developments will soon reach clinical use so that treatment-resistant epilepsy will become treatable and more patients can live safer and more fulfilling lives.

REFERENCES

1. Kwan P, Brodie MJ. Early identification of refractory epilepsy. *N Engl J Med* 2000; 341:314–319.
2. Mohanraj R, Brodie MJ. Diagnosing refractory epilepsy: response to sequential treatment schedules. *Eur J Neurol* 2006; 13:277–282.
3. Perucca E. Pharmacoresistance in epilepsy: how should it be defined? *CNS Drugs* 1998; 10:171–179.
4. Smith D, Defalla BA, Chadwick DW. The misdiagnosis of epilepsy and the management of refractory epilepsy in a specialist clinic. *QJM* 1999; 92:15–23.
5. Devinsky O. Patients with refractory seizures. *N Engl J Med* 1999; 340:1565–1570.
6. Chaves J, Sander JW. Seizure aggravation in idiopathic generalized epilepsy. *Epilepsia* 2005; 46(Suppl 9):133–139.
7. Genton P, Gelisse P, Thomas P *et al*. Do carbamazepine and phenytoin aggravate juvenile myoclonic epilepsy? *Neurology* 2000; 55:1106–1109.
8. Gelisse P, Genton P, Kuate C *et al*. Worsening of seizures by oxcarbazepine in juvenile idiopathic generalized epilepsies. *Epilepsia* 2004; 45:1282–1286.
9. Guerrini R, Dravet C, Genton P *et al*. Lamotrigine and seizure aggravation in severe myoclonic epilepsy. *Epilepsia* 1998; 39:508–512.
10. Perucca E, Dulac O, Shorvon S *et al*. Harnessing the clinical potential of anti-epileptic drug therapy: dosage optimisation. *CNS Drugs* 2001; 15:609–621.
11. Kwan P, Brodie MJ. Issues of medical intractability for surgical candidacy. In: Wyllie E (ed.) *The Treatment of Epilepsy: Principles and Practice*. 4th edn. Philadelphia, PA: Lippincott Williams & Wilkins, 2006.
12. Berg AT, Kelly MM. Defining intractability: comparisons among published definitions. *Epilepsia* 2006; 47:431–436.
13. Markand ON, Salanova V, Whelihan E *et al*. Health-related quality of life outcome in medically refractory epilepsy treated with anterior temporal lobectomy. *Epilepsia* 2000; 41:749–759.

14. Birbeck GL, Hays RD, Cui X *et al*. Seizure reduction and quality of life improvements in people with epilepsy. *Epilepsia* 2002; 43:535–538.
15. Schmidt D, Löscher W. Drug resistance in epilepsy: putative neurobiological and clinical mechanisms. *Epilepsia* 2005; 46:858–877.
16. Berg AT, Vickrey BG, Langfitt J *et al*. The Multicenter Epilepsy Surgery Study: recruitment and selection for surgery. *Epilepsia* 2003; 44:1425–1433.
17. Berg AT, Vickrey GB. Testa FM *et al*. How long does it take for epilepsy to become intractable? A prospective investigation. *Ann Neurol* 2006; 60:73–79.
18. Sillanpää M, Schmidt D. Natural history of treated childhood-onset epilepsy: prospective, long-term population-based study. *Brain* 2006; 129(Pt 3):617–624.
19. Engel J Jr. Update on surgical treatment of the epilepsies: summary of the Second International Palm Desert Conference on the Surgical Treatment of the Epilepsies (1992). *Neurology* 1993; 43:1612–1617.
20. McIntosh AM, Wilson SJ, Berkovic SF. Seizure outcome after temporal lobectomy: current research practice and findings. *Epilepsia* 2001; 42:1288–1307.
21. Wiebe S, Blume WT, Girvin JP *et al*; the Effectiveness and Efficacy of Surgery for Temporal Lobe Epilepsy Study Group. A randomised, controlled trial of surgery for temporal lobe epilepsy. *N Engl J Med* 2001; 345:311–318.
22. Engel J Jr, Wiebe S, French J *et al*. Practice parameter: temporal lobe and localized neocortical resections for epilepsy: report of the Quality Standards Subcommittee of the American Academy of Neurology, in Association with the American Epilepsy Society and the American Association of Neurological Surgeons. *Neurology* 2003; 60:538–547.
23. Zabara J. Inhibition of experimental seizures in canines by repetitive vagal stimulation. *Epilepsia* 1992; 33:1005–1012.
24. Loewy AD, Burton H. Nuclei of the solitary tract: efferent projections to the lower brain stem and spinal cord. *J Comp Neurol* 1978; 181:421–450.
25. Handforth A, DeGiorgio CM, Schachter SC, *et al*. Vagus nerve stimulation therapy for partial-onset seizures: a randomized active-control trial. *Neurology* 1998; 5:48–55.
26. Vagus Nerve Stimulation Study Group. A randomized controlled trial of chronic vagus nerve stimulation for treatment of medically intractable seizures. *Neurology* 1995; 45:224–230.
27. Morris GL, Mueller WM; the Vagus Nerve Stimulation Study Group (E01–E05). Long-term treatment with vagus nerve stimulation in patients with refractory epilepsy. *Neurology* 1999; 53:1731–1735.
28. Hui AC, Lam JMK, Wong KS *et al*. Vagus nerve stimulation for refractory epilepsy: long term efficacy and side-effects. *Chin Med J* 2004; 117:58–61.
29. Kwan P, Brodie MJ. Combination therapy in epilepsy: when and what to use? *Drugs* 2006; 66:1817–1829.
30. Kwan P, Sills GJ, Brodie MJ. The mechanisms of action of commonly used antiepileptic drugs. *Pharmacol Ther* 2001; 90:21–34.
31. Rogawski MA, Löscher W. The neurobiology of antiepileptic drugs. *Nat Rev Neurosci* 2004; 5:553–564.
32. Deckers CLP, Czuczwar SJ, Hekster YA *et al*. Selection of antiepileptic drug polytherapy based on mechanisms of action: the evidence reviewed. *Epilepsia* 2000; 41:1364–1374.
33. Kwan P, Brodie MJ. Epilepsy after the first drug fails: substitution or add-on? *Seizure* 2000; 9:464–468.
34. Mawer CE, Pleuvry BJ. Interactions involving new antiepileptic drugs. *Pharmacol Ther* 1995; 68:209–231.
35. Czuczwar SJ, Borowicz KK. Polytherapy in epilepsy: the experimental evidence. *Epilepsy Res* 2002; 52:15–23.
36. Lindberger M, Alenius M, Frisen L *et al*. Gabapentin versus vigabatrin as first add-on for patients with partial seizures that failed to respond to monotherapy: a randomized, double-blind, dose titration study. *Epilepsia* 2000; 41:1289–1295.
37. Brodie MJ, Yuen AWC; 105 Study Group. Lamotrigine substitution study: synergism with sodium valproate? *Epilepsy Res* 1997; 26:423–432.
38. Pisani F, Otero G, Russo MF *et al*. The efficacy of valproate-lamotrigine comedication in refractory complex partial seizures: evidence for a pharmacodynamic interaction. *Epilepsia* 1999; 40:1141–1146.
39. Rowan AJ, Meijer JWA, de Beer-Pawlikowski N *et al*. Valproate ethosuximide combination therapy for refractory absence seizures. *Arch Neurol* 1983; 40:797–802.
40. Cereghino JJ, Brock JT, Van-Meter JC *et al*. The efficacy of carbamazepine combination in epilepsy. *Clin Pharmacol Ther* 1975; 18:733–741.
41. Brodie MJ, Mumford JP; 012 Study Group. Double-blind substitution of vigabatrin and valproate in carbamazepine-resistant partial epilepsy. *Epilepsy Res* 1999; 34:199–205.

42. Leach JP, Brodie MJ. Synergism with GABA-ergic drugs in refractory epilepsy. *Lancet* 1994; 343:1650.
43. Stephen LJ, Sills GJ, Brodie MJ. Lamotrigine and topiramate may be a useful combination. *Lancet* 1998; 351:958–959.
44. Besag FMC, Berry DJ, Pool F *et al*. Carbamazepine toxicity with lamotrigine: pharmacokinetic or pharmacodynamic interaction? *Epilepsia* 1998; 39:183–187.
45. Barcs G, Walker EB, Elger CE *et al*. Oxcarbazepine placebo-controlled, dose ranging trial in refractory partial epilepsy. *Epilepsia* 2000; 41:1597–1607.
46. Lammers MW, Hekster YA, Keyser A *et al*. Monotherapy or polytherapy for epilepsy revisited: a quantitative assessment. *Epilepsia* 1995; 36:440–446.
47. Patsalos PN, Perucca E. Clinically important drug interactions in epilepsy: general features and interactions between antiepileptic drugs. *Lancet Neurol* 2003; 2:347–356.
48. Radulov LL, Wilder BJ, Leppik IE *et al*. Lack of interaction of gabapentin with carbamazepine or valproate. Epilepsia 1995; 35:155–161.
49. Brodie MJ, Wilson EA, Wesche DL *et al*. Pregabalin drug interaction studies: lack of effect on the pharmacokinetics of carbamazepine, phenytoin, lamotrigine and valproate in patients with partial epilepsy. *Epilepsia* 2005; 46:1407–1413.
50. Patsalos PN. Clinical pharmacokinetics of levetiracetam. *Clin Pharmacokinet* 2004; 43:707–724.
51. May TW, Korn-Merker E, Rambeck B. Clinical pharmacokinetics of oxcarbazepine. *Clin Pharmacokinet* 2003; 42:1023–1042.
52. Bialer M, Doose DR, Murthy B *et al*. Pharmacokinetic interactions of topiramate. *Clin Pharmacokinet* 2004; 43:763–780.
53. Kwan P, Brodie MJ. Refractory epilepsy: mechanisms and solutions. *Expt Rev Neurotherapeutics* 2006; 6:397–406.
54. Kwan P, Brodie MJ. Clinical trials of antiepileptic medications in newly diagnosed patients with epilepsy. *Neurology* 2003; 60(Suppl 4):S2–S12.
55. Kwan P, Brodie MJ. Emerging drugs for epilepsy. *Expt Opin Emerging Drugs* 2007; 12:407–422.
56. Rundfeldt C, Netzer R. The novel anticonvulsant retigabine activates M-currents in Chinese hamster ovary-cells tranfected with human KCNQ2/3 subunits. *Neurosci Lett* 2000; 282:73–76.
57. Solyom S, Tarnawa I. Non-competitive AMPA antagonists of 2,3-bonzodiazepine type. *Curr Pharm Des* 2002; 8:913–939.
58. Ben-Menachem E, Biton V, Jatuzis D *et al*. Efficacy and safety of oral lacosamide as adjunctive therapy in adults with partial-onset seizures. *Epilepsia* 2007; 48:1308–1317.
59. Kwan P, Brodie MJ. Potential role of drug transporters in the pathogenesis of medically intractable epilepsy. *Epilepsia* 2005; 46:225–235.
60. Van Vliet EA, van Schaik R, Edelbroek PM *et al*. Inhibition of the multidrug transporter P-glycoprotein improves seizure control in phenytoin-treated chronic epileptic rats. *Epilepsia* 2006; 47:672–680.
61. Fisher RS, Ho J. Potential new methods for antiepileptic drug delivery. *CNS Drugs* 2002; 16:579–593.
62. Bialer M, Johannessen SI, Kupferberg HJ *et al*. Progress report on new antiepileptic drugs: a summary of the Sixth Eilat Conference (EILAT VI). *Epilepsy Res* 2002; 51:31–71.
63. Boison D, Scheurer L Tseng JL *et al*. Seizure suppression in kindled rats by intraventricular grafting of an adenosine releasing synthetic polymer. *Exp Neurol* 1999; 160:164–174.
64. Kokaia M, Aebischer P, Brundin P *et al*. Seizure suppression in kindling epilepsy by intracerebral implants of GABA- but not by noradrenaline-releasing polymer matrices. *Exp Brain Res* 1994; 100:385–394.
65. Valtonen S, Timonen U, Toivanen P *et al*. Interstitial chemotherapy with carmustine-loaded polymers for high-grade gliomas: a randomized double-blind study. *Neurosurgery* 1997; 41:44–48.
66. Theodore WH, Fisher RS. Brain stimulation for epilepsy. *Lancet Neurol* 2004; 3:111–118.
67. Velasco F, Velasco M, Velasco AL *et al*. Electrical stimulation of the centromedian thalamic nucleus in control of seizures: long-term studies. *Epilepsia* 1995; 36:63–71.
68. Kerrigan JF, Litt B, Fisher RS *et al*. Electrical stimulation of the anterior nucleus of the thalamus for the treatment of intractable epilepsy. *Epilepsia* 2004; 45:346–354.
69. Osorio I, Frei MG, Sunderam S *et al*. Automated seizure abatement in humans using electrical stimulation. *Ann Neurol* 2005; 57:258–268.
70. Morrel M. Brain stimulation for epilepsy: can scheduled or responsive neurostimulation stop seizures? *Curr Opin Neurol* 2006; 19:164–168.
71. Schindler K, Leung H, Elger CE *et al*. Assessing seizure dynamics by analysing the correlation structure of multi-channel intracranial EEG. *Brain* 2007; 130:65–77.

72. US National Institutes of Health. www.clinicaltrials.gov. Accessed 10 December 2006.
73. Kossoff E, Krauss GL, McGrogan JR *et al*. Efficacy of the Atkins diet as therapy for intractable epilepsy. *Neurology* 2003; 61:1789–1791.
74. Brodie MJ, Kwan P. Staged approach to epilepsy management. *Neurology* 2002; 58(Suppl 5):S2–S8.
75. Kwan P, Brodie MJ. Effectiveness of first antiepileptic drug. *Epilepsia* 2001; 42:1255–1260.
76. Brodie MJ, Kwan P. The star systems: overview and use in determining antiepileptic drug choice. *CNS Drugs* 2001; 15:1–12.
77. Trevathan E, Gilliam F. Lost years. Delayed referral for surgically treatable epilepsy. *Neurology* 2003; 61:432–433.
78. Pellock JM, Brodie MJ. Felbamate: an update. *Epilepsia* 1997; 38:1261–1264.
79. McDonagh J. Stephen LJ, Dolan F *et al*. Peripheral retinal dysfunction in patients taking vigabatrin. *Neurology* 2003; 61:1690–1694.
80. Stephen LJ, Brodie MJ. Seizure freedom with more than one antiepileptic drug. *Seizure* 2002; 11:349–351.
81. Berg AT, Shinnar S, Levy SR *et al*. Defining early seizure outcomes in pediatric epilepsy: the good, the bad and the in-between. *Epilepsy Res* 2001; 43:75–84.
82. Arts WFM, Geerts AT, Brouwer OF *et al*. The early prognosis of epilepsy in childhood: the prediction of a poor outcome: the Dutch study of epilepsy in childhood. *Epilepsia* 1999; 40:726–734.
83. Dlugos DJ, Sammel MD, Strom BL *et al*. Response to first drug trial predicts outcome in childhood temporal lobe epilepsy. *Neurology* 2001; 57:2259–2264.
84. Camfield P, Camfield C. Nova Scotia pediatric epilepsy study. In: Jallon P, Berg A, Dulac O *et al*. (eds) *Prognosis of Epilepsies*. Montrouge, France: John Libbey, Eurotext, 2003, pp. 113–126.

9

Treatment of women with childbearing potential and beyond

Cynthia L. Harden

INTRODUCTION

The treatment of women of childbearing potential with epilepsy and those who are beyond their childbearing years with epilepsy requires special consideration. This chapter discusses practical management of this age group in terms of medication choices for pregnancy, dose considerations when using oral contraception, the risks of hormone replacement and monitoring for reproductive and sexual dysfunction. Fortunately, much new information is available to guide therapy in order to optimize the quality of life for women with epilepsy and will be presented herein.

HORMONAL CONTRACEPTION

RISKS OF CONTRACEPTIVE FAILURE FOR WOMEN WITH EPILEPSY

Women with epilepsy can use hormonal contraception with the expectation of effective contraception, keeping in mind some caveats regarding dosing and drug interactions. In the general population, oral contraceptive (OC) pills, when used without missing doses, are highly reliable, having an annual failure rate of <1% [1]. Realistically, however, the annual failure rate is 2–7% [2]. The increased failure rate of OCs in the setting of anti-epileptic drug (AED) use was reported by Coulam and Annegers in 1979 [3]. They evaluated pregnancy occurrence in 82 women with epilepsy: 41 were taking OCs and AEDs together (955 patient-months) compared with 41 women with epilepsy taking OCs alone (2278 patient-months). There were three OC failures in the group taking AEDs, but no OC failures in the comparison group. In the three pill-failure patients, seizures were well controlled, indicating that medication compliance was not a factor. The derived annual failure rate for OCs in women taking AEDs is about 6%, derived from the 41 women who took OCs with AEDs.

Therefore, the failure rate with usual OC use is similar to the failure rate often cited for OC use in the setting of concomitant AEDs. This finding does not pre-empt the need to consider interactions with AEDs and hormonal contraceptives; however, it does indicate that OC use in the setting of AED use still provides pregnancy prevention at among the highest rates of any available contraceptive method.

Cynthia L. Harden, MD, Professor of Neurology, Epilepsy Division Chief, Department of Neurology, University of Miami, Miami, USA

CYTOCHROME P450 3A4 ENZYME-INDUCING AEDs

The interaction producing OC failure in women with epilepsy is attributed to the induction of hepatic cytochrome P450 enzymes, specifically the 3A4 isoenzyme system. Induction of the 3A4 system increases the metabolism of both the oestrogenic and progestogenic components of hormonal contraceptives and reduces their circulating levels by as much as 50% [4, 5]. This occurs with phenobarbital, carbamazepine, phenytoin and oxcarbazepine since they are potent CYP3A4 inducers (Table 9.1). The newer AEDs, specifically felbamate, topiramate and lamotrigine, are less-potent inducers of CYP3A4 [6] and have differential effects on the oestrogenic and progestogenic components of OCs (Table 9.1). The interactions between the newer AEDs and OCs are discussed below.

In a study of healthy women on a low-dose OC formulation containing 30-μg ethinyl estradiol, concomitant felbamate at 2400 mg per day produced a decrease in the area under the plasma concentration–time curve (AUC) of the progesterone component by 42%. Estradiol levels did not decline significantly; furthermore, no participant receiving OCs had evidence of ovulation [7].

Topiramate reduced the AUC of the oestrogenic component of OCs in a dose-related manner in two studies, both using a frequently prescribed OC containing 35 μg of ethinyl estradiol [8, 9]. In the first report of this interaction, which evaluated topiramate at 200 mg, 400 mg and 800 mg per day, all doses reduced ethinyl estradiol AUC significantly compared with baseline, with declines in AUC of 18% following 200 mg/day, 22% with 400 mg/day and 30% at 800 mg/day [8]. This finding differs from a later report in which the ethinyl estradiol AUC declined by 12% at 50 mg of topiramate per day, increased by 5% at 100 mg per day and declined by 11% at 200 mg per day [9]. The conclusion of the authors was that doses of topiramate from 50 mg to 200 mg per day produced no significant change in ethinyl estradiol levels. Neither study showed any effect on the progestin component.

Oxcarbazepine at 1200 mg/day was studied in healthy female volunteers who were taking an OC containing 50 μg of ethinyl estradiol and 250 μg of levonorgestrel [10]. Both components had a reduced AUC of 47% with oxcarbazepine use. There are no reports on the effects of lower doses of oxcarbazepine and OCs, so it is unclear whether there is a dose-related effect of oxcarbazepine on OC metabolism.

The degree of decrease in either the oestrogenic or progestin level that permits pregnancy is unknown, making it difficult to estimate how the OC dose should be adjusted to restore maximum efficacy. Each component of the OC acts via a different mechanism to prevent pregnancy: the oestrogenic component suppresses ovulation and the progestin component

Table 9.1 Effect of AEDs on oral contraceptives

AEDs that lower the effectiveness of oral contraceptives	AEDs that have no effect on oral contraceptives
Potent effects	Valproic acid
Carbamazepine	Gabapentin
Phenytoin	Levetiracetam
Phenobarbital	Tiagabine
Oxcarbazepine – studied at 1200 mg per day	Vigabatrin
Weak effects	Zonisamide
Felbamate – induces progestin only	Pregabalin
Topiramate – induces oestrogen only	
Lamotrigine – induces progestin only	

induces production of thick cervical mucus, which interferes with sperm passage and also alters the endometrium so that it is not receptive to the blastocyst. The more clinically important of these two actions is unknown, but both mechanisms need to fail to allow pregnancy.

Although the inducing AEDs reduce the hormonal levels of OCs to variable degrees, the recommendation for the use of higher-dose OCs, and, importantly, avoiding low-dose OCs, should be applied for all women taking 3A4-inducing AEDs. Until further information is available, the most conservative recommendations for the use of hormonal contraception for women receiving enzyme-inducing AEDs are: OCs should contain at least 50 μg of ethinyl estradiol; depomedroxyprogesterone acetate injections should be given at more frequent intervals (10 weeks rather than the usual 12 weeks); and consider an additional method of contraception [11].

AEDs AND DEVICES THAT DO NOT INDUCE CYTOCHROME P450 3A4 ENZYMES

Valproic acid, gabapentin, levetiracetam, tiagabine, vigabatrin, zonisamide and pregabalin do not induce cytochrome P450 3A4 enzymes. The vagus nerve (VN) stimulator has no effect on drug metabolism. No interaction with OCs would be expected with the use of these AEDs or with the VN stimulator (Table 9.1).

LAMOTRIGINE USE REQUIRES SPECIAL CONSIDERATION WHEN USED WITH ORAL CONTRACEPTIVES

When adjusted for dose and body weight, lamotrigine levels were found to be reduced by 50% in a study of 22 women taking lamotrigine and an ethinyl estradiol and levonorgestrel combined OC, compared with women taking lamotrigine alone [12]. Further evaluation demonstrated that it is the ethinyl estradiol component that produces the interaction – the progestin component has no effect on lamotrigine levels [13]. It is thought that the mechanism of this interaction is induction of uridine diphosphate–glucuronosyltransferase (UGT) 1A4 by ethinyl estradiol, which is the main metabolic enzyme for lamotrigine.

This interaction should be considered in managing seizures in women with epilepsy. When ethinyl estradiol-containing OCs are added to the regimen of a woman with epilepsy taking lamotrigine, the level of lamotrigine may decline to a sufficient degree in some patients to increase the risk of seizures. When OCs are discontinued in a woman taking lamotrigine, lamotrigine levels can increase by 100% and result in toxicity. Women with epilepsy taking lamotrigine should therefore have levels checked before and after starting OCs. The dose of lamotrigine may need to be adjusted, guided by serum lamotrigine levels, as well as clinical monitoring for seizure control and toxicity.

The lamotrigine–OC interaction is further complicated by rising lamotrigine levels. This rise occurs during the OC placebo or pill-free week, which in most regimens occurs every fourth week. Lamotrigine levels during the placebo or pill-free week increase by 27% on the third placebo day, 63% on the fifth and 116% on the seventh placebo day, relative to lamotrigine levels during OC administration [14]. This finding suggests that for women who report lamotrigine-related CNS side-effects during the placebo or pill-free week, a small reduction in lamotrigine dose after the second placebo day may be helpful. These authors also report an effect of lamotrigine on OCs, specifically that lamotrigine is associated with a small decrease in levels of the progestin used in this study, levonorgestrel, with the AUC reduced by 19% and maximum concentration by 12% [14] (see Table 9.1).

Because lamotrigine is often an effective and well-tolerated AED with preliminary evidence of a relatively low risk of teratogenicity [15], the concomitant use of OCs and lamotrigine should not be categorically ruled out, because metabolism of lamotrigine and its induction is highly variable between individuals. However, the considerations discussed above must be taken into account during its use.

PLANNING PREGNANCY

In women with epilepsy, planning pregnancy is very important. Once a woman is pregnant, it will be too late to make significant changes in AED therapy. Counselling on birth control methods, risk of teratogenicity and how to minimize it, and seizure control during pregnancy should occur early in the relationship between a woman with epilepsy and her treating physician [16, 17]. Women of childbearing potential should receive at least 4 mg of folate per day, which is the recommended dose for all women [16]. The need for higher doses, although they are frequently used (up to 4 mg/day) has not been proven. Women actively planning pregnancy should be slowly withdrawn from polytherapy to one AED at the lowest effective dose, if at all possible, and consideration should be given to removing valproate (see below). If seizures are ongoing, the AED strategy should be re-assessed. If she has not seen an epilepsy specialist, a referral should be considered for AED optimization. If the woman is a good candidate for epilepsy surgery, she should be referred (see Chapter 2) with the hope of becoming seizure free and having AEDs withdrawn. If she has been seizure free for over 1 year, withdrawal of AEDs prior to pregnancy could be considered. Any AED adjustment (and particularly AED withdrawal) should be completed 6 months prior to attempts at conception, to ensure that any seizure exacerbation does not occur during the pregnancy itself.

PREGNANCY

Teratogenicity of AEDs

Although the increased teratogenic risk of intrauterine AED exposure has long been recognized, the risk of major congenital malformations (MCMs) attributable to each AED due to first trimester exposure is still emerging, particularly for the newer AEDs. MCMs are defined as structural abnormalities with medical, surgical or cosmetic importance. These include cardiac malformations (ventricular septal defect, coarctation of the aorta, tetralogy of Fallot, aortic valve stenosis, hypoplasia of mitral valve), neural tube defects (spina bifida, myelomeningocele, anencephaly), craniofacial defects (cleft lip and palate), microcephaly, congenital megacolon and urogenital malformations. Organogenesis is complete by 13 weeks of gestation, indicating that AED-related MCMs occur with first trimester exposure. By contrast, minor anomalies are more subtle and difficult to diagnose. However, midface hypoplasia and distal digit and nail hypoplasia are specific minor anomalies that have been reliably associated with intrauterine AED exposure.

Prospective pregnancy registries have been recently established, with the goal of ascertaining risks of the newer and older AEDs in an expedited manner. A number of academically based registries now exist throughout the world, in North America, Europe, the UK and Australia. The Lamotrigine Pregnancy Registry, sponsored by GlaxoSmithKline, has also been ongoing for more than a decade. Although the pregnancy registries differ in their methodology regarding when and how they survey for MCMs, and in their exact inclusion criteria, one finding has been present across the registries: an elevated risk of MCMs associated with valproate.

Results from the North American Antiepileptic Drug Pregnancy Registry indicate a 10.7% risk of MCMs with valproate monotherapy [18]. Furthermore, the first report from this registry was that phenobarbital monotherapy is associated with 6.5% risk for MCMs [19]. Interestingly, the elevated risk with phenobarbital has not been reproduced in other registries since phenobarbital is infrequently used in other developed nations and is not reported in the registries. In the North American registry, the elevated MCM rates for valproate and phenobarbital were significantly higher than those associated with the three other most frequently used AEDs combined at 2.9% and with that of their comparator group, the local general population in Boston, Massachusetts at 1.62% [18, 19].

Results from the Australian Registry of Antiepileptic Drugs in Pregnancy showed that the malformation rate following valproate monotherapy exposure was 17.1%, which was significantly greater than that with other AEDs combined at 2.4% [20]. The UK Epilepsy and Pregnancy Register results indicate that valproate is associated with a higher rate of major congenital malformations at 6.2% than carbamazepine at 2.2% [21]. There was also a trend towards fewer major congenital malformations with lamotrigine (3.2%) than with valproate. The incidence of MCMs in children not exposed to AEDs but born to mothers with epilepsy in this registry was 3.5%. Furthermore, the registry confirmed previous evidence of a significantly greater risk of MCMs with polytherapy at 6.0% compared with monotherapy at 3.7%.

The Swedish Medical Birth Registry survey showed a rate of MCMs for valproate of 9.7%, while for carbamazepine it was 4% [22]. This finding was reproduced in the Finnish National Medical Birth Registry with a valproate MCM rate 10.7% compared with those of untreated women (2.8%) [23]. In this report, only the use of valproate, either as monotherapy or in polytherapy significantly increased the rate of malformations above that of the untreated women; no other AEDs as monotherapy or in polytherapy imparted an increased teratogenic risk. These data showing the increased risk of MCMs with valproate compared with other treatments are summarized in Table 9.2.

The GlaxoSmithKline (GSK) International Lamotrigine Pregnancy Registry (11-year study) reported an MCM rate of 2.9% detected within the first month of life (12 out of 414 births) with first trimester monotherapy exposure [15], which is consistent with rates found in other registries. Subjects were enrolled by healthcare professionals worldwide, prior to knowledge of fetal tests.

Information on the outcome of the largest cohort of oxcarbazepine monotherapy exposure is from the Finnish registry, where there was one urogenital malformation in 99 pregnancies [23].

A recent report from the UK Epilepsy and Pregnancy Register on levetiracetam exposure during pregnancy as monotherapy and polytherapy provides at least preliminary evidence of risk: there were no MCMs or minor malformations in the 39 monotherapy exposures, and three MCMs and five minor malformations in the 78 levetiracetam as polytherapy exposures [24]. Therefore, information on levetiracetam, as with most of the other newer AEDs except

Table 9.2 Registry reports showing a significantly increased risk of major congenital malformations with valproate monotherapy

Site of registry	Malformation rate with valproate %	Malformation rate with comparator
North America [18]	10.7	Three other most frequently used AEDs combined 2.9%
		Local general population 1.62%
Australia [20]	17.1	Carbamazepine, phenytoin, lamotrigine only as monotherapy or in combinations 2.4%
United Kingdom [21]	6.2	Carbamazepine 2.2%, lamotrigine 3.2% (trend only)
Sweden [22]	9.7	Carbamazepine 4%
Finland [23]	10.7	Any other comparator group in study: all other monotherapy or polytherapy excluding valproate had no increased risk above untreated women

lamotrigine, must be considered as preliminary until information on more pregnancy outcomes is accrued.

Therefore, an elevated risk of MCMs with valproate use during pregnancy has been confirmed in multiple prospective surveys worldwide and, if possible, its use during pregnancy should be avoided. Clearly, some women will need to stay on valproate for seizure control and if other treatments are intolerable or ineffective; these women should be informed about the increased risk of teratogenicity. Further, changing AEDs during pregnancy is not advocated due to risks of the introduced AED causing allergy and other serious side-effects or incompletely controlled seizures, and because the most acute period of organogenesis is usually completed by the time the pregnancy is confirmed.

Neurocognitive Risks

Clear evidence for the neurocognitive effects of intrauterine exposure to AEDs is difficult to obtain, since multiple influences on intellectual outcome must be taken into consideration in such studies. The most important influence on cognitive outcome in a child is the maternal intelligence quotient (IQ), and, secondarily, the social environment. Furthermore, children must be followed and evaluated years after birth. Several carefully performed studies have been performed to assess this risk.

AED-related minor anomalies are associated with adverse neurocognitive outcome [25]. In a study of the association between physical anomalies and Wechsler Intelligence Scale for Children (WISC) scores on 76 children whose mothers took AEDs in pregnancy, midfacial or digit hypoplasia correlated significantly with decreased verbal IQ, performance IQ and full-scale IQ. There were too few exposures for any single AED to meaningfully compare the outcomes between AEDs. No decrease in IQ was found in association with major malformations. The authors conclude that the presence of either of these two minor malformations, midface or digital hypoplasia, should prompt a developmental evaluation.

The first report regarding an association between intrauterine exposure with a specific AED and cognitive outcome was in 1995 [26] on a cohort of adult men in Denmark who were exposed to phenobarbital *in utero*. Phenobarbital was not used for epilepsy – in fact maternal epilepsy was an exclusion criteria; it was generally used for hypertension or as a sedative. The cohort was studied at approximately age 30, and verbal IQ was significantly decreased, by a mean of 7 points, in phenobarbital-exposed men compared with matched controls. Exposure that included the third trimester was a risk factor for this decreased verbal IQ, which suggests that the risk of adverse neurocognitive effects is not confined to the first trimester, as is the exposure that causes MCMs.

Two studies have shown a risk of significantly lower verbal IQ with valproate exposure compared with other AED exposure or to children not exposed to AEDs [27, 28]; one of these studies showed no risk of impaired intelligence with carbamazepine use [28]. Valproate, therefore, has particular risk during pregnancy, for both MCMs and adverse neurocognitive outcome. Further, poorly controlled convulsive seizures pose a neurocognitive risk: five or more convulsive seizures are associated with a significantly lower verbal IQ in the offspring [27].

Risk of Seizures to the Pregnancy

Seizures have been reported to cause fetal heart rate depression, fetal hypoxia with resultant acidosis and fetal intracranial haemorrhage [29–31]. Intrauterine death related to fetal intracranial hemorrhage occurring after a single seizure has been reported [29]. Spontaneous abortion, fetal hypoxia, bradycardia and antenatal death have been associated with both partial and generalized convulsive status epilepticus, possibly related to maternal trauma and placental hypoperfusion [16, 32]. However, a recent report from the EURAP Epilepsy

Pregnancy Registry regarding seizure control during pregnancy found that in 36 cases of status epilepticus during pregnancy, of which 12 were convulsive, only one stillbirth occurred (during a convulsive status) and there were no maternal mortalities [33]. Although statistically-derived risks to the pregnancy from seizure-related complications are difficult to determine, seizures themselves impart an increased risk of fetal loss and injury. The neurocognitive outcome study previously cited [27] found that five or more convulsive seizures were associated with lower verbal IQ in the offspring. This information provides another compelling reason to prevent seizures during pregnancy that is not directly related to trauma or vascular compromise during a seizure itself. It has not been clearly shown, however, that seizures during pregnancy increase the risk of MCMs.

Seizure Change during Pregnancy

When seizures are well controlled, it is highly likely that they will continue to remain so during pregnancy [33, 34]. This information is useful for clinicians in advising patients about the risks of pregnancy, and indicates that achieving seizure control in general, prior to pregnancy, is important for having the safest possibly pregnancy. In the EURAP Study Group report on seizure control during pregnancy, which used the first trimester as a reference for seizure control during the rest of the pregnancy, 1093 out of 1718 subjects enrolled had unchanged seizure frequency throughout pregnancy; 1013 (92.7%) of the 1093 were seizure free and remained so throughout the pregnancy [33]. Overall, 15.9% improved throughout pregnancy and 17.3% deteriorated; 3.1% went in both directions during pregnancy. Seizure occurrence was associated with localization-related epilepsy, polytherapy and oxcarbazepine therapy. AED doses were more often increased in patients with seizures, and those using lamotrigine or oxcarbazepine as monotherapy [33]. The risks for increased seizures during pregnancy are therefore contributed to by epilepsies that are already more difficult to control, requiring polytherapy, and by probable decline in levels of AEDs during pregnancy.

MANAGEMENT OF AED DOSING DURING PREGNANCY

ALTERATIONS OF AED LEVELS

Decreased AED levels during pregnancy occur due to increased drug clearance and some degree of haemodilution. However, the decrease in total levels of AEDs during pregnancy is counterbalanced by an increase in the percentage of free (unbound by protein) fraction and therefore bioactive fraction of AEDs due to decreased plasma protein binding and decreased albumin concentration during pregnancy [17]. Therefore, the free fraction, which is an indication of brain concentrations, often remains stable, preventing the need for dose adjustment. If possible, for drugs that are highly protein bound (the older AEDs valproate, and phenytoin as well as the new AED tiagabine), free levels rather than total levels should be obtained pre-pregnancy, and this is the value that should be maintained during pregnancy. It is not necessary to maintain total levels at pre-pregnancy rates, and attempting to do so may in fact cause toxicity and unnecessary exposure to higher levels in the fetus.

Valproate, Phenobarbital, Phenytoin and Carbamazepine Levels during Pregnancy

For valproate, the free fraction declines little while the total level markedly declines during pregnancy [35]. Free and total levels of phenobarbital decline significantly, by up to 50% over the course of the pregnancy [36]. Total carbamazepine levels decline slightly with an insignificant decline in the free fraction during pregnancy [33]. Total phenytoin levels decline markedly, up to 40% [33, 35], while the free fraction declines less, at about 20% of preconception values [33].

Lamotrigine Levels during Pregnancy

Serum lamotrigine levels decrease variably during pregnancy, by up to 60–90% [37, 38], and levels need to be checked frequently, beginning early in the pregnancy. The increased clearance of lamotrigine can occur within the first several weeks of the pregnancy, and return to baseline within 2 weeks post-partum. Therefore, the dose adjustment of lamotrigine can be required early in the pregnancy and dramatic dose increases of several multiples of the preconception dose may be required during the pregnancy, with a rapid downward escalation after delivery. However, some women have very little change in their lamotrigine level during pregnancy. This is probably due to the genetic polymorphism of the UDP-glucuronosyltransferase enzymes (UGT enzymes), which are the main metabolic enzymes for lamotrigine and are induced by reproductive hormones during pregnancy, similar to the induction by OCs. Individualized degrees of UGT induction during pregnancy result from genetic variation in UGT isoenzymes and this has a widely disparate effect on lamotrigine metabolism. Since protein binding of lamotrigine is only about 55%, changes in the free fraction would not be expected to be proportionately great enough to affect seizure control or adverse effects. A recent study determined that seizure frequency can increase if the serum concentration during the second trimester falls below 65% of the pre-pregnancy levels [38]. The authors recommended a dose increase under these circumstances. A conservative recommendation for managing lamotrigine dosing during pregnancy is to check levels every 2–4 weeks during pregnancy.

Oxcarbazepine Levels during Pregnancy

Two reports are available on the alteration of oxcarbazepine levels during pregnancy [39, 40]. Both studies are small, reporting on five [39] and nine [40] subjects. However, both reports document a decline in levels during pregnancy [39, 40] by approximately 30% in the first trimester and up to 36% by the second trimester [40]. Again, as with lamotrigine, the decline in levels is highly variable between subjects; this may be due to glucuronide conjugation utilized for the primary metabolism of both drugs, which is induced during pregnancy. The relatively low protein binding of oxcarbazepine, at 40%, makes changes in free fraction during pregnancy unlikely to be of clinical significance.

Recommendations for Managing AED Dosing during Pregnancy

Owing to the changes in pharmacokinetics of anti-epileptic medication as described above, seizure frequency as well as AED levels should be monitored carefully during pregnancy, and the AED dose adjusted to achieve a serum level appropriate for the patient to maintain seizure freedom. Carbamazepine overall has the least alteration in levels during pregnancy. Although complete information about changes in levels of the newer AEDs during pregnancy is not available, it can be assumed the levels will decline somewhat during pregnancy due to the mechanisms described previously. Therefore, levels of all AEDs (and free levels where appropriate), including the newer AEDs, should be checked prior to conception and during the pregnancy. A level at which the patient is seizure free, if known through preconception testing, can be used as a target level upon which to base dosing.

A reasonable approach for women with well-controlled seizures is to check AED levels at baseline (before conception), and at 1- to 3-month intervals with dose adjustments to maintain an effective level. Levels should be performed more frequently when lamotrigine is used, due to the marked increase in clearance for some women, and as needed for women with recurrent seizures. Since phenytoin is 90–95% protein bound and the free fraction greatly increases relative to the total level during pregnancy, free levels of phenytoin should be followed during pregnancy rather than only total levels. Valproate is also highly protein bound, and if possible, free levels should also be obtained during pregnancy.

Risk of Epilepsy in the Offspring

A frequent concern expressed to clinicians from women with epilepsy is the chance of their child having epilepsy. Outside of some known inheritable syndromes, the overall risk of children developing epilepsy if one parent has epilepsy has been cited as ranging from 2% to 5% [41]. However, the risk of developing epilepsy is higher if the mother has epilepsy (8.5%) compared with the father having epilepsy (2.4%) [42]. It is likely that the elevated risk of children of mothers developing epilepsy will be increasingly accounted for by a genetic contribution, as the genetic variants that cause or permit epilepsy are discovered.

Breastfeeding

The advantages of breastfeeding a newborn baby are undisputed and include transfer of maternal antibodies, improved cognitive development [43] and emotional bonding between mother and child. AED levels are present in breast milk at concentrations that vary with the particular drug being used, and represent continued exposure of the newborn to systemic AEDs. Phenytoin and valproate are highly protein bound, and carbamazepine moderately so, therefore these AEDs are not transferred in high concentrations in breast milk [44]. A small study of four mother–infant pairs shows that breast-fed infants of mothers taking lamotrigine have serum concentrations of lamotrigine in the infant at a level similar to that seen in the mother, as the glucuronidation metabolic pathway is immature in infants [45]. Although no short-term adverse effects were observed in the infants in that study, breast-fed infants of mothers taking lamotrigine and all AEDs should be monitored with assessment of lethargy, adequate feeding and development. The concentrations of levetiracetam and topiramate have been found to be approximately equal in milk and plasma [46, 47]. However, the serum levels of these AEDs in breast-fed infants are low. The protein binding of lamotrigine, topiramate and levetiracetam is low, permitting transfer into breast milk, but the infant metabolism is an additional factor that must be considered regarding the resulting infant serum level. Breastfeeding is an option for women with epilepsy being treated with AEDs, and the American Academy of Neurology recommends that it is not contraindicated [48]. However, much more information is needed about the immediate risks and long-term effects of neonatal and infant exposure to AEDs through breast milk.

Vitamin K

An intramuscular injection of 1 mg vitamin K is given to all newborns to prevent haemorrhagic disease of the newborn. As AEDs that induce the hepatic CYP enzymes can induce vitamin K metabolism and therefore reduce the effectiveness of vitamin K-dependent clotting factors, oral augmentation of vitamin K by giving the mother phytonadione at 10 mg per day from 36 weeks' gestation until birth has been suggested as a practice option for women taking hepatic enzyme-inducing AEDs to prevent haemorrhagic disease of the newborn [48]. Whether only women who take CYP enzyme-inducing AEDs, all women who take any AEDs or no women who take AEDs should be prescribed oral vitamin K supplementation in the last few weeks of pregnancy is unclear. One report that compared the rate of bleeding complications in 667 neonates born to women taking CYP enzyme-inducing AEDs, none of whom took vitamin K during pregnancy, with 1334 well-matched neonates born to women not taking AEDs found no difference in bleeding complications that could be attributed to AED use [49]. Vitamin K supplementation in women with epilepsy taking AEDs remains a varied practice; this evidence suggests that it does not decrease the risk of haemorrhagic disease of the newborn. Oral vitamin K supplementation is a safe intervention, and it is often given on this basis, although the preventive benefit is unproven.

POLYCYSTIC OVARY SYNDROME AND INFERTILITY

Most women with epilepsy can successfully bear children. However, population-based studies have found reduced birth rates to both men and women with epilepsy. In a large Finnish cohort of patients with newly diagnosed epilepsy, birth rates were lower than in the general population for both men (hazard ratio [HR], 0.58) and women (HR, 0.88) [50]. It is not clear to what extent reduced fertility among people with epilepsy is due to biological disease- or treatment-related factors or to psychosocial causes. A biological contribution to the reduced birth rates to women with epilepsy is plausible, since epilepsy is associated with reproductive endocrine dysfunction in women, specifically increased frequency of anovulatory cycles [51] and polycystic ovary syndrome (PCOS) [52].

One mechanism by which epilepsy is related to reproductive dysfunction is that abnormal mesial temporal lobe neurophysiological activity, such as spikes originating in the temporal lobe, affect the nearby hypothalamus, which regulates gonadotropin secretion. The finely tuned, pulsatile secretion of luteinizing hormone (LH) has been shown to be disrupted by interictal spikes in men and women [53, 54]. Therefore, alterations in the hypothalamic–pituitary–gonadal axis induced by paroxysmal activity in nearby brain structures are thought to be an important factor contributing to reproductive dysfunction in persons with epilepsy.

Proposed causes of PCOS include primarily adrenal, ovarian, pituitary or metabolic dysfunction; we are focused herein on the central nervous system cause, specifically dysfunction of the hypothalamic–pituitary–gonadal axis. An important aspect of hypothalamic–pituitary–gonadal axis disregulation by contiguous ictal and interictal physiological activity may be increased gonadotropin-releasing hormone (GNRH) secretion, which contributes to or causes PCOS. Increased GNRH secretion preferentially increases the LH to follicle-stimulating hormone (FSH) ratio [55]. Consistent with this postulated effect, elevated LH:FSH ratios have been documented in women with epilepsy [51]. LH stimulates ovarian steroidogenesis, and an increased LH:FSH ratio will produce follicles that do not fully mature but become numerous and cystic. Immature follicles are deficient in aromatase, the enzyme that produces oestrogen in the ovary by converting it from its precursor, testosterone. In this manner, the PCOS ovarian follicle is altered to produce excessive androgens.

Women with epilepsy have higher rates of PCOS than the general population [52], which is a frequent cause of infertility. The current definition of PCOS is the presence of two of the following three factors: (i) polycystic ovaries; (ii) oligo-/anovulation; and/or (iii) clinical or biochemical evidence of hyperandrogenism [56]. Other frequently present features of PCOS include an elevated LH:FSH ratio and insulin resistance with or without obesity [57, 58].

The contribution of valproate to the occurrence of PCOS in women with epilepsy remains unclear, especially since the cause of PCOS itself is mysterious. It is clear that valproate also causes several of the primary features of PCOS. Valproate causes increased androgen levels [59–62] and probably cystic ovaries [57, 60] in women with epilepsy. The association between valproate and anovulation has not been consistently found [59, 62, 63] but, when present, could contribute to difficulty conceiving. The association of valproate with PCOS is confounded by an increased occurrence of PCOS in women with epilepsy in general; similar rates of PCOS in women with epilepsy taking carbamazepine, valproate or no AEDs have been reported, around 11% for each group [52]. Valproate itself inhibits aromatase and can block the conversion of testosterone to oestrogen, and in this manner, along with effects on testosterone metabolism itself, contribute to hyperandrogenism [64, 65]. Another well-known adverse effect of valproate now clearly emerging as an endocrinopathy is weight gain, which occurs in up to 50% of patients [59]. Valproate-induced weight gain has recently been associated with increased insulin and leptin levels, and consequent decreased ghrelin and adiponectin levels [66]. Again, the presence of weight gain and obesity is a feature, although not a necessary one, of PCOS, providing a further parallel between primary PCOS and the effects of valproate treatment.

Since valproate is an effective AED for many persons with epilepsy, the decision to use it or continue to use it in the face of concerns about the risk of endocrine dysfunction is complex. For women with evidence of reproductive dysfunction, such as anovulation, hyperandrogenism or PCOS itself, valproate should be judiciously considered as it may exacerbate these abnormalities. Weight gain due to valproate use may also be a reason for discontinuation for both men and women.

Studies have shown that women with epilepsy have a risk of early onset of perimenopausal symptoms such as hot flushes and infrequent menses, occurring significantly more often than expected in the late fourth or early fifth decade of life [67]. A recent report shows that high seizure frequency is a risk for earlier than expected menopause [68]. Women with epilepsy who have had only rare seizures (e.g. fewer than 20 in a lifetime) have less risk for earlier menopause and are more likely to have an age at menopause of 50 to 51 years, normal for the general population. However, women with epilepsy who have frequent seizures, occurring at least monthly, may experience earlier menopause, about age 46 to 47 years (Table 9.3). This is an example of reproductive dysfunction and possible infertility caused by the epilepsy itself, not associated with the use of any specific AED [68].

The potential for epilepsy and its treatment to cause reproductive dysfunction merits ongoing vigilance by clinicians for the occurrence of menstrual regularity, and for signs and symptoms of PCOS or perimenopause in women with epilepsy.

CATAMENIAL EPILEPSY

Exacerbation of seizure frequency in relationship to the menstrual cycle is termed catamenial epilepsy. This term does not refer to a specific seizure type or epilepsy syndromic classification and therefore is probably somewhat misappropriated. A current working definition of catamenial epilepsy is a two-fold increase in average daily seizure frequency that occurs at three different times of the menstrual cycle: (i) most commonly, immediately premenstrually and at the onset of menses when estradiol and progestin levels decline; (ii) around ovulation when estradiol and progestin levels increase; and (iii) during an inadequate luteal phase, which is characterized by low progesterone levels [69]. The correlation of times of seizure exacerbation during the menstrual cycle fits well with the known effects of these reproductive hormones on neural excitability. Specifically, oestrogen promotes neuronal excitability in women with epilepsy [70] and progesterone is an anti-convulsant, via its metabolism to allopregnanolone, which is a potent positive allostearic modulator of receptor for γ-amino-butyric acid (GABA), a powerful brain inhibitory neurotransmitter [71–73].

The two-fold increase in seizure frequency as a cut-off point for catamenial vs. non-catamenial seizure exacerbation was derived from evaluating a large number of monthly seizure patterns in women with partial epilepsy. A daily seizure increase of 1.6–1.8 times

Table 9.3 Menopausal age correlated with seizure frequency. Adapted from [68]

Seizure frequency	Number of patients	Mean age	Mean age at last menses*
<20 seizures in lifetime	15	55	49.9
>20 seizures in lifetime; <1 seizure per month	25	54	47.7
>1 seizure per month	28	52	46.7
*Significantly different between groups ($P=0.04$).			

during perimenstrual days, at ovulation or during the luteal phase compared with other days in the menstrual cycle reliably distinguished between women with seizure exacerbations at those times and those without [70]. Therefore, the findings suggest that an approximately two-fold increase in seizure frequency during these times of the menstrual cycle is an appropriate amount of seizure increase to constitute a catamenial seizure exacerbation. It is estimated that up to 40% of women with partial epilepsy have catamenial seizure exacerbations [74].

The hormonal fluctuations during normal menstrual cycling and during anovulatory menstrual cycling explain catamenial seizure exacerbations to some extent, but probably not completely. As low progesterone levels during the luteal phase or progesterone withdrawal prior to the onset of menses are associated with catamenial seizure occurrence, the treatment approach for catamenial seizures has involved progesterone augmentation. One of the first attempts to use a progestin was with medroxyprogesterone acetate, given either orally or by intramuscular injection in a small group of women with poorly controlled seizures [75]. Half of the 14 women treated had a marked seizure reduction of 35–71%; these were women whose menses ceased while taking medroxyprogesterone. Since this synthetic progestin is not active at the GABA receptor, it may be that the main therapeutic mechanism was via cessation of normal hormonal cycling.

The first report of natural progesterone was in eight women with epilepsy who had anovulatory cycles or low progesterone during the luteal phase [76]. Seizure frequency declined by 70% during treatment, and side-effects were infrequent; several women experienced fatigue and depression at increased doses. In a second trial of 25 women with temporal lobe epilepsy and catamenial seizure exacerbations, using progesterone lozenges at 200 mg three times a day during the luteal phase reduced seizure frequency by approximately 50% overall [77]. Focal and generalized seizures were both improved. The long-term results of this study were later reported; 23 women remained on the treatment for 3 years with sustained seizure reduction and three of the women were seizure free [78]. These small, open studies suggest that natural progesterone can be a useful treatment for women with epilepsy and currently, a randomized, double-blind, placebo-controlled trial for women with epilepsy of reproductive age is under way.

Other treatments for catamenial seizure exacerbations include acetozolamide, oral contraceptives (OCs), intermittent benzodiazepines and intermittent increases in AEDs. Acetazolamide has long been used for the treatment of catamenial seizures, although the evidence for its effectiveness is largely anecdotal. Acetazolamide is a sulfonamide carbonic anhydrase inhibitor, and the anti-seizure mechanism is thought to be related to increased brain bicarbonate accumulation, which has an inhibitory effect on neuronal activity [79]. A retrospective review of 20 women with catamenial epilepsy treated with acetazolamide found that seizure frequency was significantly reduced in 40% of women and seizure severity was reduced in 30% of women [80].

Although intermittent benzodiazepines have also been used to treat women with catamenial seizures for years, only clobazam (which is not available in the United States) has been studied in this population. In a study of women with pre-menstrual seizure exacerbations, intermittent clobazam produced a >50% seizure reduction in 14 of 18 evaluable cases [81]. In this study, one of the main concerns about benzodiazepine use, tolerance, was not present in nine women treated for more than 1 year [82].

Cyclic increases in patients' usual AED therapy during menstrual cycle-seizure exacerbation have not been systematically investigated. Patients seem to often initiate this approach, however, because it seems easy and does not involve adding another medication. However, this method does present the potential for confusion about the AED regimen and for AED toxicity. For phenytoin, which has a non-linear metabolism, even an intermittent dose increase could result in toxicity and, therefore, this approach is not recommended. The treatment approaches discussed above with the doses used in trials are listed in Table 9.4.

Since OCs suppress ovulation and most formulations provide a stable reproductive hormonal milieu during the 3-week treatment phase (followed by 1 week of placebo), it

Table 9.4 Treatments of catamenial epilepsy: reports of effectiveness in small open trials (*) or case reports (†)

Treatment	Dose
Medroxyprogesterone acetate*	Using the intramuscular depot formulation, 150 mg every 10–12 weeks
Natural progesterone*	100–200 mg three times a day on days 15–28 of the menstrual cycle with 2-day taper-off at onset of menses
Acetozolamide*	4 mg/kg, with a range of 8–30 mg/kg/day in one to four divided doses, not to exceed 1 g per day
Intermittent benzodiazepines*	Add low dose starting 4 days before menses, continuing for 10 days
Intermittent increase in AEDs already in regimen†	Increase dose slightly for duration as above

seems logical, based on the likely association between reproductive hormones and seizure occurrence, that OCs could be of benefit for catamenial seizure exacerbations. Outside of a few case reports showing either improved seizures or worsening seizures, no studies have been performed to evaluate this treatment [79].

Other treatment approaches to catamenial epilepsy include anti-oestrogens such as clomiphene citrate, and androgenic derivatives such as danazol and gonadotropin analogues, all of which have been used in small clinical trials. Owing to the profound reproductive alterations and the risks of adverse events inherent in these treatments, they are not practical interventions for most neurologists. A synthetic neuroactive steroid, ganaxolone, remains under investigation for the treatment of epilepsy, and may be particularly helpful for women with epilepsy of reproductive age [79].

SEXUAL DYSFUNCTION IN WOMEN WITH EPILEPSY

The prevalence of severe sexual dysfunction in women with epilepsy was first reported by Bergen *et al.* in 1992 [83]. Fifty women with epilepsy in a tertiary epilepsy care centre and a comparison group of women of similar age were queried on how often they had the desire for sex, and how often they actually had intercourse. They were asked to respond whether they had a very frequent, frequent, infrequent or very infrequent desire for sex. Equal proportions of women in both groups reported a frequent desire for sex; however, a much greater proportion of women with epilepsy than comparators had very infrequent sexual desire, with about 20% reporting that they almost 'never' had sexual desire. The investigators found no correlation to age, AEDs used, duration of epilepsy or seizure type. This study revealed that many women with epilepsy have normal sexuality; however, significantly more women with epilepsy have markedly decreased sexual desire than would be expected in the general population. In a separate evaluation of sexuality in 57 women with epilepsy of reproductive age, decreased sexual functioning on self-reported questionnaires was associated with phenytoin use, with mild depression, and with low levels of estradiol and dehydroepiandrosterone sulphate [84].

Orgasmic dysfunction in women with epilepsy has also been reported in several studies. Jenson *et al.* in 1990 studied sexuality in 48 women with epilepsy and compared their results with their own previously reported data on sexuality in persons with diabetes mellitus and healthy controls [85]. Sexual desire did not differ between the three groups; however, 19% of the women with epilepsy had orgasmic dysfunction compared with 11% of the diabetes mellitus group and 8% of the controls ($P = 0.081$). None of the women with epilepsy had out-of-range testosterone levels, either free or total, or testosterone-binding globulin levels

[85]. Women with epilepsy reported inadequate orgasmic satisfaction significantly more than controls in a report by Duncan *et al.* in their study of 195 women with epilepsy from a hospital-based clinic [86]. In another study of self-reported sexual functioning and sexual arousability in 116 women with epilepsy, anorgasmia was also reported by one-third of 17 women with primary generalized epilepsy and 18 of 99 women with localization-related epilepsy. Compared with historical controls, this group of women did not have reduced sexual experience, but reported less sexual arousability and more sexual anxiety [87].

Decreased sexual functioning in women with epilepsy may also be related to physiological dysfunction related to epilepsy or its treatment. This possibility is raised by a unique set of experiments in which genital blood flow was measured in women and men with temporal lobe epilepsy as they watched either erotic or sexually neutral videos [88]. Genital blood flow was significantly decreased in persons with epilepsy compared with controls; the authors proposed that disruption of relevant regions of cortex by epileptic activity, specifically limbic and frontal areas, could be the cause of sexual dysfunction. An effect of specific AEDs could not be assessed in these studies because of small numbers of subjects.

Bioactive testosterone correlates with degree of sexual interest in women with epilepsy as in normal women. This may be an important factor for sexuality in women with epilepsy. For example, low levels have been correlated with decreased sexual interest in women with right-sided temporal lobe epilepsy [89].

Although the issue has not been completely explored, AEDs may have an effect on sexual functioning for persons with epilepsy as well. In one provocative report, changing to lamotrigine was associated with improved sexual functioning in 141 women and men with epilepsy, including those who were initiated on monotherapy or switched to monotherapy from another AED [90].

Impaired sexual functioning that includes decreased desire and orgasmic dissatisfaction in women with epilepsy is likely contributed to by multiple factors. There is evidence for a physiological impairment of sexual functioning related to epilepsy or its treatments, as well as to low testosterone levels. Treatment approaches include assessment of the quality of sexuality for women with epilepsy, and evaluating free testosterone levels for further intervention.

PERIMENOPAUSE AND MENOPAUSE

Women with epilepsy report increased seizure frequency with perimenopause [91]. Thirty-nine women with epilepsy in perimenopause, as manifested by irregular menses and hot flushes, were surveyed regarding change in seizure frequency as they became perimenopausal. Most of the women (63%) reported an increase in seizure frequency as they became perimenopausal, although their medication had not been changed. Women who had a history of a catamenial seizure exacerbation, specifically pre-menstrual increase in seizure frequency, had an even greater risk for increased seizure frequency during perimenopause (Figure 9.1). Conversely, women with a catamenial seizure pattern were more likely to have a decrease in overall seizure frequency when they became postmenopausal, defined as 1 year without menses [91]. This change in seizure frequency during these life changes may be related to hormonal changes during perimenopause and menopause, specifically a relative increase in the oestrogen:progesterone ratio in early perimenopause. These findings indicate that for women with epilepsy, perimenopause is a life epoch that merits careful monitoring for seizure change and, if necessary, medication adjustment. Furthermore, at postmenopause, women with catamenial epilepsy exacerbations may experience a decrease in seizures.

The Women's Health Initiative (WHI) reported in 2002 that hormone replacement therapy (HRT) in the commonly used form of conjugated equine oestrogens and medroxyprogesterone acetate was associated with an increased risk for breast cancer and stroke [92]. These results

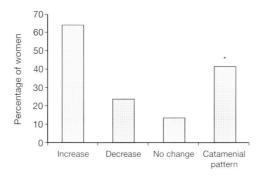

Figure 9.1 Seizure patterns in perimenopausal women with epilepsy [91]. *Significantly associated with an increase in seizures ($P=0.02$).

were surprising in the light of the long use of this compound, effective in the treatment of both the vasomotor symptoms ('hot flushes') and vaginal dryness associated with menopause. After a survey in which women with epilepsy reported an increase in seizures with HRT use [91], a randomized, double-blind, placebo-controlled trial using two dosages of conjugated equine oestrogens and medroxyprogesterone acetate was performed to evaluate the effect of HRT on seizure frequency [93]. This study found a dose-related increase in seizure frequency during the treatment period compared with baseline among women with partial epilepsy. Therefore, women with epilepsy have a risk of increased seizure frequency with the use of this standard HRT regimen. For women with epilepsy experiencing menopausal symptoms, a brief intervention of HRT using estradiol with natural progesterone would be an alternative treatment, although the safety of this alternate regimen has not been specifically evaluated.

CONCLUSION

The treatment of women with epilepsy of childbearing potential and beyond has been refined and improved with the advent of new information. One major advance has been the development of worldwide pregnancy registries which have provided clear information about the risk of valproate during pregnancy. More complete information about the other AEDs, including the newer AEDs, is expected in the near future. More information about the neurocognitive effects of AEDs will be forthcoming as the results of the NEAD study emerge. This study group is evaluating the long-term cognitive effects of intrauterine exposure to lamotrigine, phenytoin, carbamazepine and valproate in children born to mothers with epilepsy. Information about the outcome at 2 years of age, and eventually 3 years and 6 years of age is expected. The first report from this study group confirmed the risk of adverse pregnancy outcomes with valproate [94]. A randomized, double-blind, placebo-controlled study of natural progesterone for the treatment of women with epilepsy between ages 13 and 45 is under way and will provide more definitive information about the efficacy of this intervention.

An emerging area of interest is the effects of AEDs on the developing brain, which is relevant for both *in utero* and neonatal exposure. In the developing mammalian brain, AEDs interfere with cell proliferation and migration, synaptogenesis and plasticity [95]. Phenytoin, phenobarbital, valproate, diazepam, clonazepam and vigabatrin increase apoptosis (physiologic cell death) in the developing brain, while topiramate at therapeutic doses, and levetiracetam at any dose, do not have this effect [95]. These adverse effects have obvious relevance for the treatment of women with epilepsy of childbearing potential, and translation from laboratory to the clinic is anticipated.

REFERENCES

1. *Physician's Desk Reference* 2005. (Prescribing information for Ortho Tri-cyclen® Lo Tablets.) Montvale, NJ: Thomson PDR.
2. Trussel J. Contraceptive failure in the United States. *Contraception* 2004; 70:89–96.
3. Coulam CB, Annegers JF. Do anticonvulsants reduce the efficacy of oral contraceptives? *Epilepsia* 1979; 20:519–525.
4. Back DJ, Bates M, Bowden A *et al*. The interaction of phenobarbital and other anticonvulsants with oral contraceptive steroid therapy. *Contraception* 1980; 22:495–503.
5. Crawford P, Chadwick, DJ, Martin C *et al*. The interaction of phenytoin and carbamazepine with combined contraceptive steroids. *Br J Clin Pharmacol* 1990; 30:892–896.
6. Anderson GD. Pharmacogenetics and enzyme induction/inhibition properties of antiepileptic drugs. *Neurology* 2004; 63(Suppl 4):S3–S8.
7. Saano V, Manfield CR, Reidenberg P *et al*. Effects of felbamate on the pharmacokinetics of a low-dose combination oral contraceptive. *Clin Pharmacol Ther* 1995; 58:523–531.
8. Rosenfeld WE, Doose DR, Walker SA *et al*. Effect of topiramate on the pharmacokinetics of an oral contraceptive containing norethindrone and ethinyl estradiol in patients with epilepsy. *Epilepsia* 1997; 38:317–323.
9. Doose DR, Wang SS, Padmanabhan M *et al*. Effect of topiramate or carbamazepine on the pharmacokinetics of an oral contraceptive containing norethindrone and ethinyl estradiol in healthy obese and non-obese female subjects. *Epilepsia* 2003; 44:540–549.
10. Fattore C, Cipolla G, Gatti G *et al*. Induction of ethinyl estradiol and levonorgestrel metabolism by oxcarbazepine in healthy women. *Epilepsia* 1999; 40:783–787.
11. Crawford P. Interactions between antiepileptic drugs and hormonal contraception. *CNS Drugs* 2002; 16:263–272.
12. Sabers A, Ohman I, Christensens J *et al*. Oral contraceptives reduce lamotrigine plasma levels. *Neurology* 2003; 61:570–571.
13. Reimers A, Helde G, Brodtkorb E. Ethinyl estradiol, not progestogens, reduces lamotrigine serum concentration. *Epilepsia* 2005; 46:1414–1417.
14. Sidhu J, Job S, Singh S *et al*. The pharmacokinetic and pharmacodynamic consequences of the co-administration of lamotrigine and a combined oral contraceptive in healthy female subjects. *Br J Clin Pharmacol* 2006; 61:191–199.
15. Cunnington M, Tennis P. Lamotrigine and the risk of malformations in pregnancy. *Neurology* 2005; 64:955–960.
16. Zahn C. Neurologic care of pregnant women with epilepsy. *Epilepsia* 1998; 39(Suppl 8):S26–S31.
17. Kalviainen R, Tomson T. Optimizing treatment of epilepsy during pregnancy. *Neurology* 2006; 67(Suppl 4):S59–S63.
18. Wyszynski DF, Nambisan M, Surve T *et al*. Increased rate of major malformations in offspring exposed to valproate during pregnancy. *Neurology* 2005; 64:961–965.
19. Holmes LB, Wyszynski DF, Lieberman E. The AED (antiepileptic drug) pregnancy registry: a 6-year experience. *Arch Neurol* 2004; 61:673–678.
20. Vajda FJ, Eadie MJ. Maternal valproate dosage and foetal malformations. *Acta Neurol Scand* 2005; 112:137–143.
21. Morrow JI, Russell A, Guthrie E *et al*. Malformation risks of antiepileptic drugs in pregnancy: a prospective study from the UK Epilepsy and Pregnancy Register. *J Neurol Neurosurg Psychiatry* 2005; 77:193–198.
22. Wide K, Winbladh B, Kallen B. Major malformations in infants exposed to antiepileptic drugs in utero, with emphasis on carbamazepine and valproic acid: a nation-wide, population-based register study. *Acta Paediatr* 2004; 93:174–176.
23. Artama M, Auvinen A, Raudaskoski T *et al*. Antiepileptic drug use of women with epilepsy and congenital malformations in offspring. *Neurology* 2005; 64:1874–1878.
24. Hunt S, Craig J, Russell A *et al*. Levetiracetam in pregnancy: preliminary experience from the UK Epilepsy and Pregnancy Register. *Neurology* 2006; 67:1876–1879.
25. Holmes LB, Coull BA, Dorfman J *et al*. The correlation of deficits in IQ with midface and digit hypoplasia in children exposed in utero to anticonvulsant drugs. *J Pediatr* 2005; 146:118–122.
26. Reinisch JM, Sanders SA, Mortensen EL *et al*. In utero exposure to phenobarbital and intelligence deficits in adult men. *JAMA* 1995; 274:1518–1525.

27. Vinten J, Adab N, Kini U *et al*. Neuropsychological effects of exposure to anticonvulsant medication in utero. *Neurology* 2005; 64:949–954.

28. Gaily E, Kantola-Sorsa E, Hiilesmaa V *et al*. Normal intelligence in children with prenatal exposure to carbamazepine. *Neurology* 2004; 62:28–32.

29. Minkoff H, Schaffer RM, Delke I *et al*. Diagnosis of intracranial hemorrhage in utero after a maternal seizure. *Obstet Gynecol* 1985; 65:S22–S24.

30. Teramo K, Hiilesmaa V, Bardy A *et al*. Fetal heart rate during a maternal grand mal epileptic seizure. *J Perinat Med* 1979; 7:3–6.

31. Hiilesmaa VK, Bardy A, Teramo K. Obstetric outcome in women with epilepsy. *Am J Obstet Gynecol* 1985; 152:499–504.

32. Nulman I, Laslo D, Koren G. Treatment of epilepsy in pregnancy. *Drugs (New Zealand)* 1999; 57:535–544.

33. The EURAP Study Group. Seizure control and treatment in pregnancy: observations from the EURAP Epilepsy Pregnancy Registry. *Neurology* 2006; 66:354–360.

34. Tomson T, Lindbom U, Ekqvist B *et al*. Epilepsy and pregnancy: a prospective study of seizure control in relation to free and total plasma concentrations of carbamazepine and phenytoin. *Epilepsia* 1994; 35:122–130.

35. Yerby MS, Friel PN, McCormick K. Antiepileptic drug disposition during pregnancy. *Neurology* 1992; 42(Suppl 5):12–16.

36. Battino D, Binelli S, Bossi L *et al*. Changes in primidone/phenobarbital ratio during pregnancy and the puerperium. *Clin Pharmacokinet* 1984; 9:252–269.

37. Tran TA, Leppik IE, Blesi K *et al*. Lamotrigine clearance during pregnancy. *Neurology (United States)* 2002; 59:251–255.

38. Pennell PB, Peng L, Newport DJ *et al*. Lamotrigine in pregnancy. Clearance, therapeutic drug monitoring, and seizure frequency. *Neurology* 2007; Nov 28 (Epub ahead of print).

39. Mazzucchelli I, Ontal FY, Ozkara C *et al*. Changes in the disposition of oxcarbazepine and its metabolites during pregnancy and the puerperium. *Epilepsia* 2006; 47:504–509.

40. Christense J, Savers A, Sidenius P. Oxcarbazepine concentrations during pregnancy: a retrospective study in patients with epilepsy. *Neurology* 2006; 67:1497–1499.

41. Beck-Mannagetta G, Janz D. Syndrome-related genetics in generalized epilepsy. *Epilepsy Res Suppl* 1991; 4:105–111.

42. Ottman R, Annegers JF, Hauser WA *et al*. Higher risk of seizures in offspring of mothers than of fathers with epilepsy. *Am J Hum Genet* 1988; 43:257–264.

43. Angelsen NK, Vik T, Jacobsen G *et al*. Breast feeding and cognitive development at age 1 and 5 years. *Arch Dis Child* 2001; 85:183–188.

44. Pennell PB. Antiepileptic drug pharmacokinetics during pregnancy and lactation. *Neurology* 2003; 61(Suppl 2):S35–S42.

45. Liporace J, Kao A, D'Abreu A. Concerns regarding lamotrigine and breast-feeding. *Epilepsy Behav* 2004; 5:102–105.

46. Johannessen SI, Helde G, Brodtkorb E. Levetiracetam concentrations in serum and in breast milk at birth and during lactation. *Epilepsia* 2005; 46:775–777.

47. Ohman I, Vitols S, Luef G *et al*. Topiramate kinetics during delivery, lactation, and in the neonate: preliminary observations. *Epilepsia* 2002; 43:1157–1160.

48. Practice parameter: management issues for women with epilepsy (summary statement). Report of the Quality Standards Subcommittee of the American Academy of Neurology. *Neurology* 1998; 51:944–948.

49. Kaaja E, Kaaja R, Matila R *et al*. Enzyme-inducing antiepileptic drugs in pregnancy and the risk of bleeding in the neonate. *Neurology* 2002; 58:549–553.

50. Artama M, Isojärvi JI, Raitanen J *et al*. Birth rate among patients with epilepsy: a nationwide population-based cohort study in Finland. *Am J Epidemiol* 2004; 159:1057–1063.

51. Morrell MJ, Giudice L, Flynn KL *et al*. Predictors of ovualtory failure in women with epilepsy. *Ann Neurol* 2002; 52:704–711.

52. Bauer J, Jarre A, Klingmuller M *et al*. Polycystic ovary syndrome in patients with focal epilepsy: a study in 93 women. *Epilepsy Res* 2000; 41:163–167.

53. Drislane FW, Coleman AE, Schomer DL *et al*. Altered pulsatile secretion of luteinizing hormone in women with epilepsy. *Neurology* 1994; 44:306–310.

54. Herzog AG, Drislane FW, Schomer DL *et al.* Abnormal pulsatile secretion of luteinizing hormone in men with epilepsy: relationship to laterality and nature of paroxysmal discharges. *Neurology* 1990; 40:1557–1561.

55. Knobil E. The neuroendocrine control of the menstrual cycle. *Recent Prog Horm Res* 1980; 36:53–88.

56. Hart R, Hickey M, Franks S. Definitions, prevalence and symptoms of polycystic ovaries and polycystic ovary syndrome. *Best Pract Res Clin Obstet Gynaecol* 2004; 18:671–683.

57. Legro RS, Kunselman AR, Dodson WC *et al.* Prevalence and predictors of risk for type 2 diabetes mellitus and impaired glucose tolerance in polycystic ovary syndrome: a prospective, controlled study in 254 affected women. *J Clin Endocrinol Metab* 1999; 84:165–169.

58. Rasgon N. The relationship between polycystic ovary syndrome and antiepileptic drugs. *J Clin Psychopharmacol* 2004; 24:322–334.

59. Isojarvi JI, Laatikainen TJ, Pakarinen AJ *et al.* Polycystic ovaries and hyperandrogenism in women taking valproate for epilepsy. *N Engl J Med* 1993; 329:1383–1388.

60. Isojarvi JIT, Laatikainen TJ, Knip M *et al.* Obesity and endocrine disorders in women taking valproate for epilepsy. *Ann Neurol* 1996; 39:579–584.

61. Mikkonen K, Vainionpaa LK, Pakarinen AJ *et al.* Long-term reproductive endocrine health in young women with epilepsy. *Neurology* 2004; 62:445–450.

62. Morrell MJ, Isojarvi J, Taylor AE *et al.* Higher androgens and weight gain with valproate compared with lamotrigine for epilepsy. *Epilepsy Res* 2003; 54:189–199.

63. Murialdo G, Galimberti CA, Magri F *et al.* Menstrual cycle and ovary alterations in women with epilepsy on antiepileptic therapy. *J Enodcrinol Invest* 1997; 20:519–526.

64. Harden CL. Polycystic ovaries and polycystic ovary syndrome in epilepsy: evidence for neurogonadal disease. *Epilepsy Curr* 2005; 5:142–146.

65. Tauboll E, Gregoaszczuk EL, Kolodziej A *et al.* Valproate inhibits the conversion of testosterone to estradiol and acts as an apoptotic agent in growing porcine ovarian follicular cells. *Epilepsia* 2003; 44:1014–1021.

66. Greco R, Latini G, Chiarelli F *et al.* Leptin, ghrelin, and adiponectin in epileptic patients treated with valproic acid. *Neurology* 2005; 65:1808–1809.

67. Klein P, Serje A, Pezzullo JC. Premature ovarian failure in women with epilepsy. *Epilepsia* 2001; 42:1584–1589.

68. Harden CL, Koppel BS, Herzog AG *et al.* Seizure frequency is associated with age of menopause in women with epilepsy. *Neurology* 2003; 61:451–455.

69. Herzog AG, Klein P, Ransil BJ. Three patterns of catamenial epilepsy. *Epilepsia* 1997; 38:1082–1088.

70. Scharfman HE, MacLusky NJ. The influence of gonadal hormones on neuronal excitability, seizures, and epilepsy in the female. *Epilepsia* 2006; 47:1423–1444.

71. Reddy DS. Physiological role of adrenal deoxycorticosterone-derived neuroactive steroids in stress-sensitive conditions. *Neuroscience* 2006; 138:911–920.

72. Frye CA, Bayon LE. Seizure activity is increased in endocrine states characterized by decline in endogenous levels of the neurosteroid 3 alpha,5 alpha THP. *Neuroendocrinology* 1998; 68:272–280. Erratum in: *Neuroendocrinology* 1998; 68:436.

73. Hsu FC, Smith SS. Progesterone withdrawal reduces paired-pulse inhibition in rat hippocampus: dependence on GABA(A) receptor alpha4 subunit upregulation. *J Neurophysiol* 2003; 89:186–198.

74. Herzog AG, Harden CL, Liporace J *et al.* Frequency of catamenial seizure exacerbation in women with localization-related epilepsy. *Ann Neurol* 2004; 56:431–444.

75. Mattson RH, Cramer JA, Caldwell BV *et al.* Treatment of seizures with medroxyprogesterone acetate: preliminary report. Neurology 1984; 34:1255–1258.

76. Herzog AG. Intermittent progesterone therapy of partial complex seizures in women with menstrual disorders. *Neurology* 1986; 36:1607–1610.

77. Herzog AG. Progesterone therapy in women with complex partial and secondary generalized seizures. *Neurology* 1995; 45:1660–1662.

78. Herzog A. Progesterone therapy in women with epilepsy: a 3-year follow-up. *Neurology* 1999; 52:1917–1918.

79. Foldvary-Schaefer N, Falcone T. Catamenial epilepsy: pathophysiology, diagnosis, and management. *Neurology* 2003; 61(Suppl 2):S2–S15.

80. Lim LL, Foldvary N, Mascha E *et al.* Acetazolamide in women with catamenial epilepsy. *Epilepsia* 2001; 42:746–749.

81. Feely M, Calvert R, Gibson J. Clobazam in catamenial epilepsy: a model for evaluating anticonvulsants. *Lancet* 1982; 2:71–73.
82. Feely M, Gibson J. Intermittent clobazam for catamenial epilepsy: tolerance avoided. *J Neurol Neurosurg Psychiatry* 1984; 47:1279–1282.
83. Bergen D, Daugherty S, Eckenfels E. Reduction of sexual activities in females taking antepileptic drugs. *Psychopathology* 1992; 25:1–4.
84. Morrell MJ, Flynn KL, Done S *et al*. Sexual dysfunction, sex steroid hormone abnormalities, and depression in women with epilepsy treated with antiepileptic drugs. *Epilepsy Behav* 2005; 6:360–365.
85. Jensen P, Jensen SB, Sorensen PS *et al*. Sexual dysfunction in male and female patients with epilepsy: a study of 86 outpatients. *Arch Sex Behav* 1990; 19:1–14.
86. Duncan S, Blacklaw J, Beastall GH *et al*. Sexual function in women with epilepsy. *Epilepsia* 1997; 38:1074–1081.
87. Morrell MJ, Guldner GT. Self-reported sexual function and sexual arousability in women with epilepsy. *Epilepsia* 1996; 37:1204–1210.
88. Morrell MJ, Sperling MR, Stecker M *et al*. Sexual dysfunction in partial epilepsy: a deficit in physiologic sexual arousal. *Neurology* 1994; 44:243–247.
89. Herzog AG, Coleman AE, Jacobs AR *et al*. Relationship of sexual dysfunction to epilepsy lateralization and reproductive hormone levels in women. *Epilepsy Behav* 2003; 4:407–413.
90. Gil-Nagel A, Lopez-Munoz F, Serratosa JM *et al*. Effect of lamotrigine on sexual function in patients with epilepsy. *Seizure* 2006; 15:142–149.
91. Harden CL, Pulver MC, Jacobs AR. The effect of menopause and perimenopause on the course of epilepsy. *Epilepsia* 1999; 40:1402–1407.
92. Rossouw JE, Anderson GL, Prentice RL *et al*.; the Writing Group for the Women's Health Initiative Investigators. Risks and benefits of estrogen plus progestin in healthy post-postmenopausal women: principal results of the Women's Health Initative randomized, controlled trial. *JAMA* 2002; 288:321–333.
93. Harden CL, Herzog AG, Nikolov BG *et al*. Hormone replacement therapy in women with epilepsy: a randomized, double-blind, placebo-controlled study. *Epilepsia* 2006; 47:1447–1451.
94. Meador KJ, Baker GA, Finnell RH *et al*; NEAD Study Group. In utero antiepileptic drug exposure: fetal death and malformations. *Neurology* 2006; 67:407–412.
95. Kaindl AM, Asimiadou S, Manthey D *et al*. Antiepileptic drugs and the developing brain. *Cell Mol Life Sci* 2006; 63:399–413.

10

Treatment of the elderly with epilepsy

Joseph I. Sirven

INTRODUCTION

Older adults have increased steadily in number and proportion of the total world population. In the United States, the population aged 65 and older numbered 35 million in 2000 and is expected to more than double by 2050 [1]. The older population was 12% of the total population in 2000 and will increase to 20% by 2050 [1]. The increase in the size of America's older population is accompanied by rapid growth in the 'oldest old' or the population aged 85 and older [1]. The oldest old comprised 12.1% of the older adult population in 2001, up from 9.9% in 1991 [1]. The population aged 85 and older is currently the fastest-growing segment of the older population and is expected to grow faster than any other age group. The United States Census Bureau projections suggest that the oldest old population could grow from about 4 million in 2000 to 19 million by 2050. By 2050, nearly 24% of the older population is projected to be age 85 and older [1]. The size of this segment of the population is especially important for the future of healthcare systems because those individuals older than 85 years tend to be in poorer health and require more services than the 'younger' old individuals.

The issue of older adults is most apparent when it pertains to neurological illnesses. Older patients tend to suffer from a disproportionate number of neurological conditions, including seizures and epilepsy. It is important to understand that there are several aspects of seizures in older adults that tend to be more or less confined to this age group and require special consideration in order to deliver the best care and ensure quality of life.

Older patients with seizures can be differentiated from younger ones based on five separate variables that are unique to older adults. These are: (i) epidemiology; (ii) aetiology; (iii) seizure presentation; (iv) pharmacokinetic and pharmacodynamic differences; and (v) psychosocial concerns. This chapter will explore these areas and discuss in detail diagnosis, management, therapy and the psychosocial concerns relating to the older adult with epilepsy.

EPIDEMIOLOGY/AETIOLOGY

Seizures can be classified into two main categories for both younger and older adults. Seizures can occur acutely and may be the presenting symptom of an underlying illness such as a haemorrhage or neoplasm, or they can simply be a condition unto themselves (e.g. epilepsy). This chapter will deal primarily with recurrent unprovoked seizures and epilepsy.

Joseph I. Sirven, MD, Professor, Department of Neurology, Mayo Clinic College of Medicine, Scottsdale, Arizona, USA

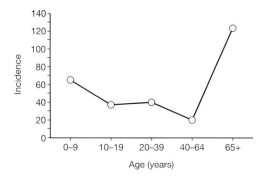

Figure 10.1 Age-specific average annual incidence of epilepsy per 100 000 population. Adapted from [2].

Figure 10.1 details the incidence of epilepsy according to age [2]. It is interesting to note that epilepsy has a peak incidence in older age groups. The annual incidence of epilepsy is 134 per 100 000 in those aged 65 years or older [2–7]. In contrast, the incidence of Alzheimer's-type dementia is approximately 123 per 100 000 [8]. Epilepsy increases with age, with an exponential increase in incidence for every decade of life after the age of 65 [2]. Thus, a seizure in the older adult is more often the rule than the exception.

EPILEPSY AETIOLOGY IN THE ELDERLY

The aetiology of seizures in older adults has been studied in a number of epidemiological investigations. Figure 10.2 shows the results from an Olmsted County population study. Cerebrovascular disease is the most common aetiological factor associated with epilepsy in individuals over the age of 65 [2, 8]. Other conditions accounting for epilepsy included neurodegenerative diseases, neoplasms, trauma, congenital abnormalities and infection [2, 8]. A majority of epilepsy cases in older adults are cryptogenic (no known cause), probably reflecting an unidentified variable associated with the ageing process that leads to an increased risk for the development of epilepsy.

EPILEPSY RISK FACTORS IN THE ELDERLY

There are several risk factors that can increase the potential for seizures in older adults. These include: stroke; dementia of all types; trauma, particularly with haemorrhage (three-

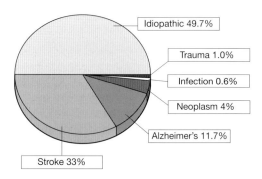

Figure 10.2 Aetiology of epilepsy in the elderly. Adapted from [8].

fold); alcohol usage; infection; low-grade neoplasms; and depression [2, 9–19]. Of these risk factors, cerebrovascular diseases, neurodegenerative conditions such as Alzheimer's dementia, and low-grade neoplasms are frequently associated with seizures in older adults and should always be considered in the differential diagnosis in patients who are having repeated spells.

Status Epilepticus

The incidence of status epilepticus (SE) in the elderly is almost twice that of the general population [19–22]. Thirty per cent of acute seizures in older adults present as status epilepticus. Concurrent medical conditions are more likely to complicate therapy and worsen prognosis. Mortality of status epilepticus in older adults is the highest of any age group and reported to be 38–50% [19–22]. SE aetiologies include stroke, remote symptomatic seizures, subtherapeutic serum anti-epileptic drug concentrations, hypoxia, metabolic disorders, alcohol-related, tumour, infection, anoxia, haemorrhage, trauma, and idiopathic [19–22]. If one were to combine remote symptomatic stroke cases with acute stroke cases, stroke accounts for 40% of elderly patients with SE. Thus, cerebrovascular disease is the most common cause of SE in the elderly. Non-convulsive SE is the most common form of SE in critically ill patients. Despite its frequency, non-convulsive status is easily mistaken as delirium, which can lead to delayed diagnosis or misdiagnosis [23].

SEIZURE SEMIOLOGY IN THE ELDERLY

Although seizures are a frequent occurrence in older adults, epilepsy is often perceived as an uncommon diagnosis of later life. There are several possibilities that explain this observation. The most obvious reason is that seizures are not recognized because of the non-specific nature by which they present in older adults. Older patients tend to have more frontal and parietal lobe foci as opposed to the more commonly recognized temporal lobe foci of younger adults [14, 16, 21, 23–25]. Because of the frontal and parietal lobe foci, older adults will commonly report auras of dizziness. Unfortunately, dizziness is a common and non-specific symptom and is reported with a variety of medical conditions, including neurological, cardiac or other organ system dysfunction. Therefore, when a patient reports dizziness, it is often misdiagnosed or overlooked.

Simple partial seizures (seizures without alteration in awareness) often manifest with focal motor and/or sensory components which can easily be misinterpreted as tremors and numbness commonly seen in older adults [26]. Complex partial seizures (seizures with alteration of awareness) can present as altered mentation, staring, blackouts or confusion, which is at times subtle. When elderly people present with these symptoms, they are often misdiagnosed as having an acute confusional state, the onset of dementia, a medication effect or some other condition, and seizures will often be overlooked in the differential diagnosis [26, 27].

Because seizures are under-recognized, there is often a delay in the diagnosis. One study by Sheth and colleagues [23] investigated ambulatory patients with acute ictal confusion at both the University of Wisconsin and Mayo Clinic, Arizona. Twenty-two older patients with acute ictal confusion were identified to assess how quickly a correct diagnosis was made. Ictal confusion was not recognized for up to 5 days. Of the 22 patients, 20 had partial complex partial SE and two had newly diagnosed primary generalized SE. Motor movements were not present in either group, although reduced mood state and ictal neglect were noted in some patients. Fifteen patients had 2 to 10 previous episodes of protracted ictal confusion. Once identified, treatment reversed confusion and eventually patients were discharged to home, although a small minority of patients demonstrated persistent reduction in their baseline cognition. The study concluded that protracted ictal confusion is often not considered in the ambulatory older patient, resulting in a delay in diagnosis. Electroencephalographic and video-electroencephalographic studies performed while the patient is experiencing symptoms are crucial to early diagnosis and timely management.

Further complicating diagnosis is the prolonged post-ictal state seen in aged patients. One investigation reported that 14% of adults over the age of 65 had a prolonged post-ictal state, and in some cases the post-ictal state was more than 24 h for a 1-minute seizure [7, 24, 28]. Todd's paralysis is also more common in older adults, often leading to a misdiagnosis of a transient ischaemic attack (TIA) or a cerebrovascular event [24, 28]. Most worrying about seizure presentation is the issue of falls. Seizures in both younger and older individuals may be associated with loss of posture, leading to a fall, but the consequences may be much more devastating in the elderly. Falls in the elderly have been noted by several investigators to be associated with functional dependence and may lead to nursing home admissions [29–33].

Differential Diagnosis

Seizures often mimic a number of other common conditions. These conditions include syncope, TIA, transient global amnesia (TGA) and vertigo. Several diagnostic tests may be useful in differentiating seizures from other conditions. Yet, the most important aspect of evaluation is considering seizures in the differential diagnosis and obtaining a clear, detailed history.

Diagnostic tests help to narrow the differential diagnosis. The gold standard for diagnosis is a witnessed description of the event; however, because older adults are more likely to live alone, their seizures are more likely to be unwitnessed. Complicating this issue is the fact that accurate self-reporting may not be possible in some individuals due to memory deficits. Tests commonly performed are magnetic resonance imaging (MRI), electroencephalography and laboratory tests. Other tests which are germane to older adults include cardiovascular testing, ambulatory electrocardiogram and tilt-table testing. Table 10.1 outlines how test results can help in diagnosing epilepsy.

The diagnosis of seizures is based on clinical history. A clinician should be suspicious of epilepsy if a seizure is directly observed or if transient episodes of either loss of consciousness or altered consciousness, stereotypic changes in speech, sensation or movement occur. This is particularly true if there is a history of a structural neurological abnormality such as neoplasm, stroke or encephalomalacia.

Evaluation of a Patient with a Presumed Seizure

An approach to the diagnosis of seizures in the older adult generally begins by considering whether the event could have been a seizure. If the answer is yes, then an electroencephalogram (EEG) should be obtained. EEGs are useful in identifying whether there are abnormalities, and if so, whether they are focal or generalized. In most cases where a cause is not immediately apparent, an MRI scan should be obtained to rule out a structural lesion such as tumour, stroke or other lesion. If the EEG shows generalized abnormalities (including diffuse background slowing), it is essential to look for a metabolic cause by obtaining serum sodium, glucose, liver enzymes and complete blood count for signs of infection. Some metabolic causes of epilepsy can also produce focal seizures. Evaluation should include a medication review as several medications can cause seizures. A lumbar puncture is not done routinely unless a seizure occurred in the setting of a fever or there is a suspicion of meningitis. If a metabolic infectious or toxic cause is found, then eliminating that agent or treating the underlying condition will essentially treat the seizures. If the EEG does not show any change, but the events continue to occur, then video-electroencephalography and ambulatory electroencephalography are the best options to try to capture events.

Table 10.1 Diagnostic testing for epilepsy in older adults

Test modality	Establishes diagnosis of epilepsy	Suggestive of epilepsy	Non-specific
Routine EEG	Recording an electrographic seizure	Interictal spike or sharp waves	Focal or generalized slowing, amplitude asymmetry, wicket waves, SREDA
Video-EEG	Recording an electrographic seizure	Interictal spike or sharp waves	Focal or generalized slowing, amplitude asymmetry
MRI	None	Any cortically based lesion (neoplasm, cerebral infarctions, encephalomalacia, haemorrhage, abscess)	Subcortical unidentified bright objects, subcortical infarctions
Laboratory evaluations	None	Systemic infections of any type, hyponatraemia, hypernatraemia, hypoglycaemia, hyperglycaemia hypocalcaemia, hypoxia, positive toxicology for stimulant agents	Elevated liver function studies, hypokalaemia, hyperkalaemia
Electrocardiogram	None	Paroxysmal tachycardia, arrhythmias	Persistent bradycardia, tachycardia, arrhythmias

SREDA, subclinical rhythmic electrical discharges of adulthood.

Electroencephalography

Evaluation of older patients with electroencephalography does not differ from that of younger patients; however, there are a number of EEG changes that are commonly seen in the elderly but are not indicative of epilepsy. These changes include slowing of the background alpha rhythm accompanied by a decrease in amplitude. Slow EEG frequencies such as delta and theta can increase with age [34–42]. Slowing of the background is often non-specific when it occurs diffusely, but it may implicate a central nervous system (CNS) structural lesion if it occurs focally. EEG patterns of uncertain significance can occur with age, such as small sharp spikes, or subclinical rhythmic electrical discharges of adulthood (SREDA), the latter occurring exclusively in older adults [40, 41]. Of note, epileptiform transients can be seen in patients with diseases other than epilepsy such as dementia, stroke, neoplasms and prion diseases [43]. Nevertheless, capturing epileptiform transients on an EEG in a patient with a relevant history strongly suggests epilepsy (see Table 10.1). The gold standard for diagnosing epilepsy on EEG is the actual recording of a seizure. New technologies now make recording feasible by the use of video-electroencephalography recording or ambulatory EEG. Therefore, when the diagnosis is in question, either of these two modalities should be pursued in the diagnosis. Persistent episodes warrant monitoring, especially if they impact quality of life.

Imaging

Imaging studies such as MRI and computerized tomography (CT) should be performed as part of the initial evaluation of all older patients with epilepsy to identify and treat aetiologies such as CNS haemorrhage, tumour and abscess. MRI is the procedure of choice because it is superior to CT in detecting all pathological processes except subarachnoid haemorrhage [44]. CT should be used only in emergency situations or when MRI is contraindicated. Contrast enhancement should be employed in both modalities because it improves detection of tumours and infection.

There are age-related changes seen commonly on MRI. These findings include diffuse atrophy defined as cerebral volume loss manifesting as dilatation of ventricles and foci, and periventricular hyperintensities [44–50]. When any of these radiological signs are found, they are not readily attributable to the aetiology of epilepsy, but rather contribute to non-specific findings commonly associated with longstanding hypertension or small-vessel atherosclerosis. Therefore, one must be careful in ascribing causes of seizures when obtaining imaging.

THERAPY

Therapy is initiated when the risk of recurrence is high and the risk of injury from a seizure outweighs the risk of AED toxicity. Older patients tend to have a higher risk of seizure recurrence after a single seizure. In one study by Luhdorf and colleagues [4], 75% of 151 older patients studied proceeded to have a second seizure. Therefore, as patients grow older, the risk of subsequent seizures rises, and is greater than that of younger patients [4, 10, 23, 50]. Often, medications can be initiated after one seizure if the presenting seizure was SE, there is an underlying cause such as a cortical infarction with haemorrhage, cortical tumour, or the presence of focal or generalized epileptiform discharges on EEG. After a decision is made to initiate medication, it will be important to choose the most appropriate AED. The reader is referred to other chapters in this book for a more detailed review of AEDs. The following discussion on AEDs will pertain only to those issues that are unique to the older adult.

Simple partial, complex partial, secondary generalized tonic–clonic and myoclonic are the most common seizure types in the aged [3, 25]. Therefore, agents that are approved for use for those seizure types are the best choices as initial therapy. First-line therapy for simple partial and complex partial seizures includes carbamazepine, gabapentin, levetiracetam, lamotrigine, phenobarbital, pregabalin, phenytoin, tiagabine, topiramate, valproic acid and zonisamide. Primary agents approved for generalized tonic–clonic events include phenytoin, topiramate, levetiracetam, lamotrigine, valproic acid and zonisamide. Primary agents available for myoclonic seizures include benzodiazepines, felbamate, levetiracetam, topiramate, valproic acid and zonisamide. The choice of any of these agents is appropriate. Adverse effects and drug interactions are more important than efficacy variables in deciding which agent to utilize [24, 28, 51–53].

AEDs IN OLDER ADULTS

As previously discussed, older adults have more co-morbidities and multiple pathologies than the younger adult. Because of this, patients are often taking other medications, and the treatment of seizures can lead to complex polypharmacy. Moreover, older adults are more susceptible to cognitive adverse effects. It appears that the elderly therefore have a narrowed therapeutic window, and are not able to tolerate the higher end of what would be considered the therapeutic range in younger patients (e.g. phenytoin levels over 15 or carbamazepine levels over 10). Thus, one has to be cautious with dosing of an AED in individuals older than 65, and in general, lower doses should be used initially [51, 54–58]. Compliance with the drug regimen coupled with serum AED levels that are not representative of this age group should all be considered when managing AED therapy.

ADVERSE EFFECTS

Adverse effects are an important factor associated with the choice of AED in older adults. In the mid-1980s, the Veteran's Administration (VA) Cooperative Studies were performed to evaluate AEDs in adults with epilepsy. In these studies, patients were stratified into three age groups – 18–40, 40–64, and over the age of 65. The results were that more older adult patients dropped out of these studies due to intolerability of adverse effects. In fact, there were more side-effects reported in the older adult group than any of the other two age groups [53]. Therefore, adverse effects are a critical consideration when selecting an AED.

BONE HEALTH

One of the more worrying adverse effects is the impact of AEDs on osteoporosis and bone health. The rationale for this concern is that brittle bones may lead to fractures. Because seizures are associated with falling, there is a concern that falls may lead to a devastating outcome [33]. Falls in the older adult are associated with significant mortality and morbidity. Injuries from falls are the sixth leading cause of death in patients over the age of 65, and falls account for 66% of all injuries. Twenty-five per cent of individuals who are hospitalized for a fall die within 1 year [31, 32]. The most common fractures are those of the distal forearm and hip fractures. Hip fractures are notoriously difficult to manage, accounting for 15% of hospital mortality and 33% of 1-year mortality [31–33]. Enzyme-inducing AEDs (phenytoin, phenobarbital, carbamazepine and primidone) have been found to impact bone health. Pack and colleagues found a fourfold increase in risk of femoral neck fractures in patients with epilepsy compared with age-matched controls [59]. AED use and duration of therapy significantly correlated with a bone mineral density in adults and children, and fracture rates were higher overall. There are a number of potential mechanisms by which AEDs can affect bone health, but none has been proven to account for these findings. Caution in prescribing enzyme-inducing agents in older adults is advised, particularly when there is a history of osteoporosis.

COGNITIVE SIDE-EFFECTS

Cognitive issues are a major concern when prescribing AEDs in the elderly, as cognitive decline may be mistaken for dementia. Drugs that are a particular risk for cognition include phenytoin, phenobarbital and topiramate, but other drugs may also cause or worsen cognitive dysfunction. If a patient appears cognitively impaired, and is on a sedating AED, it is reasonable to attempt a trial of a more cognitively favourable AED such as lamotrigine.

OTHER ISSUES

Haematological concerns are an important adverse effect. Valproic acid, carbamazepine, phenytoin and felbamate are associated with a reduction in white blood cell count and/or platelet function. Nephrolithiasis can occur with topiramate and zonisamide. Patients at risk have either a prior history of nephrolithiasis or a positive first-degree relative.

Tremor and/or parkinsonian symptoms can be seen with valproic acid use. Lastly, hyponatraemia occurs with either carbamazepine or oxcarbazepine. Therefore, patients who are sodium depleted, have fluid/electrolyte abnormalities or are receiving diuretics should be careful when utilizing these agents. The elderly are at increased risk of hyponatraemia with these agents (up to 6–7%), and their electrolytes should be monitored on a routine basis.

DRUG INTERACTIONS

Drug interactions are a common concern with AEDs in older adults. A Minneapolis, Minnesota survey of older adults found that two-thirds of people over the age of 60 take prescription medications. Moreover, outpatients took an average of seven medications at one time and up to 19 per year [55]. Not surprisingly, one has to evaluate potential adverse drug interactions when prescribing an agent.

Alteration in liver function is responsible for a majority of drug interactions. Therefore, attempting to find compounds that are not metabolized through the liver can be beneficial in older patients who are on polypharmacy. Enzyme-inducing agents – phenytoin, carbamazepine, phenobarbital and primidone – are the most problematic in regard to drug interactions due to the induction of cytochrome P450 enzyme. Induction will increase clearance of many drugs metabolized through the liver, which includes a number of drugs commonly prescribed to the elderly, for hypercholesterolaemia, hypertension and depression. Higher doses of these other drugs will be necessary to produce the same therapeutic effect, which can increase the cost of concomitant therapy. Unfortunately, doses are often not increased appropriately, leading to under-treatment. Thus, avoiding these agents may be beneficial. Further information on which drugs are affected can be found in Chapter 13.

OTHER PHARMACOKINETIC ISSUES

The elderly differ from younger individuals in a number of important ways. They have reduced hepatic and renal clearance of drugs. This is part of the reason why lower doses are necessary, and is particularly important for completely renally cleared drugs such as gabapentin, levetiracetam and pregabalin. The elderly's capacity to absorb drugs through the gastrointestinal tract may also be delayed or variable. The metabolism of phenytoin deserves specific note, since this is a drug prescribed to many elderly and nursing home patients. In the elderly, metabolism through cytochrome P450 may be saturated at lower concentrations than in younger individuals, within the therapeutic range, after which serum concentrations may rise precipitously, leading to toxicity [52].

BEST EVIDENCE FOR CHOOSING AEDs IN THE OLDER ADULT

There are few trials to support the choice of one medication for all older patients with epilepsy. However, some comparative head-to-head trials of AEDs in older adults have been conducted. Craig and colleagues compared valproic acid with phenytoin. A total of 166 patients over the age of 65 with adult-onset seizures were randomized to either valproic acid or phenytoin. The median age of patients was 78 years. The investigators found that 78% of valproic acid patients and 76% of phenytoin patients were seizure free at 6 months [60]. Moreover, there were no cognitive differences that were noted between the two AEDs. This study was important in that this was one of the first trials to study older adult patients in a comparative, randomized trial. It was also the first trial to suggest that alternative agents other than phenytoin can be used as first-line therapy in older patients.

Recently, a VA Cooperative geriatric epilepsy study was completed. Rowan and colleagues [25] evaluated the tolerability and efficacy of gabapentin and lamotrigine vs. carbamazepine in older adult patients. They randomized 593 individuals of age 60 years and older in a double-blind, double-placebo parallel study in patients with newly diagnosed seizures. Patients were assigned to one of the three treatment groups: gabapentin 1500 mg per day, lamotrigine 150 mg per day and carbamazepine 600 mg per day. The primary outcome measure was retention in the trial for a 12-month period. The mean age of their patients was 72 years, with individuals taking an average of seven co-medications. They reported early terminations of lamotrigine (44%), gabapentin (51%) and carbamazepine (64%). Terminations for adverse events included 12% for lamotrigine, 21% for gabapentin and 31% for carbamazepine. There were no significant differences in seizure-free rates at 12 months. The authors concluded that the main limiting factor in patient retention was adverse drug reactions. Patients taking lamotrigine or gabapentin did better than those taking carbamazepine. They recommended that lamotrigine and gabapentin should be considered as initial therapy for older patients with newly diagnosed epilepsy. Similarly, Brodie and colleagues compared carbamazepine with lamotrigine in older adults and found that lamotrigine was equivalent in efficacy and better tolerated than carbamazepine [61]. Other than these two studies, there are no randomized controlled trials (RCTs) evaluating AEDs in older adults.

Despite the paucity of RCT evidence, there appears to be an emerging consensus regarding general principles of AED use in older adults. Table 10.2 shows risk and benefits for various AEDs. Older adults tend to respond at lower doses than younger ones. It is important that one initiates AEDs at lower doses than one would for a younger adult. It is also important to simplify dosing regimens to accentuate compliance. If a patient reports an adverse event,

Table 10.2 Risks/benefits of specific epilepsy therapies in the older adult

Therapy	*Benefits*	*Risks*
Carbamazepine	Efficacy	Hyponatraemia, potential drug interactions, osteoporosis
Felbamate	Efficacy, lack of impact on cognition, alerting effect	Weight loss, risk of aplastic anaemia and hepatic failure, drug interactions, multiple daily doses
Gabapentin	Limited drug interactions, multiple indications, minimal cognitive impact	Limited efficacy, multiple daily doses
Lamotrigine	Limited drug interactions, minimal cognitive impact, efficacy	Rash potential, insomnia
Levetiracetam	Limited drug interactions, minimal cognitive impact, efficacy	Exacerbates depression, insomnia
Oxcarbazepine	Efficacy	Hyponatraemia, dizziness
Phenytoin	Efficacy, once-daily dosing	Imbalance, multiple drug interactions, risk of cognitive impairment, osteoporosis, potential for toxicity from zero-order kinetics, variable absorption in the very old
Phenobarbital	Efficacy, once-daily dosing	Sedation, cognitive impairment, depression, osteoporosis
Pregabalin	Minimal drug interactions, multiple indications	Limited efficacy, multiple daily dose, peripheral oedema
Surgery	Potentially curative	Serious surgical risks, including infection, haemorrhage, cognitive complaints
Tiagabine	Minimal drug interactions	Limited efficacy, multiple daily doses
Topiramate	Efficacy, migraine treatment, paucity of drug interactions	Cognitive complaints, glaucoma, nephrolithiasis, weight loss
Zonisamide	Efficacy, once-daily dose, paucity of drug interactions	Nephrolithiasis, weight loss
Vagus nerve stimulation	Compliance assured, approved for depression	Surgical risk, limited efficacy
Valproic acid	Efficacy, migraine treatment	Tremor

it is important to listen to that patient and try to provide supportive care by identifying the offending agent. It is essential to always determine the overall need for each medication. One must not be afraid to adjust or discontinue medications. AED formulations, including extended-release preparations and agents with longer half-lives, may be of particular benefit in older adults due to the minimal number of daily doses that are required. Extended-release formulations can also be useful in decreasing peak-related adverse effects and improving efficacy with higher blood levels. Some older adults have dysphagia so variable formulations such as sprinkles, liquids and parenterals can be utilized and may be beneficial in these individuals who have difficulty with swallowing.

THERAPEUTIC MONITORING WITH SERUM AED LEVELS

Measuring AED concentrations is important in epilepsy management for two reasons: (i) assessment of compliance and (ii) ascertaining toxicity. Monitoring AED levels becomes even more important in the aged because older patients may have memory problems or fail to comply with the drug regimen. Pharmacokinetic changes associated with advanced age include variable absorption, reduced renal and hepatic clearance and reduced serum albumin, which may contribute to more variability in the relationship between dose and serum concentration. Over- or under-dosing may be prevented by checking serum AED concentrations. However, there are problems in utilizing published serum level ranges for AEDs. AED levels represent younger patient data and therefore may not be applicable to older adults [54, 56]. There is evidence that older adults may be more sensitive to the sedative and cognitive effects of benzodiazepines than younger patients with similar drug concentrations. The narrowed therapeutic window may place them at a greater risk for toxicity if one strictly adheres to AED levels. Therefore, when checking serum concentrations, one must remember that these are likely to be useful in identifying non-compliance and pharmacokinetic issues, but should not be over-interpreted when defining an optimal therapeutic level. It follows that levels that appear to be low may actually be appropriate for the older adult. Clinical presentation rather than laboratory values should be guiding AED dose decisions.

VAGUS NERVE STIMULATION

Vagus nerve stimulation (VNS) has been approved in the treatment of epilepsy (see Chapter 3). In this procedure, the carotid sheath is opened and two spiral electrodes are wrapped around the vagus nerve and connected to an infraclavicular generator pack. In experienced surgical hands, the procedure has a duration of less than 1 hour. The implanted device is a programmable stimulator, with the stimulation programmed in advance so that patients may turn the device on or off at any time by placing a magnet against the implant site. The mechanism of the anti-epileptic effect of the vagus nerve stimulator is not known. The efficacy of the procedure compares favourably with medication. The average seizure reduction is 31% at 3 months with 50–60% of patients achieving at least a 50% reduction by 1 year [62]. Adverse effects are few, consisting of hoarseness, coughing and paraesthesias. There may be an impact on sleep. Three studies have addressed VNS in older adults. All have found that there are no unique adverse effects associated with older adults with epilepsy.

Recently, the vagus nerve stimulator has been approved for use for refractory depression. Considering that depression is a common condition found in older adults, this may be a useful device in the older adult population in patients who have both epilepsy and depression. More studies are needed to address whether VNS has increased efficacy over drugs in older adults. VNS is a reasonable choice in individuals who have failed to respond to medications, and there are no increased surgical complications associated with its use in the older adult group.

RESECTIVE SURGERY FOR EPILEPSY IN OLDER ADULTS

In 15–20% of all epilepsy patients, seizures are not completely controlled by medical therapy. Some of these patients can be candidates for surgical treatment. In younger adults, temporal lobectomy, the most common surgical procedure for epilepsy, is readily performed in most settings and its efficacy and safety have been well documented. However, the percentage of older adults that are refractory to all medications is unknown. The VA Cooperative Studies found that the proportion of older adults with intractable epilepsy is small [55]. This study addressed epilepsy of younger onset, which is pathophysiologically distinct from older-onset epilepsy. Because older adults are different, one cannot assume that their response to resective surgery is the same as younger adults.

Four studies have investigated resective epilepsy surgery in older vs. younger adults [63–67]. Sirven and colleagues [62, 63] evaluated a total of 340 patients aged 50 years and younger and compared them with 30 patients older than 50 years, all of whom had anterior temporal lobectomy for refractory epilepsy. Seizure outcome, neuropsychological test scores and change in driving status were analysed. Age and duration of epilepsy related independently to outcome, but laterality of interictal sharp waves, an early epilepsy risk factor, and presence of tumour were not. Sixteen patients (52%) in the older group and 257 patients (75.6%) in the younger group ($P<0.008$) were seizure free. Post-operative neuropsychological outcome and driving status were similar in both the older and younger patients. The study concluded that older patients can indeed have successful epilepsy surgery; however, there is an increased risk of neuropsychological adverse effects.

Grivas and colleagues [65] evaluated 52 patients older than 50 years who underwent temporal lobectomy between 1991 and 2002. The mean age of operation was 55 years with the mean duration of epilepsy at 33 years. They found that 37 older patients attained complete seizure control (71%) and only 10 patients had rare post-operative seizures (19%). The same rate of seizure control was attained by the patients older than age 60 at the time of surgery. These results were not significantly different from those in the younger patient cohort. A trend toward better seizure control was noted in 16 patients with an epilepsy duration of less than 30 years and in 20 patients with a seizure frequency of fewer than five per month. Four per cent of older patients had permanent neurological morbidity, primarily hemiparesis and dysphasia. Hemianopsia occurred in 6% of patients. Neuropsychological testing revealed low pre-operative performances and some gradual deterioration after surgery. The authors concluded that the results of surgery for temporal lobectomy are promising in patients older than 60 years of age, despite a long seizure history.

Similarly to the Sirven study, they found that the risk of complications is somewhat higher compared with that in a younger control group. The finding of lower post-operative neuropsychological performance is a cause for concern. The debate will probably continue as to whether epilepsy surgery should be performed in older adults. Clearly, more care must be taken with epilepsy surgery evaluations before any decision is made to proceed with a resective procedure. Nevertheless, some individuals can benefit from surgery.

WHEN TO DISCONTINUE TREATMENT

One of the more common consultation questions that neurologists face is when an AED can be stopped in older adults. Unfortunately, there are no clear answers to this question. There have been studies that have evaluated discontinuation of AEDs in younger patients, but these have not specifically addressed the older adult population [68]. No definitive guidelines or evidence exists to clearly define when to discontinue seizure medications in older adults. Some general suggestions can be made to help the clinician. It is best to confirm the diagnosis of seizures. Often, medications are initiated for conditions which may appear to be epilepsy and may have been incorrectly diagnosed. Confirming the diagnosis of epilepsy ensures that the agent is being utilized appropriately. A patient should be seizure free for a minimum of 2–5 years to maximize the chance of success. It is important to have normal imaging. The EEG should lack epileptiform sharp waves. There must be no history of status epilepticus. More studies are needed to address this important clinical scenario.

MENOPAUSE

Although treatment of epilepsy in women is addressed elsewhere, it is important to consider the impact of menopause on seizure management. During menopause, ovarian follicles involute resulting in an abrupt decline of oestrogen and progesterone. Seizures can become less predictable. In a retrospective study of 42 menopausal women, a catamenial pattern of epilepsy was associated with increased seizures during perimenopause, but ultimately fewer seizures were noted after menopause. This study suggested that oestrogen replacement therapy might be associated with increased seizures. Epilepsy is not a contraindication for hormone replacement therapy [69], but women need to be advised to watch for a change in their seizure pattern. Selective oestrogen receptor modulators may be a better alternative in this population. Interestingly, one study reported that some women began to have seizures during menopause and suggested that menopause may be a risk factor for epilepsy [70]. Therefore, at this time it is unclear if menopause is beneficial or detrimental to the management of seizures.

PSYCHOSOCIAL CONCERNS

Psychosocial concerns in older adults are often similar to those of the younger epilepsy patient. Most disturbing is the loss of independence. Seizures may lead to falls and fractures, which can have a profound consequence in older adults. Driving is a major concern in older patients. There is no specific statute that addresses older patients with epilepsy; however, six states require mandatory reporting of seizures to their state motor vehicle bureau. These six states include California, Delaware, Nevada, New Jersey, Oregon and Pennsylvania. Moreover, California has special rules and regulations for patients who may have cognitive impairment. It is essential that older adults are continuously monitored for any changes in their medical condition which can adversely affect their ability to drive a car. One has to take extra care in making informed decisions and balancing public health risk vs. the preservation of independence for a patient's quality of life. Although investigators have begun to address the impact of AEDs on performance on driving simulation, no definitive results have emerged.

CONCLUSIONS

The study of seizures in older adults is at a nascent stage. There has been progress in that this population is being investigated as a distinct group. There are a few general consensus points for the clinician treating the older patient with seizures. Diagnosis is not always easy because seizures in the aged mimic many other conditions. One must always keep seizures in the differential diagnosis when diagnosing paroxysmal events. If seizures are diagnosed, they are likely to recur, and are most commonly associated with cerebrovascular events. Treatment should be pursued using AEDs at low doses with slow titration schedules, keeping in mind that adverse events lead to treatment failure. Invasive treatment options such as electrical stimulation and resective surgery can be employed for intractable seizures but one must use caution regarding adverse effects.

A number of clinical questions are left unanswered at this time due to paucity of evidence. It is unclear which aspect of the ageing process makes the older adult more prone to seizure recurrence. Are there preventative measures against the development of epilepsy in the older adult? What is the most cost-efficient algorithm for diagnosing epilepsy? What is the appropriate dose of an AED for the aged? Are there unknown systemic side-effects of AEDs that should be studied, such as imbalance or gait difficulties? Finally, when is it safe to discontinue AEDs in this population? With time, we hope that these questions can be answered.

REFERENCES

1. Rogers C. America's older population. United States Census Bureau. Accessibility verified at: www.census.gov/population/estimates/nation (accessed 9 May 2006).
2. Hauser WA, Annegers JF, Kurland LT. Incidence of epilepsy and unprovoked seizures in Rochester, Minnesota: 1935–1984. *Epilepsia* 1993; 34:453–468.
3. Hauser WA. Seizure disorders: the changes with age. *Epilepsia* 1992; 33(Suppl 4):S6–S14.
4. Luhdorf K, Jensen LK, Plesner AM. Epilepsy in the elderly: incidence, social function, and disability. *Epilepsia* 1989; 30:389–399.
5. Sanders JWA, Hart YM, Johnson AL *et al*. Natural General Practice Study of Epilepsy: newly diagnosed epileptic seizures in general population. *Lancet* 1990; 336:1267–1270.
6. Loiseau J, Loiseau P, Duche B *et al*. A survey of epileptic disorders in southwest France: seizures in elderly patients. *Ann Neurol* 1990; 27:233–237.
7. Tallis R, Hall G, Craig I *et al*. How common are epileptic seizures in old age? *Age & Ageing* 1991; 20:442–448.
8. Hauser WA. *Epidemiology of seizures and epilepsy in the elderly*. Boston: Butterworth-Heinemann, 1997, pp. 7–18.
9. Annegers JF, Shirts SB, Hauser WA *et al*. Risk of seizure recurrence after an initial unprovoked seizure. *Epilepsia* 1986; 27:43–50.
10. Annegers JF, Hauser WA, Lee JR *et al*. Incidence of acute symptomatic seizures in Rochester, Minnesota: 1935–1984. *Epilepsia* 1995; 36:327–333.
11. Hauser WA, Ramirez-Lassepas M, Rosenstein R. Risk for seizures and epilepsy following cerebrovascular insults (Abstract). *Epilepsia* 1984; 26:666.
12. Lancsman ME, Golimstok A, Norscini J *et al*. Risk factors for developing seizures after a stroke. *Epilepsia* 1993; 34:141–143.
13. Kilpatrick CJ, Davis SM, Tress BM *et al*. Early seizures after acute stroke. Risk of late seizures. *Arch Neurol* 1992; 49:509–511.
14. So EL, Annegers JF, Hauser WA *et al*. Population-based study of seizure disorders after cerebral infarction. *Neurology* 1996; 46:350–355.
15. Tallis R. Epilepsy in old age. *Lancet* 1990; 336:295–296.
16. Giroud M, Gras P, Fayolle H *et al*. Early seizures after acute stroke: a study of 1,640 cases. *Epilepsia* 1994; 35: 959–964.
17. Ettinger AB, Shinnar S. New-onset seizures in an elderly hospitalized population. *Neurology* 1993; 43:489–492.
18. Loiseau P. Pathologic processes in the elderly and their association with seizures. In: Rowan AJ, Ramsey RE (eds) *Seizures and Epilepsy in the Elderly*. Boston: Butterworth-Heinemann, 1997, pp. 63–68.
19. Ramsey RE, Pryor F. Epilepsy in the elderly. *Neurology* 2000; 55(Suppl 1):S9–S14.
20. Hauser WA, Cascino GD, Annegers JF *et al*. Incidence of status epilepticus and associated mortality (Abstract). *Epilepsia* 1994; 33(Suppl 8):33.
21. Thomas P, Lebrun C, Chatel M. De novo absence status epilepticus as a benzodiazepine withdrawal syndrome. *Epilepsia* 1993; 34:355–358.
22. Thomas RJ. Seizures and epilepsy in the elderly. *Arch Intern Med* 1997; 157:605–617.
23. Sheth RD, Drazkowski JF, Sirven JI *et al*. Protracted ictal confusion in elderly patients. *Arch Neurol* 2006; 63:529–532.
24. Tinuper P. The altered presentation of seizures in the elderly. In: Rowan AJ, Ramsey RE (eds) *Seizures and Epilepsy in the Elderly*. Boston: Butterworth-Heinemann, 1997, pp. 123–130.
25. Rowan AJ, Ramsay RE, Collins JF, Pryor F; the VA Cooperative Study 428 Group. New onset geriatric epilepsy: a randomized study of gabapentin, lamotrigine and carbamazepine. *Neurology* 2005; 64:1868–1873.
26. Hopkins A, Garman A, Clarke C. The first seizure in adult life: value of clinical features, electroencephalography and computerized tomographic scanning in prediction of seizure recurrence. *Lancet* 1988; 1:721–726.

27. Towne AR, Pellock JM, Ko D *et al.* Determinants of mortality in status epilepticus. *Epilepsia* 1994; 5:27–34.
28. Stolarek JH, Brodie A, Brodie MJ. Management of seizures in the elderly: a survey of UK Geriatricians. *J R Soc Med* 1995; 88:686–689.
29. Blake AJ, Morgan K, Bendall MJ *et al.* Falls by elderly people at home: prevalence and associated factors. *Age & Ageing* 1988; 17:365–372.
30. O'Loughlin JL, Robitaille Y, Boivin JF *et al.* Incidence of and risk factors for falls and injurious falls among the community-dwelling elderly. *Am J Epidemiol* 1993; 137:342–354.
31. Tinnetti ME, Speechley M, Ginter SF. Risk factors for falls among elderly persons living in the community. *N Engl J Med* 1988; 319:1701–1707.
32. Tinnetti ME, Williams CS. Falls, injuries due to falls, and the risk of admission to a nursing home. *N Engl J Med* 1997; 337:1279–1284.
33. Vestergaard P, Tigaran S, Rejnmark L *et al.* Fracture risk in epilepsy. *Acta Neurol Scand* 1999; 99:269–275.
34. Ehle AL, Johnson PC. Rapidly evolving EEG changes in a case of Alzheimer's disease. *Ann Neurol* 1977; 34:593–595.
35. Lee K, Pedley T. Electroencephalography and seizures in the elderly. In: Rowan AJ, Ramsay RE (eds) *Seizures and Epilepsy in the Elderly*. Boston: Butterworth-Heinemann, 1997, pp. 139–158.
36. Muller HF, Kral VA. The EEG in advanced senile dementia. *J Am Geriatr Soc* 1967; 15:415–426.
37. Otomo E. Electroencephalography in old age: dominant alpha rhythm. *Electrencephalogr Clin Neurophysiol* 1966; 21:489–491.
38. Roubicek J. The electroencephalogram in the middle aged and the elderly. *J Am Geriatr Soc* 1977; 25:145–152.
39. Silverman AJ, Busse EW, Barnes RH. Studies in the process of aging: electroencephalographic findings in 400 elderly subjects. *Electroencephalogr Clin Neurophysiol* 1955; 7:67–77.
40. Westmoreland BF, Klass DW. A distinctive rhythmic EEG discharge of adults. *Electroencephalogr Clin Neurophysiol* 1981; 51:186–191.
41. Westmoreland BF. Benign variants and patterns of uncertain clinical significance. In: Daly DD, Pedley TA (eds) *Current Practice of Clinical Electroencephalography*. 2nd edn. New York: Raven Press, 1990, pp. 243–252.
42. White JC, Langston JW, Pedley TA. Benign epileptiform transients of sleep: clarification of the small sharp spike controversy. *Neurology* 1977; 27:1061–1068.
43. Chatrian GE, Shaw CM, Leffman H. The significance of periodic lateralized epileptiform discharges in EEG. An electrographic, clinical, and pathological study. *Electroencephalogr Clin Neurophysiol* 1964; 17:177–193.
44. Zimmerman R. Diagnostic methods II: imaging studies. In: Rowan AJ, Ramsay RE (eds). *Seizures and Epilepsy in the Elderly*. Boston: Butterworth-Heinemann, 1997, pp. 159–177.
45. Zimmermann RD, Fleming CA, Lee BC *et al.* Periventricular hyperintensity as seen by magnetic resonance: prevalence and significance. *AJNR* 1986; 7:13–20.
46. Drayer BP. Imaging of the aging brain. Part I. Normal findings. *Radiology* 1988; 166:785–796.
47. Heier LA, Bauer CJ, Schwartz L *et al.* Large Virchow–Robin spaces: MR–clinical correlation. *AJNR* 1989; 10:929–936.
48. Heier LA. White matter disease in the elderly: vascular etiologies. *Neuroimaging Clin North Am* 1992; 2:441–445.
49. Bradley WG, Waluch V, Brandt-Zawadski M *et al.* Patchy periventricular white matter lesions in the elderly: a common observation during NMR imaging. *Noninvasive Med Imag* 1984; 1:35–41.
50. Awad IA, Spetzler RF, Hodak JA *et al.* Incidental subcortical lesions in the elderly. Correlation with age and cerebral vascular risk factors. *Stroke* 1986; 6:1084–1090.
51. Haider A, Tuchek J, Haider S. Seizure control: how to use the new antiepileptic drugs in older patients. *Geriatrics* 1996; 51:42–45.
52. Bergey, GK Initial treatment of epilepsy: special considerations in treating the elderly. *Neurology* 2004; 63:S40–S48
53. Mattson RH, Cramer JA, Collins JF. Department of Veterans Affairs Epilepsy Cooperative Study No 264. A comparison of valproate with carbamazepine for the treatment of complex partial seizures and secondarily generalized tonic–clonic seizures in adults. *N Engl J Med* 1992; 327:765–771.
54. Cameron H, Macphee GJ. Anticonvulsant therapy in the elderly – a need for placebo controlled trials. *Epilepsy Res* 1995; 21:149–157.

55. Cloyd JC, Lackner TE, Leppik IE. Antiepileptics in the elderly. Pharmacoepidemiology and pharmacokinetics. *Arch Fam Med* 1994; 3:589–598.

56. Leppik IE. Metabolism of antiepileptics medications: newborn to elderly. *Epilepsia* 1992; 33(Suppl 4):S32–S40.

57. McLean MJ. New antipiletic medications: pharmacokinetic and mechanistic considerations in the treatment of seizures and epilepsy in the elderly. In: Rowan AJ, Ramsey RE (eds) *Seizures and Epilepsy in the Elderly*. Boston: Butterworth-Heinemann, 1997, pp. 239–307.

58. Tallis R. Antiepileptic drug trials in the elderly: rationale, problems, and solutions. In: Rowan AJ, Ramsey RE (eds) *Seizures and Epilepsy in the Elderly*. Boston: Butterworth-Heinemann, 1997, pp. 311–320.

59. Pack AM, Morrell, MJ, Marcus R *et al*. Bone mass and turnover in women with epilepsy on antiepileptic drug monotherapy. *Ann Neurol* 2005; 57:252–257.

60. Craig I, Tallis R. Impact of valproate and phenytoin on cognitive function in elderly patients: results of a single-blind randomized comparative study. *Epilepsia* 1994; 35:381–390.

61. Brodie MJ, Overstall PW, Giorgi L. Multicentre double-blind, randomized comparison between lamotrigine and carbamazepine in elderly patients with newly diagnosed epilepsy. *Epilepsy Res* 1999; 37:81–84.

62. Sirven JI; VNS in the Elderly Study Group. Vagus nerve stimulation therapy for epilepsy in older adults. *Neurology* 2000; 54:1179–1182.

63. Sirven JI, Malamut BL, O'Connor MJ *et al*. Temporal lobectomy outcome in older versus younger adults. *Neurology* 2000; 54:2166–2170.

64. Malamut BL, Cloud B, Sirven JI *et al*. Neuropsychological and psychosocial outcome after unilateral temporal lobectomy over age 45 (Abstract). Neurology 1998; 50(Suppl 4):A202.

65. Grivas A, Schramm J, Kral T *et al*. Surgical treatment for refractory temporal lobe epilepsy in the elderly: seizure outcome and neuropsychological sequelae compared with a younger cohort. *Epilepsia* 2006; 47:1364–1372.

66. McLachlan RS, Chovaz CJ, Blume WT *et al*. Temporal lobectomy for intractable epilepsy in patients over age 45 years. *Neurology* 1992; 42:662–665.

67. Cascino GD, Sharbrough FW, Hirschorn KA *et al*. Surgery for focal epilepsy in the older patient. *Neurology* 1991; 41:1415–1417.

68. Medical Research Council Antiepileptic Drug Withdrawal Study Group. Randomised study of antiepileptic drug withdrawal in patients in remission. *Lancet* 1991; 337:1175–1180.

69. Harden CL, Pulver MC, Ravdin L *et al*. The effect of menopause and perimenopause on the course of epilepsy. *Epilepsia* 1999; 40:1402–1407.

70. Abassi F, Krumholtz A, Kittner SJ *et al*. Effects of menopause on seizures in women with epilepsy. *Epilepsia* 1999; 40:205–210.

Section IV

Idiopathic epilepsy

11

The treatment of idiopathic generalized epilepsy

Mar Carreño

INTRODUCTION

Idiopathic generalized epilepsies (IGEs) comprise a wide variety of generalized syndromes including variable combinations of absence, myoclonic and generalized tonic–clonic seizures. Within the IGEs, distinct entities are distinguished, based primarily on the predominant seizure types and the age of onset. Some syndromes are very well individualized, while others have less-clear boundaries [1]. As a group, IGEs have the highest rate of complete seizure control with anti-epileptic medication. Sodium valproate (VPA) is usually considered the drug of first choice; however, due to its teratogenicity [2, 3], VPA may not be suitable for women of childbearing age, and lamotrigine (LTG) has established itself as an interesting option in this special population of patients. Cosmetic and hormonal adverse effects of VPA may also make LTG preferable to VPA as the first-choice drug in young girls with IGE. Lamotrigine is also a very useful drug in IGE which does not respond to VPA, especially when used as add-on therapy to VPA. Other new AEDs that are proving to be efficacious include levetiracetam (LVT), topiramate (TPM) and zonisamide (ZNS). Some of the old AEDs still have an important role in the management of IGE. These include clobazam (CLB), clonazepam (CLZ) and ethosuximide (ETX) [4]. In this chapter, the available evidence regarding efficacy of the range of anti-epileptic drugs in the different syndromes of IGE will be reviewed, including the recommendations given by the American Academy of Neurology and the International League Against Epilepsy (ILAE).

There are several problems in obtaining good evidence-based data in idiopathic generalized epilepsy [5]:

- The fact that seizures in IGE are often readily controlled with monotherapy presents a problem in performing the type of controlled trial that will produce class I evidence, as the Food and Drug Administration in the USA will only approve one AED in monotherapy if a trial demonstrates superiority compared with another treatment (placebo, active control). In addition, this trial design is felt to be unethical, and recruitment for these trials in the USA is often difficult.
- Because of the good response to AEDs, it is difficult to demonstrate superior efficacy of a new AED over an established treatment. Large randomized trials are required to find a significant difference, and it is not easy to recruit such a large number of patients.
- Seizure frequency in IGE is generally much lower than that seen in patients who have refractory complex partial seizures. For this reason, if inclusion criteria require a high

Mar Carreño, MD, PhD, Director, Epilepsy Unit, Hospital Clínic de Barcelona, Barcelona, Spain

number of seizures, recruitment to sufficiently power the study may be difficult even in refractory patients.

- New anti-epileptic drugs felt to have broad spectrum are used to treat patients with IGE before formal indications are granted. This means that limited numbers of patients are available for well-designed clinical trials, and recruitment for such trials is challenging.
- IGE is less common than focal epilepsies in the adult population. Since the majority of the well-designed trials have been performed in adults, good-quality evidence is sparse for the treatment of IGE.
- A very relevant fact for clinical practice is that very few trials have examined the efficacy of AEDs in specific epilepsy syndromes, which is most important for the clinician and patient. Some of the more recently performed clinical trials focus on certain types of seizures (e.g. generalized tonic–clonic or myoclonic seizures) and include patients who may display several other seizure types, belonging to different epilepsy syndromes.
- Clinical and electroencephalogram (EEG) criteria for absence and idiopathic myoclonic seizures are reasonably well established; however, unless strict EEG criteria are used, patients with partial epilepsy and secondarily generalized tonic–clonic seizures may be included in some trials aimed at evaluating the efficacy of AEDs in primary generalized tonic–clonic seizures. Patients with atypical absence or symptomatic myoclonic seizures may also be included in trials recruiting refractory IGE patients.
- As in partial epilepsies, assessment of efficacy of AEDs involves counting seizures. Frequency of generalized tonic–clonic seizures is easy to assess, but absence and myoclonic seizures are less obvious to the patient and the observer and their frequency is more difficult to assess. However, not all studies in absence seizures have included electroencephalography to monitor 3-Hz spike and wave activity as a surrogate marker, and, in myoclonic seizures, patient self-reporting is still the mainstay, with all its limitations.
- It is unclear if results from trials including refractory IGE patients can extrapolate to the common patient with more responsive IGE.

This chapter focuses on well-controlled trials or large uncontrolled trials from which evidence-based recommendations for the treatment of IGE can be obtained. Selected class III and class IV data (Tables 11.1 and 11.2) will also be mentioned to illustrate the potential spectrum of action of a given AED. Recently, rigorous reviews of published data have been

Table 11.1 Categories of evidence [95]

Ia	Evidence from meta-analysis of randomized controlled trials
Ib	Evidence from at least one randomized controlled trial
IIa	Evidence from at least one controlled study without randomization
IIb	Evidence from at least one other type of quasi-experimental study
III	Evidence from non-experimental descriptive studies, such as comparative studies, correlation studies and case-controlled studies
IV	Evidence from expert committee reports or opinions and/or clinical experience of respected authorities
Level A	Based on class I evidence (efficacy or lack of efficacy)
Level B	Based on class II evidence or extrapolated from class I evidence (probably effective or ineffective)
Level C	Based on class III evidence (possibly effective or ineffective)
Level D	Based on class IV evidence
Level U	Inadequate or conflicting knowledge

Table 11.2 Categories of evidence used in the International League Against Epilepsy (ILAE) guidelines [10]

Class	Criteria
I	An RCT, or meta-analysis of RCTs, in a representative population that meets all six criteria: • Primary outcome variable: efficacy or effectiveness • Treatment duration: ≥48 weeks and information on ≥24-week seizure freedom data (efficacy) or ≥48-week retention data (effectiveness) • Study design: double-blind • Superiority demonstrated, or if no superiority demonstrated, the study's actual sample size was sufficient to show non-inferiority of no worse than a 20% relative difference in effectiveness/efficacy • Study exit: not forced by a predetermined number of treatment-emergent seizures • Appropiate statistical analysis
II	An RCT or meta-analysis meeting all the class I criteria except that: • No superiority was demonstrated and the study's actual sample size was sufficient only to show non-inferiority at a 21–30% relative difference in effectiveness/efficacy OR • Treatment duration: ≥24 weeks but <48 weeks
III	An RCT or meta-analysis not meeting the criteria for any class I or class II category (e.g. an open-label study or a double-blind study with either a detectable inferiority boundary of >30% or forced-exit criteria)
IV	Evidence from non-randomized, prospective, controlled or uncontrolled studies, case series or expert reports

RCT, randomized controlled trial.

performed in an attempt to provide guidelines. The American Academy of Neurology recently published two reports on reviews of the efficacy and tolerability of the new AEDs, for both recent-onset and refractory epilepsy [6–9]. In addition, the ILAE has also released treatment guidelines about evidence-based efficacy and effectiveness of AEDs as initial monotherapy for epileptic seizures and syndromes [10].

These guidelines use a level-of-evidence classification approach based on the United States Agency for Health Care and Policy Research and the American Academy of Neurology scoring system. Grading of recommendations included levels A (effective or ineffective), B (probably effective or ineffective) and C (possibly effective or ineffective). Requirements for each level of evidence vary depending on the guideline (Tables 11.1, 11.2 and 11.3).

TREATMENT OF CHILDHOOD ABSENCE EPILEPSY

Childhood absence epilepsy (CAE) typically requires treatment because the seizures are frequent and interfere with normal cognitive functioning.

INTERNATIONAL LEAGUE AGAINST EPILEPSY GUIDELINES (NEWLY DIAGNOSED EPILEPSY)

According to the ILAE guidelines, the absence of class I and class II randomized controlled trials (RCTs) for children with absence seizures implies a marked deficiency in adequately powered, seizure type-specific, published studies for this category, and no AEDs reach the highest level of evidence (level A or B) for efficacy/effectiveness for children with absence seizures (level C).

Table 11.3 Recommendations on treatment of specific IGE syndromes in AAN and ILAE guidelines

Syndrome	AAN (new AEDs in newly diagnosed epilepsy)	AAN (new AEDs in refractory epilepsy)	ILAE (all AEDs in newly diagnosed epilepsy)	
Juvenile myoclonic epilepsy	No level A or B recommendation	No level A or B recommendation	VPA, CLZ, LTG, LVT, TPM and ZNS may have some efficacy as initial monotherapy	Class IV studies (recommendation level D)
Absence epilepsy	LTG is effective in children with newly diagnosed absence seizures. Class II studies (recommendation level B)	No level A or B recommendation for refractory absence epilepsy	ETX, LTG, VPA possibly efficacious/effective for children with absence seizures. May be considered as initial monotherapy, individualized prescription encouraged	Class III studies (recommendation level C)
GTC seizures	No recommendation for new-onset GTC seizures (insufficient data to make a recommendation for the syndromes individually). LTG, TPM and OXC are effective in a mixed population of newly diagnosed partial and GTC seizures	TPM may be used for the treatment of refractory GTC seizures in adults and children (recommendation level A)	*Adults* CBZ, LTG, OXC, PHB, PHT, TPM, VPA possibly efficacious/effective as initial monotherapy for adults with GTC seizures CBZ, OXC and PHT may precipitate or aggravate GTC seizures and more commonly other generalized seizure types in patients with GTC seizures and these drugs should be used with caution in these patients	Class III studies (recommendation level C) Class IV studies
			Children CBZ, PHB, PHT, TPM and VPA are possibly efficacious/effective for children with GTC seizures and may be considered for initial monotherapy. Individualized treatment encouraged	Class III studies (recommendation level C)
			CBZ, OXC, PHT may precipitate or aggravate GTC seizures and, more commonly, other generalized seizure types in patients with GTC seizures	Class IV studies

CBZ, carbamazepine; CLZ, clonazepam; ETX, ethosuximide; GTC, generalized-onset tonic–clonic; LVT, levetiracetam; OXC, oxcarbazepine; PHB, phenobarbital, PHT, phenytoin; TPM, topiramate; VPA, valproate; ZNS, zonisamide.

Based on RCT efficacy and effectiveness evidence, ETX, LTG and VPA are possibly efficacious/effective for children with absence seizures (level C):

- ETX had similar efficacy/effectiveness to VPA.
- LTG had superior efficacy to placebo and slower onset of efficacy compared with VPA.
- VPA had similar efficacy/effectiveness to ETX and faster onset of efficacy compared with LTG.

Based on these data, the ILAE recommends that ETX, LTG and VPA may be considered as candidates for initial monotherapy in children with newly diagnosed or untreated absence seizures. Among these three AEDs, no clear first-choice AED exists based only on efficacy or effectiveness criteria.

AMERICAN ACADEMY OF NEUROLOGY GUIDELINES (NEW AEDs ONLY)

American Academy of Neurology (AAN) guidelines evaluating efficacy of new AEDs state only that LTG is effective in children with newly diagnosed absence seizures (level B recommendation).

ETHOSUXIMIDE

After ETX was described as effective in absence epilepsy in 1958, a number of open-label, non-comparative studies where ETX was added to existing treatment followed. However, at that time epilepsy syndromes were still poorly defined and trial methodology was not well developed. The overall seizure-free rate for these studies was 52%. There is one single-blinded, comparative, non-randomized study with placebo in untreated patients [11]. One week of placebo preceded 8 weeks of treatment with ETX. Fourteen of the 37 recruited patients had, in addition to clinically defined absence seizures, other seizure types. Absence seizures were controlled in seven patients. All these studies were poorly designed and they did not clearly show the percentage of patients with absence seizures which responded to ETX [12].

SODIUM VALPROATE

Sodium valproate has been assessed in several open, non-comparative studies, in which the seizure-free rate has varied from 88% to 95% [13–16]. Seven children with absence seizures were treated with VPA, and all but one became seizure free [17]. Twenty-four-hour electroencephalography was performed before and during treatment. A dose–response relationship was suggested by the authors regarding reduction of spike–wave discharges, but the number of patients was too small to draw any conclusions [12].

Two single-blind, placebo-controlled trials with VPA have been published [12]. Both included a period of placebo followed by a 10-week period of treatment with VPA. In the study by Villarreal et al., involving 25 adult patients with absence seizures (some with other seizure types and some receiving other AEDs), 10-week treatment with VPA resulted in 75% or greater reduction in spike and wave EEG discharges in 46% of patients [18]. Nineteen patients had fewer absence seizures, which seemed to correlate with serum levels reaching 50–60 µg/ml. Another study, involving mainly children with refractory seizures, showed that 82% of children had at least a 75% reduction in the number of absence seizures. There was no correlation between plasma levels of VPA and response [19].

A double-blind study comparing ETX with VPA looked at a treatment-naive group and a group of patients who were refractory to treatment with ETX [20]. The main outcome measure was the frequency and duration of 3-Hz spike and wave discharges with 12-h electroencephalography. A crossover design was used, in which VPA and ETX were switched if the previously treatment-naive untreated group failed to achieve 100% control or the refractory group failed to achieve 80% of seizure control. There was a good response to treatment with either drug in the newly diagnosed group that was accompanied by reductions in spike and wave discharges. In the refractory group, 3 of 15 patients responded to VPA and 4 of the 14 patients responded to ETX. There was no statistically significant difference in efficacy between ETX and VPA or in reduction of spike and wave discharges. Pitfalls of these studies include the small number of patients and the fact that the design was not a true crossover, as patients who responded to the initial drug were not crossed over [12].

An add-on, comparative study of ETX and VPA in 35 patients with mainly absence seizures found no significant differences between the drugs [21]. By counting attacks (without EEG monitoring), they found improvement in 81% of patients in the VPA group and 71% of patients in the ETX group. Another comparative, randomized, but not blinded, study found no significant difference in efficacy between the drugs [22]. Increased efficacy with the combination of ETX and VPA combination treatment was claimed in a small open-label study where neither drug alone proved effective [23]. This was thought to be due partly to a pharmacokinetic interaction, because VPA inhibits the metabolism of ETX, increasing the serum concentrations.

Common clinical practice is to choose VPA in patients with both absence and generalized tonic–clonic (GTC) seizures. And because 50% of patients with childhood absence epilepsy will develop GTC seizures, it can be argued that VPA is preferable because of its broader spectrum [1].

An ongoing study (National Institutes of Health CAE trial) is analyzing the comparative efficacy and tolerability of VPA, LTG and ETX in patients with newly diagnosed absence seizures.

BENZODIAZEPINES

The benzodiazepine that has been more studied in the treatment of absence epilepsy is clonazepam [12]. CZP was found to be superior to placebo in a single-blind, crossover study with 10 refractory patients. Eight of 10 patients became seizure free [24].

LAMOTRIGINE

One double-blind, placebo-controlled study of patients (aged 3–15) was not a pure initial monotherapy trial, but rather a conditional, randomized conversion to placebo double-blind trial [25]. In the study, 45 patients entered an open-label dose-escalation phase of LTG lasting 5–25 weeks followed by a 4-week double-blind placebo-controlled phase in which patients with well-controlled absence seizures were randomized either to continue LTG at their current dose or to be weaned to placebo. Overall, 28 patients were randomized to LTG ($n = 14$) or placebo ($n = 14$). The proportion of patients remaining seizure free during the double-blind treatment phase was greater for LTG (61%) compared with placebo (21%) ($P = 0.03$). The AAN rated the evidence provided by this study as class II, due to the enriched design. ILAE guidelines consider this class III evidence due to the design and short duration of the double-blind phase.

One study of LTG as first-line therapy included 20 children with childhood absence seizures. After a mean follow-up of 10.8 months, 11 of 20 were seizure free, with another four having a greater than 50% decrease in seizure frequency [26]. LTG and VPA were compared in an open-label study involving 38 patients who were randomized to either VPA ($n = 19$) or LTG ($n = 19$) and followed for 1 year. At the end of 12 months, no statistical difference in seizure-free rates was found between the two groups, although VPA acted faster in achieving seizure freedom [27].

One meta-analysis [28] examined AED efficacy and effectiveness for children with absence seizures. This compared ETX, VPA and LTG with a focus on four end-points: proportion of seizure-free children at 1, 6 and 18 months after randomization; children with ≥50% reduction in seizure frequency; normalization of the EEG; and adverse effects.

The majority of data used in this meta-analysis were from class III studies. The meta-analysis found insufficient evidence to inform clinical practice.

TOPIRAMATE

A small open-label trial of TPM in five children with typical absence (untreated or unsuccessfully treated) reported one previously untreated child becoming seizure free, two improved at low dose (6 mg/kg/day) but not at higher doses, and two children (one previously untreated) showed no significant improvement [29].

LEVETIRACETAM

In an open-label study, LVT was administered to four patients with childhood absence epilepsy (as initial monotherapy in one and as add-on therapy in three). Three patients became seizure free and one patient had 50–75% seizure reduction. Clinical improvement was accompanied by a reduction or disappearance of generalized spike and wave discharges [30].

ZONISAMIDE

Because of its multiple mechanisms of action, ZNS is thought to be a potentially broad-spectrum agent with efficacy for seizure types other than partial seizures. A recent retrospective, chart review study examined 15 patients with absence seizures, most of whom (89%) had received previous AED therapy [31]. Of these patients, 51% reported seizure freedom with ZNS. This study, however, does not provide details as to whether the absences were typical or atypical, and no syndromic classification is provided. Several abstracts provide some suggestion that ZNS may have some efficacy for absence seizures [32, 33]. In summary, there are no well-controlled studies and many of the published reports are preliminary reports of small numbers of patients.

COMMON CLINICAL PRACTICE

First-line drugs to treat absence epilepsy are ETX, VPA and LTG, alone or in combination. Maximum tolerated doses must be reached before switching to a second monotherapy. When choosing the first drug, it is important to consider if the patient has only absence seizures or has other generalized seizure types in addition. Sodium valproate controls absences in 75% of patients and also has the advantage of controlling generalized tonic–clonic seizures (70%) and myoclonic jerks (75%). LTG may control absences in possibly 50–60%, but may worsen myoclonic jerks [34]. ETX controls 70% of absences but it is undesirable as monotherapy if the patient has other types of generalized seizures. Small doses of LTG added to VPA may have a dramatic beneficial effect. CLZ and CLB are second-line drugs for absence epilepsy; their use is limited by their adverse effects (mainly somnolence) and the development of tolerance in a significant proportion of patients. CLZ may be useful as adjunctive drug especially in absences with myoclonic components. Carbamazepine (CBZ), vigabatrin (VGB), gabapentin (GBP) and tiagabine (TGB) are contraindicated because they may exacerbate absence seizures. Phenytoin (PHT) and phenobarbital (PB) are contraindicated because of their usual inefficacy. The place of TPM, LVT and ZNS is still unknown. Gradual withdrawal of medication is recommended in patients with absence seizures who are seizure free for 1–2 years and have a normalized EEG. EEG confirmation of the seizure-free state is needed during this withdrawal period [35].

TREATMENT OF JUVENILE ABSENCE EPILEPSY

Trial data regarding juvenile absence epilepsy (JAE) are scarce; however, JAE is regarded as similar to CAE, and VPA and ETX are suggested as effective treatments. One case series of patients with JAE and CAE found that 85% of the JAE patients responded to VPA, ETX or both [36]. In this series, the response was better in JAE than in CAE. Combination with myoclonic seizures did not affect the response to therapy. As GTC seizures are common in patients with JAE, VPA is usually considered the drug of choice. In the rare instances where the absences in this syndrome do not respond to VPA, or when there is concern about teratogenicity, LTG can be given, as shown in a study including patients with absence seizures starting during both childhood and adolescence [37], although onset of action may be slower compared with VPA [27].

TREATMENT OF IGE WITH GTC SEIZURES ONLY

The syndrome of primary GTC seizures presents the clinician with nosologic, diagnostic and treatment difficulties. Some patients with IGE appear to have GTC seizures alone and the 1989 ILAE epilepsy classification individualized epilepsy with grand mal seizures on awakening and epilepsies with specific modes of precipitation [38]. The evolving classification of IGE uses more inclusive terms such as IGE with GTC seizures only [39] and IGE with pure grand mal seizures [40]. This common syndrome is typically characterized by GTC seizures only and is probably the same as GTC seizures on awakening, in which seizures are not limited to the morning. When other seizure types exist in these IGEs, the seizures can clinically include mixed features, giving rise to confusing names [1].

The assumption is that such GTC seizures will respond to AEDs that have been demonstrated to be of benefit in partial and secondary generalized seizures. It is difficult to assess the evidence for this group, because many studies for GTC seizures have not specifically included patients with IGE or have included patients with IGE who, in addition to GTC seizures, had other seizure types and probably a variety of IGE syndromes. Because GTC seizures overlap with other IGE syndromes, the use of some drugs, for example PHT or CBZ, could result in suboptimal control [12]. This view is reflected in the recently released guidelines from the ILAE [10]. Greater understanding of this syndrome as an entity and subsequent drug studies will improve evidence for optimum treatment.

ILAE GUIDELINES (NEWLY DIAGNOSED EPILEPSY)

ILAE guidelines state that CBZ, LTG, OXC, PH, PHT, TPM and VPA are possibly efficacious/ effective as initial monotherapy for adults with GTC seizures and may be considered for initial therapy in selected situations (recommendation level C). In children with GTC seizures, CBZ, PB, PHT, TPM, and VPA are possibly efficacious/effective and may be considered for initial monotherapy. No clear first choice exists; individualized prescription is encouraged. However, the guidelines state that CBZ, OXC and PHT may also precipitate or aggravate GTC seizures and, more commonly, other generalized seizure types in patients with primary GTC seizures and therefore these drugs should be used with caution in these patients.

AAN GUIDELINES (NEW AEDs ONLY)

The AAN guidelines state that TPM is effective for the treatment of refractory GTC seizures in adults and children (recommendation level A). A small study with LTG used as add-on therapy in patients with refractory IGE and a combination of seizure types is mentioned in the guidelines. However, LTG is not mentioned in the 'summary of evidence' of the guidelines.

SODIUM VALPROATE

A recent review of generalized epilepsy with GTC seizures only [41] suggested that counselling to patients with primary GTC seizures should be the same as in JME. The patient needs to avoid clear triggering factors such as sleep deprivation, photic stimulation and excessive alcohol intake. The pharmacological sensitivity is probably the same as in JME, with a selective efficacy of VPA [42]. One review on treatment options in IGE does not clearly separate this syndrome from JME and other IGE syndromes and stresses the first-line place of VPA [43]. One meta-analysis found no evidence to support the use of VPA vs. CBZ as the treatment of choice for patients with GTC seizures as part of generalized epilepsy. However, the number of patients in the GTC seizure subgroup was small and confidence intervals were wide, so the authors considered that they had not been able to exclude the existence of an important therapeutic difference [44].

PHENOBARBITAL

There is one case series suggesting efficacy for PB for patients with idiopathic GTC seizures that began in childhood and persisted into adulthood [45].

LAMOTRIGINE

LTG showed potential in the treatment of primary GTC seizures on the basis of pre-clinical data, case reports and case series, open-label and randomized, double-blind, active-comparator clinical trials that enrolled patients with newly diagnosed primary or secondarily GTC seizures. Biton *et al.* evaluated the efficacy and tolerability of adjunctive LTG in primary GTC seizures in a randomized, double-blind, placebo-controlled trial [46]. Patients with a diagnosis of epilepsy with GTC seizures (with or without other types of generalized seizures) who were receiving one or two anti-epileptic drugs at study entry were eligible. Patients were required to have at least three primary GTC seizures during the 8-week baseline period. Patients with partial seizures were excluded on the basis of seizure history and screening EEGs. The study comprised a baseline phase, an escalation phase, during which study medication was titrated to a target dose, and a 12-week maintenance phase, during which doses of LTG/placebo and concomitant AEDs were maintained. Of the 121 randomized patients aged between 2 and 55 years, 117 (58 lamotrigine, 59 placebo) entered the escalation phase and received study medication. It is important to mention that 31% of patients had absence seizures, 29% had myoclonic seizures and 9% had tonic seizures in addition to GTC seizures.

During the escalation and maintenance phases combined, median per cent reduction in primary GTC seizure frequency was 66.5% with LTG compared with 34.2% with placebo ($P = 0.006$). The corresponding numbers for LTG and placebo were 60.6% and 32.8% ($P = 0.038$) during the escalation phase and 81.9% and 43.0% ($P = 0.006$) during the maintenance phase. During the maintenance phase, 72% of LTG-treated patients compared with 49% of placebo-treated patients experienced a $\geq 50\%$ reduction in frequency of primary GTC seizures ($P = 0.014$). A similar pattern of results was observed for all generalized seizures. The most common drug-related adverse events were dizziness (5% LTG, 2% placebo), somnolence (5% LTG, 2% placebo) and nausea (5% LTG, 3% placebo).

TOPIRAMATE

The efficacy of TPM in primary GTC seizures was shown in a double-blind, randomized, placebo-controlled trial [47]. Eighty patients (aged 3–59 years) with a diagnosis of primary GTC seizures (with or without other types of generalized seizures), who had at least three GTC seizures during an 8-week baseline phase (in spite of treatment with one or two

AEDs) were randomly assigned to treatment with either TPM ($n = 39$) or placebo ($n = 41$). Approximately 70% of patients had other types of generalized seizures (absence, myoclonic or tonic seizures). A more detailed syndromic classification was not made, but EEG findings suggestive of generalized epilepsy, without other significant findings, were required to be included in the study. TPM was titrated to target doses of approximately 6 mg/kg/day over 8 weeks and maintained for another 12 weeks. The median percentage reduction from baseline in primary GTC seizure rate was 56.7% for TPM and 9.0% for placebo ($P = 0.019$). The proportion of patients with 50% or higher reduction in primary GTC seizure rate was 22/39 (56%) and 8/40 (20%) for the TPM and placebo groups respectively ($P = 0.001$). The median percentage reduction in the rate of all generalized seizures was 42.1% for TPM patients and 0.9% for placebo patients ($P = 0.003$). The proportions of patients with 50% or higher reduction in generalized seizure rate were 18/39 (46%) and 7/41 (17%) for the TPM and placebo groups respectively ($P = 0.003$). Thirteen per cent of TPM-treated patients and 5% of placebo-treated patients became free of GTC seizures, but this difference was not statistically significant. The most common adverse events were somnolence, fatigue, weight loss, difficulty with memory and nervousness.

In an open label study [48], TPM was administered to 131 adults and children with refractory GTC seizures of non-focal origin who had completed double-blinded trials. The mean duration of open-label TPM treatment was 387 days (range 14–909 days); the mean TPM dose was 7 mg/kg/day (range 1–16 mg/kg/day). At the last study visit, the frequency of GTC seizures was reduced by ≥50% from baseline in 63% of patients and by ≥75% in 44%. Among patients treated ≥6 months, 16% were free of GTC seizures for ≥6 months despite a pre-treatment seizure frequency of one GTC seizures/week (median). Treatment with TPM was being continued in 82% of patients ($n = 107$) at the last visit. During treatment periods of up to 2.5 years, 11 (8%) patients discontinued TPM because of adverse events and seven (5%) because of inadequate seizure control.

LEVETIRACETAM

A recent study [49] explored the efficacy of LVT to treat refractory primary GTC seizures. The trial included 164 patients with a diagnosis of IGE and refractory primary GTC seizures in spite of treatment with stable doses of one or two AEDs. A minimum number of three GTC seizures during the 8-week baseline period was required to be included in the study. It was a double-blind, randomized, placebo-controlled, parallel-group and multicentre study. Patients were randomized to received add-on LVT (80 patients) or placebo (84 patients). There was a 4-week titration phase, followed by a 20-week maintenance phase and a 6-week down-titration phase. Mean percentage reduction in number of GTC seizures per week was 77.6% in the LVT group compared with 44.6% in the placebo group ($P = 0.004$). The percentage of responders (patients who experienced a reduction of at least 50% in frequency of seizures per week) during the treatment period was 72.2% in the LVT group compared with 45.2% in the placebo group ($P = 0.0005$). A significant number of patients (24.1%) became seizure free in the LVT group, compared with 8.3% in the placebo group ($P = 0.009$). The safety profile of LVT was similar to that observed in previous studies, with 1.3% withdrawing from the study because of adverse effects compared with 4.8% in the placebo group.

ZONISAMIDE

In a preliminary report on patients with refractory primary generalized epilepsy treated with ZNS [33], two of four patients with tonic–clonic seizures had a greater than 50% reduction in seizures. No mention was made of whether any patients became seizure free. In summary, although there are suggestions that ZNS may have efficacy for primary GTC seizures, there are no well-controlled studies and the published reports include small numbers of patients [5].

COMMON CLINICAL PRACTICE

When clear triggering factors such as sleep deprivation, photic stimulation or excessive alcohol intake have been identified, specific measures to avoid them should be adopted by the patient, as in JME [41]. The pharmacological sensitivity is probably the same as in JME, with VPA being the first-line treatment, together with LTG, TPM and possibly LVT. Zonisamide may be another option in the future.

TREATMENT OF JUVENILE MYOCLONIC EPILEPSY

ILAE Guidelines (Newly Diagnosed Epilepsy)

Despite being a relatively common syndrome, there are no randomized trials reporting efficacy or effectiveness as a primary outcome measure in newly diagnosed JME. VPA has long been regarded as the drug of choice to treat this condition.

> 'In the absence of class I, class II and class III RCTs for patients with JME, class IV studies suggest that CZP, LTG, LVT, TPM, VPA and ZNS may have some efficacy for patients with newly diagnosed JME. Among these AEDs, no clear first-choice AED exists for initial monotherapy in patients with newly diagnosed or untreated JME based solely on efficacy or effectiveness. Selection of the initial AED therapy for a patient with newly diagnosed JME requires integration of patient-specific, AED-specific, and nation-specific variables that can affect overall response to therapy.' [10]

AAN Guidelines (New AEDs)

No syndrome-specific recommendation is made for JME.

SODIUM VALPROATE

In spite of the lack of controlled studies of VPA on JME, this drug continues to be the choice of treatment for JME. In special populations such as women of childbearing age, VPA may be less suitable as the first option because of its potential teratogenicity [2, 3].

Evidence for VPA effectiveness in the treatment of JME mainly consists of case series that have demonstrated good responses, with seizure-free rates ranging from 54% to 93% [50–54]. Some studies have reported that seizures in some patients can be controlled with VPA doses as low as 500 mg daily [55, 56], showing that some patients with IGE are sensitive to a small dose of an effective medication. This may be important when considering the teratogenic potential of VPA, as a dose effect has been observed in some studies [3, 57]. Another study tried to show a dose–response relationship with VPA. Sixteen patients with JME were given two different doses of VPA (1000 mg or 2000 mg daily) in a randomized, double-blind, crossover study [58]. Each patient spent 6 months taking the high or low dose before switching, and there was no significant difference in seizure frequency between the two doses [12].

BENZODIAZEPINES

One trial studied the efficacy of CZP as add-on treatment in 17 patients with JME [59]. Myoclonic jerks were controlled in 15 patients and the remaining two experienced a 75% reduction in seizure frequency. However, CZP only controlled GTC seizures in 6/14 patients who had this type of seizure before entering the study. While being treated with CZP, another patient without a history of GTC seizures had a convulsion [12].

LAMOTRIGINE

It is not established whether LTG is beneficial for idiopathic myoclonic seizures such as those associated with JME [5]. Open-label studies suggest that LTG may benefit all three types of seizures in IGE: GTC, myoclonic and absence. When used in 12 patients with JME experiencing side-effects of VPA [60], LTG used in monotherapy controlled all seizure types in five patients. VPA could not be withdrawn in three patients because of re-emergence of myoclonus. Two patients had successful pregnancies while taking LTG. The authors concluded that LTG is a useful alternative in the management of JME.

Morris *et al.* [61], in an open-label study, studied 63 patients with JME who failed previous treatment with VPA. During treatment with LTG, 44% patients became free of GTC seizures, 33% free of myoclonic seizures and 60% free of absence seizures. Fourteen per cent of patients had a >50% increase in myoclonic seizures. This worsening of myoclonic seizures induced by LTG in a subset of patients with JME has been reported in several series of patients [34, 62, 63]. It is not clear if these patients have some distinguishing features or represent some genetic heterogeneity [5].

Prasad *et al.* [64] compared the efficacy of VPA, LTG, TPM, PHT or CBZ in a retrospective cohort study of 72 patients with JME. Seizure control was similar in patients taking VPA or LTG monotherapy, and VPA polytherapy was similar in terms of seizure control to LTG polytherapy. VPA, LTG and TPM, when compared with PHT or CBZ, demonstrated significantly better control of myoclonic seizures but not of GTC seizures.

LEVETIRACETAM

Open-label studies in patients with refractory primary generalized seizures suggest efficacy particularly in tonic–clonic and myoclonic seizures [65, 66]. The study by Betts *et al.* included 30 patients with refractory primary generalized epilepsy, with 43% and 30% of patients achieving seizure freedom for 6 and 12 months respectively. The series of 55 refractory patients included in the study by Krauss *et al.* [66] had 63%, 85% and 34% reduction in monthly GTC, myoclonic and absence seizures respectively [5].

A recently completed trial of LVT (3000 mg/day) in IGE in adolescents and adults fulfils class I evidence for myoclonic seizures [67]. This was a double-blind, randomized, placebo-controlled trial of 122 patients. These patients continued to have myoclonic seizures in spite of stable doses of one AED. To be included in the study, patients were required to have 8 days with myoclonus during the 8-week baseline period. Responder rate was 58.3% in the LVT group compared with 23.3% in the placebo group ($P = 0.002$). Thirteen out of 61 patients taking LVT had complete control of myoclonic seizures compared with 2 out of 60 patients taking placebo.

TOPIRAMATE

There are no class I or II data for the use of TPM in myoclonic seizures. Sixteen patients with myoclonic seizures were included in one class I study, including patients with primary GTC seizures [47]. However, no conclusions (other than lack of worsening) could be made. In the open-label portion of the study, 67% of the patients with myoclonic seizures were responders. One study reported outcome of a subset of 22 patients with JME included in two controlled trials aimed to study the efficacy and tolerability of TPM in primary GTC seizures. Eight out of 11 TPM-treated patients (73%) had at least 50% reduction in the number of GTC seizures, compared with 2/11 placebo-treated patients (18%) ($P = 0.03$). Reductions in myoclonic, absence and total generalized seizures were also observed, although TPM vs. placebo differences did not achieve statistical significance [68].

A recent study reported 28 patients who were randomized (unblinded) to VPA or TPM therapy for JME. Nineteen patients were randomized to TPM and nine patients to VPA.

Among patients completing 26 weeks of treatment, 8 of 12 (67%) in the TPM group and 4 of 7 (57%) in the VPA group were seizure free during the 12-week maintenance period. Median daily dose was 250 mg TPM or 750 mg VPA [69].

In a review of 72 consecutive patients with JME receiving VPA, LTG, TPM, PHT or CBZ [61], TPM provided good control of GTC seizures (<1 seizure per year) in three of four patients on monotherapy and 9 of 11 patients on polytherapy including TPM [5]. Relative control of myoclonic seizures (defined as <5 seizures or clusters/month) was achieved with TPM monotherapy in three of four patients and 8 of 15 patients on TPM polytherapy. TPM monotherapy did not benefit one patient with JME and absence seizures; TPM polypharmacy provided good (<5 seizures a month) control in three of five patients.

ZONISAMIDE

In a preliminary report of patients with refractory primary generalized epilepsy [33] treated with ZNS, two of three patients with myoclonic seizures had a >50% reduction in seizures. On a database review of patients with JME treated with LTG, TPM and ZNS, four patients were on ZNS [70]. Generalized tonic–clonic seizures were substantially reduced, but myoclonic seizures increased in these patients on ZNS, while absence seizures remained unchanged. One retrospective study looked into the efficacy and tolerability of ZNS in the treatment of JME [71]. Fifteen patients taking ZNS as monotherapy (13 patients) or as add-on treatment to VPA (two patients) were included in the study. Overall, 80% of patients on ZNS monotherapy showed good control, defined as ≥50% seizure reduction. Mean follow up was 12 months. Sixty-nine per cent, 62% and 38% of patients were free of GTC, myoclonic, and absence seizures, respectively.

Another recent retrospective study [72] analysed the efficacy of ZNS as add-on treatment in seven patients with refractory JME. Six patients had a history of GTC seizures. Five of six patients had ≥50% reduction in frequency of GTC seizures, with two patients becoming free of this seizure type. Six patients had active myoclonus when started on ZNS. All six patients had ≥50% reduction in myoclonus, and two became free of this seizure type. Of the four patients who were having absence seizures when ZNS was started, all four experienced ≥50% reduction in seizure frequency, and one became free of absences. These results were sustained over more prolonged follow-up in five of seven patients, with one patient improving further over time. Four patients initially had minor side-effects that resolved during the maintenance period. The authors concluded that ZNS may be effective and well tolerated as add-on therapy in patients with refractory JME.

COMMON CLINICAL PRACTICE

In JME, counselling on lifestyle is essential. The importance of regular sleep habits must be stressed, and drinks containing excessive caffeine should not be consumed in the evening. Excessive alcohol intake must be avoided also [73]. If patients are photosensitive, they should avoid relevant visual stimuli and wear dark glasses in brightly lit surroundings. Such measures will decrease the necessity of high-dose medical treatment, but the use of AEDs is still necessary [73]. As mentioned earlier, total control of seizures on VPA monotherapy may be achieved in up to 84% of patients [73]. Daily dosage in adults ranges between 1000 and 2000 mg, although some patients may be controlled on significantly lower doses and theoretically 'sub-therapeutic' blood levels. If an extended-release formulation is used, the whole daily dose may be given in the evening. CZP may also be useful, best in association with VPA. Among newer AEDs, LTG is often used in association with VPA and LVT has shown its efficacy against myoclonic and also GTC seizures. LTG is an interesting option when VPA causes significant side-effects or when there is concern about teratogenicity (women of fertile age). TPM and ZNS may be useful, especially in drug-resistant patients.

There is a widespread belief that lifelong treatment is mandatory in JME because of very frequent relapses at attempts to terminate treatment. If the decision is made for long-term maintenance of treatment, low-dose controlled-release VPA with a single evening intake may be an adequate option [73].

AGGRAVATION OF SEIZURES IN IGE

Unlike partial seizures, seizures in IGE seem to be more vulnerable to aggravation by AEDs. Aggravation may consist of increase in seizure frequency or appearance of new seizure types. Many patients with IGE who are not controlled with AEDs are not truly intractable, but instead have been treated with appropriate AEDs (pseudo-refractoriness) [1]. Before seizure exacerbation can be attributed to an AED, one has to exclude other possible factors such as spontaneous fluctuations in the number of seizures, poor compliance, co-morbid illnesses and medications, increase in precipitating factors and development of tolerance to a previously efficacious AED [74]:

CLINICAL EVIDENCE FOR AGGRAVATION OF GENERALIZED EPILEPSIES

To support the hypothesis that seizure aggravation is due to the effect of one or several AEDs, certain conditions need to be fulfilled [74]:

- Seizure aggravation is seen soon after initiation of therapy.
- An increase in dosage is followed by further seizure exacerbation.
- When the dose is lowered, seizure frequency decreases or new seizure types disappear.
- A rechallenge with the drug results again in seizure aggravation.

Most often these conditions are not fulfilled; in particular a rechallenge is usually not done, as it is deemed unethical. Evidence of seizure aggravation can also be provided by objective data, including seizure quantification in placebo-controlled trials aimed at demonstrating efficacy and tolerability of a drug. However, most controlled trials are performed in partial epilepsies, and most data on aggravation of generalized seizures are based on anecdotal case reports, case series or uncontrolled, open-label or retrospective studies. For all these reasons, one has to be cautious when interpreting these data. ILAE guidelines also make some statements regarding seizure aggravation by certain AEDs [74].

CARBAMAZEPINE

ILAE Guidelines

Class IV evidence suggests that CBZ may precipitate or aggravate GTC seizures and more commonly other generalized seizure types in patients with IGE and therefore should be used with caution in these patients [10]. Based solely on scattered reports (class IV), CBZ may precipitate or aggravate absence seizures [10]. Class IV studies indicate that CBZ may precipitate or aggravate myoclonic seizures [75–78].

CBZ may worsen absence seizures and may trigger status epilepticus in patients with absence epilepsy [79–82]. Absence seizures may also reappear or appear *de novo* with CBZ.

CBZ has also been implicated in the aggravation of generalized convulsive seizures and in precipitating absence, myoclonic and generalized status in patients with IGE [75, 83–86]. CBZ also aggravates myoclonic seizures. In a retrospective, uncontrolled study, CBZ was said to aggravate seizures in over 65% of patients with JME [40].

PHENYTOIN

ILAE Guidelines

Based on class IV studies, PHT may precipitate or aggravate GTC seizures, absence and myoclonic seizures [10] and should be used with caution in these patients [76, 77]. PHT may worsen absence and myoclonic seizures, and may provoke absence and generalized status in patients with IGE [80, 82, 86]. In one retrospective study, aggravation of seizures was reported in one-third of patients with JME to whom PHT was prescribed [40].

OXCARBAZEPINE

OXC is similar to CBZ and has been reported to cause exacerbation or appearance of new seizure types in IGE, mainly absence and myoclonus. In spite of class IV evidence, cautious use in patients with IGE is recommended in the ILAE guidelines [10].

BARBITURATES

Phenobarbital (PB) has been reported to induce *de novo* atypical absence seizures [87].
   ILAE guidelines include PB in the list of AEDs which may worsen absence seizures based on scattered, class IV reports [10].

VIGABATRIN

Vigabatrin (VGB) aggravates absence and myoclonic seizures; *de novo* myoclonic seizures, absence and convulsive status induced by VGB have been reported [85, 88]. ILAE guidelines recommend cautious use in absence epilepsy based on class IV scattered reports.

LAMOTRIGINE

Although LTG is effective in IGE and in most epileptic myoclonus, some reports have suggested that it may occasionally worsen or trigger *de novo* myoclonic seizures. In open-label studies of LTG monotherapy for JME, some patients experienced a worsening in myoclonus, which was transient in some [34]. This study is mentioned in the ILAE guidelines [10]. Five patients with IGE treated with LTG experienced exacerbation or *de novo* appearance of myoclonic jerks. In three patients, LTG exacerbated myoclonus in a dose-dependent manner with early aggravation during titration. Myoclonus disappeared when LTG dose was decreased by 25% to 50%. In two patients, LTG exacerbated myoclonic jerks in a delayed but more severe manner, with the appearance of myoclonic status that only ceased after LTG withdrawal [89].

GABAPENTIN

Gabapentin (GBP) has been implicated in worsening and *de novo* appearance of new-onset myoclonus [74]. In an open-label study of GBP as add-on therapy, new-onset myoclonus was seen in around 10% of cases. However, this series included patients with focal epilepsy [90]. Thomas *et al.*, in their series of status epilepticus induced by AEDs, included one patient with atypical absence status with eyelid myoclonia when GBP was started and CBZ increased [86]. GBP is included in the list of AEDs which may precipitate or aggravate absence seizures and myoclonic seizures according to class IV evidence in the ILAE guidelines.

TIAGABINE

As with other GABA-ergic AEDs, seizure exacerbation induced by tiagabine (TGB) has been reported, mainly in IGE [74]. This includes aggravation and *de novo* appearance of absence seizures and even absence status. TGB may also aggravate myoclonic seizures [91, 92]. TGB may precipitate or aggravate myoclonic seizures according to the ILAE guidelines (class IV studies) [10].

COMMON CLINICAL PRACTICE

In spite of poor-quality data, when treating patients with IGE, the possibility of seizure aggravation induced by AEDs has to be considered. It is critical to make a correct syndromic diagnosis and identify all seizure types. If this is not possible, a broad-spectrum AED should be used. Patients with multiple seizure types seem to be especially prone to seizure aggravation [74]. Drugs that block Na^+ channels, in addition to GABA-ergic drugs, may exacerbate absence and myoclonic seizures, so they should be avoided in these seizure types.

MEDICALLY INTRACTABLE IDIOPATHIC GENERALIZED EPILEPSY

Many patients who appear to have medically intractable IGE are not truly intractable, but have been treated with inappropriate AEDs. Another possibility is that frontal lobe epilepsy with secondary bilateral synchrony is mistaken for IGE [1]. Once these possibilities have been ruled out, a small minority of patients with IGE remain refractory to medical treatment. These patients may benefit from different drug combinations including VPA, LTG, CZP, TPM, LVT and ZNS, as shown in trials which have included patients with refractory generalized seizure types. For some patients, vagal nerve stimulation (VNS) can be a good option. It seems that VNS has similar or greater efficacy in IGE than in partial epilepsy, but this is still an off-label use [93, 94]. Ketogenic diet could also be an option, although no solid data are available to support this.

REFERENCES

1. Benbadis SR. Practical management issues for idiopathic generalized epilepsies. *Epilepsia* 2005; 46(Suppl 9):125–132.
2. Perucca E. Birth defects after prenatal exposure to antiepileptic drugs. *Lancet Neurol* 2005; 4:781–786.
3. Morrow J, Russell A, Guthrie E, Parsons L, Robertson I, Waddell R *et al*. Malformation risks of antiepileptic drugs in pregnancy: a prospective study from the UK Epilepsy and Pregnancy Register. *J Neurol Neurosurg Psychiatry* 2006; 77:193–198.
4. Patsalos PN. Properties of antiepileptic drugs in the treatment of idiopathic generalized epilepsies. *Epilepsia* 2005; 46(Suppl 9):140–148.
5. Bergey GK. Evidence-based treatment of idiopathic generalized epilepsies with new antiepileptic drugs. *Epilepsia* 2005; 46(Suppl 9):161–168.
6. French JA, Kanner AM, Bautista J, Abou-Khalil B, Browne T, Harden CL *et al*. Efficacy and tolerability of the new antiepileptic drugs II: treatment of refractory epilepsy: report of the Therapeutics and Technology Assessment Subcommittee and Quality Standards Subcommittee of the American Academy of Neurology and the American Epilepsy Society. *Neurology* 2004; 62:1261–1273.
7. French JA, Kanner AM, Bautista J, Abou-Khalil B, Browne T, Harden CL *et al*. Efficacy and tolerability of the new antiepileptic drugs I: treatment of new onset epilepsy: report of the Therapeutics and Technology Assessment Subcommittee and Quality Standards Subcommittee of the American Academy of Neurology and the American Epilepsy Society. *Neurology* 2004; 62:1252–1260.
8. French JA, Kanner AM, Bautista J, Abou-Khalil B, Browne T, Harden CL *et al*. Efficacy and tolerability of the new antiepileptic drugs II: treatment of refractory epilepsy: report of the TTA and QSS Subcommittees of the American Academy of Neurology and the American Epilepsy Society. *Epilepsia* 2004; 45:410–423.

9. French JA, Kanner AM, Bautista J, Abou-Khalil B, Browne T, Harden CL *et al*. Efficacy and tolerability of the new antiepileptic drugs I: treatment of new-onset epilepsy: report of the TTA and QSS Subcommittees of the American Academy of Neurology and the American Epilepsy Society. *Epilepsia* 2004; 45:401–409.

10. Glauser T, Ben Menachem E, Bourgeois B, Cnaan A, Chadwick D, Guerreiro C *et al*. ILAE treatment guidelines: evidence-based analysis of antiepileptic drug efficacy and effectiveness as initial monotherapy for epileptic seizures and syndromes. *Epilepsia* 2006; 47:1094–1120.

11. Browne TR, Dreifuss FE, Dyken PR, Goode DJ, Penry JK, Porter RJ *et al*. Ethosuximide in the treatment of absence (petit mal) seizures. *Neurology* 1975; 25:515–524.

12. Hitiris N, Brodie MJ. Evidence-based treatment of idiopathic generalized epilepsies with older antiepileptic drugs. *Epilepsia* 2005; 46(Suppl 9):149–153.

13. Covanis A, Gupta AK, Jeavons PM. Sodium valproate: monotherapy and polytherapy. *Epilepsia* 1982; 23:693–720.

14. Dulac O, Steru D, Rey E, Perret A, Arthuis M. Sodium valproate monotherapy in childhood epilepsy. *Brain Dev* 1986; 8:47–52.

15. Henriksen O, Johannessen SI. Clinical and pharmacokinetic observations on sodium valproate – a 5-year follow-up study in 100 children with epilepsy. *Acta Neurol Scand* 1982; 65:504–523.

16. Bourgeois B, Beaumanoir A, Blajev B, de la CN, Despland PA, Egli M *et al*. Monotherapy with valproate in primary generalized epilepsies. *Epilepsia* 1987; 28(Suppl 2):S8–S11.

17. Braathen G, Theorell K, Persson A, Rane A. Valproate in the treatment of absence epilepsy in children: a study of dose-response relationships. *Epilepsia* 1988; 29:548–552.

18. Villarreal HJ, Wilder BJ, Willmore LJ, Bauman AW, Hammond EJ, Bruni J. Effect of valproic acid on spike and wave discharges in patients with absence seizures. *Neurology* 1978; 28:886–891.

19. Erenberg G, Rothner AD, Henry CE, Cruse RP. Valproic acid in the treatment of intractable absence seizures in children: a single-blind clinical and quantitative EEG study. *Am J Dis Child* 1982; 136:526–529.

20. Sato S, White BG, Penry JK, Dreifuss FE, Sackellares JC, Kupferberg HJ. Valproic acid versus ethosuximide in the treatment of absence seizures. *Neurology* 1982; 32:157–163.

21. Suzuki M, Maruyama H, Ishibashi Y. A double-blind, comparative trial of sodium dipropylacetate and ethosuximide in epilepsy in children with pure petit mal seizures. *Igaku No Ayumi* 1972; 82:470–488.

22. Callaghan N, O'Hare J, O'Driscoll D, O'Neill B, Daly M. Comparative study of ethosuximide and sodium valproate in the treatment of typical absence seizures (petit mal). *Dev Med Child Neurol* 1982; 24:830–836.

23. Rowan AJ, Meijer JW, de Beer-Pawlikowski N, van der Geest P, Meinardi H. Valproate-ethosuximide combination therapy for refractory absence seizures. *Arch Neurol* 1983; 40:797–802.

24. Mikkelsen B, Birket-Smith E, Bradt S, Holm P, Lung M *et al*. Clonazepam in the treatment of epilepsy. A controlled clinical trial in simple absences, bilateral massive epileptic myoclonus, and atonic seizures. *Arch Neurol* 1976; 33:322–325.

25. Frank LM, Enlow T, Holmes GL, Manasco P, Concannon S, Chen C *et al*. Lamictal (lamotrigine) monotherapy for typical absence seizures in children. *Epilepsia* 1999; 40:973–979.

26. Coppola G, Licciardi F, Sciscio N, Russo F, Carotenuto M, Pascotto A. Lamotrigine as first-line drug in childhood absence epilepsy: a clinical and neurophysiological study. *Brain Dev* 2004; 26:26–29.

27. Coppola G, Auricchio G, Federico R, Carotenuto M, Pascotto A. Lamotrigine versus valproic acid as first-line monotherapy in newly diagnosed typical absence seizures: an open-label, randomized, parallel-group study. *Epilepsia* 2004; 45:1049–1053.

28. Posner EB, Mohamed K, Marson AG. Ethosuximide, sodium valproate or lamotrigine for absence seizures in children and adolescents. *Cochrane Database Syst Rev* 2005; (4):CD003032.

29. Cross JH. Topiramate monotherapy for childhood absence seizures: an open label pilot study. *Seizure* 2002; 11:406–410.

30. Di Bonaventura C, Fattouch J, Mari F, Egeo G, Vaudano AE, Prencipe M *et al*. Clinical experience with levetiracetam in idiopathic generalized epilepsy according to different syndrome subtypes. *Epileptic Disord* 2005; 7:231–235.

31. Wilfong A, Schultz R. Zonisamide for absence seizures. *Epilepsy Res* 2005; 64:31–34.

32. Andriola M, Vitale S, Firas B, Guido M. Zonisamide as adjunctive and monotherapy in absence epilepsy. *Epilepsia* 2002; 43(Suppl 7):190.

33. Biton V, Bebin M. Multicenter, open label assessment of the efficacy and safety of zonisamide as adjunctive therapy for primary generalized epilepsy. *Epilepsia* 2002; 43(Suppl 7):190.

34. Biraben A, Allain H, Scarabin JM, Schuck S, Edan G. Exacerbation of juvenile myoclonic epilepsy with lamotrigine. *Neurology* 2000; 55:1758.

35. Hirsch E, Panayiotopoulos CP. Childhood absence epilepsy and related syndromes. In: Roger J, Bureau M, Dravet C, Genton P, Tassinari CA, Wolf P (eds) *Epileptic syndromes in infancy, childhood and adolescence.* Montrouge, France: John Libbey Eurotext, 2005, pp. 315–335.

36. Wolf P, Inoue Y. Therapeutic response of absence seizures in patients of an epilepsy clinic for adolescents and adults. *J Neurol* 1984; 231:225–229.

37. Frank LM, Enlow T, Holmes GL, Manasco P, Concannon S, Chen C *et al*. Lamictal (lamotrigine) monotherapy for typical absence seizures in children. *Epilepsia* 1999; 40:973–979.

38. Proposal for revised classification of epilepsies and epileptic syndromes. Commission on Classification and Terminology of the International League Against Epilepsy. *Epilepsia* 1989; 30:389–399.

39. Engel J Jr. A proposed diagnostic scheme for people with epileptic seizures and with epilepsy: report of the ILAE Task Force on Classification and Terminology. *Epilepsia* 2001; 42:796–803.

40. Genton P, Gelisse P, Thomas P, Dravet C. Do carbamazepine and phenytoin aggravate juvenile myoclonic epilepsy? *Neurology* 2000; 55:1106–1109.

41. Genton P, Gonzalez Sanchez S, Thomas P. Epilepsy with grand mal on awakening. In: Roger J, Bureau M, Dravet C, Genton P, Tassinari C, Wolf P (eds) *Epileptic syndromes in infancy, childhood and adolescence.* John Libbey Eurotext, 2005, pp. 389–394.

42. Shian WJ, Chi CS. Epilepsy with grand mal on awakening. *Zhonghua Yi Xue Za Zhi (Taipei)* 1994; 53:106–108.

43. Sullivan JE, Dlugos DJ. Idiopathic generalized epilepsy. *Curr Treat Options Neurol* 2004; 6:231–242.

44. Marson AG, Williamson PR, Clough H, Hutton JL, Chadwick DW. Carbamazepine versus valproate monotherapy for epilepsy: a meta-analysis. *Epilepsia* 2002; 43:505–513.

45. Lerman-Sagie T, Lerman P. Phenobarbital still has a role in epilepsy treatment. *J Child Neurol* 1999; 14:820–821.

46. Biton V, Sackellares JC, Vuong A, Hammer AE, Barrett PS, Messenheimer JA. Double-blind, placebo-controlled study of lamotrigine in primary generalized tonic–clonic seizures. *Neurology* 2005; 65:1737–1743.

47. Biton V, Montouris GD, Ritter F, Riviello JJ, Reife R, Lim P *et al*. A randomized, placebo-controlled study of topiramate in primary generalized tonic–clonic seizures. Topiramate YTC Study Group. *Neurology* 1999; 52:1330–1337.

48. Montouris GD, Biton V, Rosenfeld WE. Nonfocal generalized tonic–clonic seizures: response during long-term topiramate treatment. Topiramate YTC/YTCE Study Group. *Epilepsia* 2000; 41(Suppl 1):S77–S81.

49. Berkovic SF, Knowlton RC, Leroy RF, Schiemann J, Falter U; Levetiracetam N01057 Study Group. Placebo-controlled study of levetiracetam in idiopatic generalized epilepsy. *Neurology* 2007; 69: 1751–1760.

50. Asconape J, Penry JK. Some clinical and EEG aspects of benign juvenile myoclonic epilepsy. *Epilepsia* 1984; 25:108–114.

51. Delgado-Escueta AV, Enrile-Bacsal F. Juvenile myoclonic epilepsy of Janz. *Neurology* 1984; 34:285–294.

52. Calleja S, Salas-Puig J, Ribacoba R, Lahoz CH. Evolution of juvenile myoclonic epilepsy treated from the outset with sodium valproate. *Seizure* 2001; 10:424–427.

53. Jeavons PM, Clark JE, Maheshwari MC. Treatment of generalized epilepsies of childhood and adolescence with sodium valproate ('epilim'). *Dev Med Child Neurol* 1977; 19:9–25.

54. Panayiotopoulos CP, Obeid T, Tahan AR. Juvenile myoclonic epilepsy: a 5-year prospective study. *Epilepsia* 1994; 35:285–296.

55. Karlovassitou-Koniari A, Alexiou D, Angelopoulos P, Armentsoudis P, Dimitrakoudi E, Delithanasis I *et al*. Low dose sodium valproate in the treatment of juvenile myoclonic epilepsy. *J Neurol* 2002; 249:396–399.

56. Panagariya A, Sureka RK, Sardana V. Juvenile myoclonic epilepsy – an experience from north western India. *Acta Neurol Scand* 2001; 104:12–16.

57. Vajda FJ, O'Brien TJ, Hitchcock A, Graham J, Cook M, Lander C *et al*. Critical relationship between sodium valproate dose and human teratogenicity: results of the Australian register of anti-epileptic drugs in pregnancy. *J Clin Neurosci* 2004; 11:854–858.

58. Sundqvist A, Tomson T, Lundkvist B. Valproate as monotherapy for juvenile myoclonic epilepsy: dose-effect study. *Ther Drug Monit* 1998; 20:149–157.

59. Obeid T, Panayiotopoulos CP. Clonazepam in juvenile myoclonic epilepsy. *Epilepsia* 1989; 30:603–606.

60. Buchanan N. The use of lamotrigine in juvenile myoclonic epilepsy. *Seizure* 1996; 5:149–151.
61. Morris GL, Hammer AE, Kustra RP, Messenheimer JA. Lamotrigine for patients with juvenile myoclonic epilepsy following prior treatment with valproate: results of an open-label study. *Epilepsy Behav* 2004; 5:509–512.
62. Crespel A, Genton P, Berramdane M, Coubes P, Monicard C, Baldy-Moulinier M *et al*. Lamotrigine associated with exacerbation or de novo myoclonus in idiopathic generalized epilepsies. *Neurology* 2005; 65:762–764.
63. Carrazana EJ, Wheeler SD. Exacerbation of juvenile myoclonic epilepsy with lamotrigine. *Neurology* 2001; 56:1424–1425.
64. Prasad A, Kuzniecky RI, Knowlton RC, Welty TE, Martin RC, Mendez M *et al*. Evolving antiepileptic drug treatment in juvenile myoclonic epilepsy. *Arch Neurol* 2003; 60:1100–1105.
65. Betts T, Yarrow H, Greenhill L, Barrett M. Clinical experience of marketed levetiracetam in an epilepsy clinic – a one year follow up study. *Seizure* 2003; 12:136–140.
66. Krauss GL, Betts T, Abou-Khalil B, Gergey G, Yarrow H, Miller A. Levetiracetam treatment of idiopathic generalised epilepsy. *Seizure* 2003; 12:617–620.
67. Noachtar S, Andermann E, Meyvisch P, Andermann F, Gough WB, Schiemann-Delgado J; NI66 Levetiracetam Study Group. Levetiracetam for the treatment of idiopatic generalized epilepsy with myoclonic seizures. *Neurology* 2008; 70:607–616.
68. Biton V, Bourgeois BF. Topiramate in patients with juvenile myoclonic epilepsy. *Arch Neurol* 2005; 62:1705–1708.
69. Levishon PM, Holland KD. Topiramate or valproate in patients with juvenile myoclonic epilepsy: a randomized open-label comparison. *Epilepsy Behav* 2007; 10:547–552.
70. Welty T, Martin J, Faught E. Comparisons of outcomes in patients with juvenile myoclonic epilepsy treated with lamotrigine, topiramate, zonisamide or levetiracetam (Abstract). *Epilepsia* 2002; 43(Suppl 7):239.
71. Kothare SV, Valencia I, Khurana DS, Hardison H, Melvin JJ, Legido A. Efficacy and tolerability of zonisamide in juvenile myoclonic epilepsy. *Epileptic Disord* 2004; 6:267–270.
72. O´Rourke D, Flynn C, White M, Doherty CP, Delanty N. Potential efficacy of zonisamide in refractory juvenile myoclonic epilepsy: retrospective evidence from an Irish compassionate-use case series. *Ir Med J* 2007; 100:431–433.
73. Thomas P, Genton P, Gelisse P, Wolf P. Juvenile myoclonic epilepsy. In: Roger J, Bureau M, Dravet C, Genton P, Tassinari C, Wolf P (eds) *Epileptic syndromes in infancy, childhood and adolescence*. John Libbey Eurotext, 2005, pp. 367–388.
74. Chaves J, Sander JW. Seizure aggravation in idiopathic generalized epilepsies. *Epilepsia* 2005; 46(Suppl 9):133–139.
75. Shields WD, Saslow E. Myoclonic, atonic, and absence seizures following institution of carbamazepine therapy in children. *Neurology* 1983; 33:1487–1489.
76. Perucca E, Gram L, Avanzini G, Dulac O. Antiepileptic drugs as a cause of worsening seizures. *Epilepsia* 1998; 39:5–17.
77. Guerrini R, Belmonte A, Genton P. Antiepileptic drug-induced worsening of seizures in children. *Epilepsia* 1998; 39(Suppl 3):S2–S10.
78. Genton P. When antiepileptic drugs aggravate epilepsy. *Brain Dev* 2000; 22:75–80.
79. So EL, Ruggles KH, Cascino GD, Ahmann PA, Weatherford KW. Seizure exacerbation and status epilepticus related to carbamazepine-10,11-epoxide. *Ann Neurol* 1994; 35:743–746.
80. Yang MT, Lee WT, Chu LW, Shen YZ. Anti-epileptic drugs-induced de novo absence seizures. *Brain Dev* 2003; 25:51–56.
81. Sachdeo RC, Wasserstein A, Mesenbrink PJ, D'Souza J. Effects of oxcarbazepine on sodium concentration and water handling. *Ann Neurol* 2002; 51:613–620.
82. Osorio I, Reed RC, Peltzer JN. Refractory idiopathic absence status epilepticus: a probable paradoxical effect of phenytoin and carbamazepine. *Epilepsia* 2000; 41:887–894.
83. Liporace JD, Sperling MR, Dichter MA. Absence seizures and carbamazepine in adults. *Epilepsia* 1994; 35:1026–1028.
84. Talwar D, Arora MS, Sher PK. EEG changes and seizure exacerbation in young children treated with carbamazepine. *Epilepsia* 1994; 35:1154–1159.
85. Parker AP, Agathonikou A, Robinson RO, Panayiotopoulos CP. Inappropriate use of carbamazepine and vigabatrin in typical absence seizures. *Dev Med Child Neurol* 1998; 40:517–519.

86. Thomas P, Valton L, Genton P. Absence and myoclonic status epilepticus precipitated by antiepileptic drugs in idiopathic generalized epilepsy. *Brain* 2006; 129:1281–1292.

87. Hamano S, Mochizuki M, Morikawa T. Phenobarbital-induced atypical absence seizure in benign childhood epilepsy with centrotemporal spikes. *Seizure* 2002; 11:201–204.

88. de Krom MC, Verduin N, Visser E, Kleijer M, Scholtes F, De Groen JH. Status epilepticus during vigabatrin treatment: a report of three cases. *Seizure* 1995; 4:159–162.

89. Crespel A, Genton P, Berramdane M, Coubes P, Monicard C, Baldy-Moulinier M *et al*. Lamotrigine associated with exacerbation or de novo myoclonus in idiopathic generalized epilepsies. *Neurology* 2005; 65:762–764.

90. Asconape J, Diedrich A, DellaBadia J. Myoclonus associated with the use of gabapentin. *Epilepsia* 2000; 41:479–481.

91. Knake S, Hamer HM, Schomburg U, Oertel WH, Rosenow F. Tiagabine-induced absence status in idiopathic generalized epilepsy. *Seizure* 1999; 8:314–317.

92. Skardoutsou A, Voudris KA, Vagiakou EA. Non-convulsive status epilepticus associated with tiagabine therapy in children. *Seizure* 2003; 12:599–601.

93. Ng M, Devinsky O. Vagus nerve stimulation for refractory idiopathic generalised epilepsy. *Seizure* 2004; 13:176–178.

94. Holmes MD, Silbergeld DL, Drouhard D, Wilensky AJ, Ojemann LM. Effect of vagus nerve stimulation on adults with pharmacoresistant generalized epilepsy syndromes. *Seizure* 2004; 13:340–345.

Section V

Complicating conditions

12

Treatment of the hospitalized patient with new-onset seizures

Karine J. Abou Khaled, Lawrence J. Hirsch

INTRODUCTION

Seizures are not uncommon in hospitalized patients, particularly in the critically ill. Seizure types seen in these patients include simple motor or sensory, complex partial (characterized by alteration of awareness), generalized tonic–clonic, subclinical seizures and non-convulsive status epilepticus (NCSE). Many seizures in hospitalized patients are provoked by an acute derangement in systemic homeostasis (as with electrolyte abnormalities, hypoglycaemia or hypoperfusion) or are symptomatic of an acute insult to cerebral function (as in acute stroke or intracranial haemorrhage). Unprovoked seizures can also occur, and by definition are seizures that occur in the absence of an acute provoking event [1]. The approach to evaluating and treating seizures in a hospitalized patient differs from the long-term outpatient care of patients with epilepsy. Evaluation of new-onset seizures in this situation should focus on identifying acutely life-threatening causes requiring emergent action, followed by finding correctable underlying systemic derangements, in turn followed by understanding the co-morbidities which may affect treatment decisions and risk for ongoing seizures. Treatment must be tailored to each clinical situation. The most important questions include: is an anti-epileptic medication needed; how rapidly is treatment needed; what co-morbidities and medication interactions will affect the choice of anti-convulsant; and how long should treatment be continued? The goal of this chapter is to help the clinician navigate the clinical decision-making process in the initial evaluation of seizures and their appropriate management in the hospitalized patient. Discussions will include initial evaluation, choice of anti-convulsant therapy and treatment issues in specific clinical scenarios.

APPROACH TO NEW-ONSET SEIZURES IN THE HOSPITAL

Initial diagnostic evaluation and treatment must often occur simultaneously, at least until the patient has been stabilized and there is time for more extensive consideration of the clinical situation. Caring for acute seizures in the hospital begins with basic life support measures, including ensuring the patient has a patent airway, is breathing adequately and has intact circulation. While vital signs, electrocardiography and pulse oximetry monitoring are being

Karine J. Abou Khaled, MD, NYU Comprehensive Epilepsy Center, New York, USA. Currently at Hôtel-Dieu de France Hospital, Department of Neurology, Saint Joseph University, Beirut, Lebanon

Lawrence J. Hirsch, MD, Associate Clinical Professor of Neurology, NYU Comprehensive Epilepsy Center; Department of Neurology, Columbia University, New York, New York, USA

implemented, care-givers should ensure the patient is in a safe position to prevent injury and/
or aspiration. Part of assessment of circulation is obtaining intravenous access and obtaining
blood for laboratory studies. In addition to bedside glucose testing, and electrolytes including
calcium, laboratory tests should be chosen based on what is known about the patient's other
medical conditions, including tests of renal and hepatic function. Part of the initial assessment
includes a focused review of the patient's history, including recent neurological and systemic
complaints, medications (especially those recently introduced), and drug and alcohol use. A
proposed timetable and treatment protocol for acute seizures in the hospitalized patient are
outlined in Table 12.1. Treatment should be first directed towards all potentially correctable
underlying causes, as delineated in Tables 12.2 and 12.3. Most seizures cease spontaneously
within 5 minutes, requiring no immediate intervention. If a seizure is prolonged (longer than
5 minutes), treatment with an intravenous benzodiazepine such as lorazepam is generally
indicated. Treatment of status epilepticus is discussed in detail in Chapter 14.

Once the patient has been stabilized and the initial evaluation is complete, more extensive
evaluation includes a focused physical examination to identify focal neurological deficits or
other clues to the underlying aetiology of the seizure. Following this, urgent brain imaging
is usually warranted. Non-contrast computerized tomography (CT) imaging of the head,
which can be obtained rapidly, is useful for identifying acute intracranial haemorrhage and
can identify subacute or chronic cerebral infarcts, mass lesions and hydrocephalus. Magnetic
resonance imaging (MRI) is superior in the less-emergent setting for characterizing the huge
variety of lesions that may cause seizures, including cerebral infarcts, oedema, tumours or
abscesses or other infections. Specific MRI sequences are important for certain diagnoses

Table 12.1 Evaluation and initial treatment of acute seizures in adults

Time (min)	Action
0–5	Diagnose; give oxygen; stabilize airway, breathing and circulation; obtain intravenous access; begin ECG monitoring; draw blood for electrolytes, BUN test, creatinine, glucose, magnesium, calcium, phosphate, complete blood count, liver enzymes, anti-epileptic drug levels, arterial blood gas test, troponin; toxicology screen (urine and blood)
6–10	If still seizing or not back to baseline mental status and adequate glucose not documented, give thiamine 100 mg i.v. and 50 ml of D50 i.v.
	If still seizure activity: *Lorazepam* 4 mg i.v. over 2 min; if still seizing, repeat x 1 in 5 mins
	If no rapid i.v. access give diazepam 20 mg PR or midazolam 10 mg intranasally, buccally or i.m.*
10–20	If seizures persist, or patient estimated to be at high risk for recurrence or high risk for seizure-related adverse secondary effects, begin *fosphenytoin* 20 mg/kg i.v. at 150 mg/min, with blood pressure and ECG monitoring. For ongoing seizures (i.e. status epilepticus), this step can be skipped initially, especially if proceeding to midazolam or propofol infusion, or performed simultaneously with the next step; if done simultaneously, administration rate can be slowed. *Valproic acid* i.v. 25–40 mg/kg is a reasonable alternative in specific situations (e.g. hypotensive). i.v. *Levetiracetam* 1500–4000 mg i.v. may be a reasonable option in those with contraindications to phenytoin and valproate
	Begin electroencephalography monitoring if patient does not rapidly awaken to rule out non-convulsive seizures

*The i.v. solution of diazepam can be given rectally if Diastat is not available; the i.v. solution of midazolam can be given by any of these routes.
BUN, blood urea nitrogen; ECG, electrocardiography; i.m., intramuscular; i.v., intravenous.

Table 12.2 Common aetiologies of seizures in hospitalized patients

History of epilepsy	Medication withdrawal or non-compliance
	Other
Acute neurological insult	Cerebrovascular disease: infarct, haemorrhage, vasculitis
	Intracranial haemorrhage: subarachnoid, subdural, intracerebral, other
	Infection: meningitis, encephalitis, brain abscess
	Head trauma
	Anoxia
	Brain tumours
	Demyelinating disorders
Acute systemic insult	Electrolyte imbalance: hyponatraemia, hypocalcaemia, hypomagnesaemia, hypophosphataemia (especially in alcoholics)
	Hypoglycaemia, and hyperglycaemia with hyperosmolar state; both can cause focal seizures as well
	Vitamin deficiency: pyridoxine
	Illicit drug use
	Toxins
	Hypertensive encephalopathy (also known as reversible posterior leukoencephalopathy syndrome [RPLS] or posterior reversible encephalopathy syndrome [PRES])
	Hypotension from shock or secondary to syncope
	Organ failure: uraemia, hepatic failure, cardiac failure
	Multi-system illness such as systemic lupus erythematosus
	Medications: side-effects, toxicity, withdrawal (see Table 12.3)
	Alcohol related
	Systemic infection/sepsis
	Eclampsia

Table 12.3 Medications that can lower the seizure threshold [74, 75]

Antidepressants, especially bupropion and maprotiline
Neuroleptics, especially clozapine, but also phenothiazines
Lithium
Baclofen
Phenytoin at supratherapeutic levels (including very high free levels)
Theophylline
Analgesics: meperidine, fentanyl and tramadol
Opioid withdrawal
Antibiotics: beta-lactams (imipenem, cefazolin), quinolones, isoniazid (treat with B6 for seizures related to isoniazid), metronidazole
Anti-arrhythmic medications: mexiletine, lidocaine, digoxin
Radiographic contrast agents
Immunomodulators: cyclosporine, tacrolimus, interferons
Chemotherapeutic agents: alkylating agents such as chlorambucil and busulfan

– for example, diffusion-weighted imaging (DWI) is best for identifying acute ischaemia. Fluid-attenuated inversion recovery (FLAIR) sequences are used to detect inflammatory changes or oedema. In the reversible posterior leukoencephalopathy syndrome ([RPLS], a cause of seizures associated with hypertension, particularly in transplant patients on certain immunosuppressant medications) FLAIR images may show bilateral hyperintensities in the subcortical and cortical parieto-occipital regions, and DWI images will show increased diffusion, corresponding to vasogenic oedema rather than ischaemia [2, 3].

Additional diagnostic testing should be guided by the patient's specific clinical situation. Lumbar puncture may be needed in the setting of headache, meningismus, rash or other signs of infection, immunosuppression or recent neurosurgery. Following repetitive seizures or status epilepticus, the cerebrospinal fluid (CSF) white cell count may be mildly and transiently elevated, and CSF protein might also be mildly elevated secondary to blood–brain barrier breakdown [4].

A large number of critically ill patients have non-convulsive seizures, unrecognized by care-givers, and diagnosed only by electroencephalogram (EEG) monitoring [5, 6]; at our centre, 101 of 110 intensive care unit (ICU) patients who had seizures recorded while undergoing continuous EEG monitoring had purely non-convulsive seizures that would have been missed without EEG [5]. Risk factors for non-convulsive seizures or NCSE include coma, age <18, prior convulsive seizures, acute or remote risk factors for epilepsy, oculomotor abnormalities (such as nystagmus, eye deviation and even hippus), and EEG findings of periodic lateralized epileptiform discharges (PLEDs) or burst-suppression [5, 7]. In our series of 97 patients in coma who had continuous EEG ordered, 56% had non-convulsive seizures.

ANTI-EPILEPTIC DRUG SELECTION

Anti-epileptic drug (AED) selection for hospitalized patients with new-onset seizures differs from chronic treatment of patients with epilepsy. The type and timing of therapy with AEDs should be individualized, taking into account the age of the patient, medical history, likelihood of a particular side-effect, drug interactions and risk of recurrence. Agents offering rapid protection against seizures are preferred in patients with a high risk of recurrent seizures or in critically ill patients in whom recurrent seizures would further compromise stability of brain or systemic function. Table 12.4 contains a summary of anti-epileptic agents, chief benefits and risks and recommendations for specific patient populations. Although most of the new-generation AEDs have been approved as add-on treatments, most (if not all) are efficacious when used alone [8].

The only AED that requires very slow introduction (several weeks or more to therapeutic dose) is lamotrigine. Drugs that can be loaded or started immediately at an effective dose include phenytoin, phenobarbital, valproate, levetiracetam, gabapentin, pregabalin and probably carbamazepine, oxcarbazepine, topiramate and zonisamide. Levetiracetam is now frequently used as a first-line AED in hospitalized patients because it can be initiated at an effective dose, it achieves steady therapeutic serum levels quickly, it has primarily renal elimination, minimal protein binding, no significant drug interactions and low risk of allergic reactions [9]. In patients with refractory epilepsy, LVT at a dose of 1000 mg/day has rapid onset of action with a significant increase of proportion of seizure-free patients on the first day of therapy [10]. Gabapentin and pregabalin have similar advantageous features, including 100% renal elimination with no interactions and quite rare allergic reactions [11, 12]. Initiation of gabapentin at 900 mg/day has been fairly well tolerated and proven to be as safe as reaching the same total dose over 3 days. Dizziness was the most frequent side-effect [13]. It can be titrated to maintenance dosages exceeding 3600 mg per day [12]. Rapid titration to a daily dose of 3600 mg within 24 h was also well tolerated [14]. Pregabalin has been shown to be highly effective and generally well tolerated as an add-on therapy in

Table 12.4 Anti-epileptic drugs: clinically relevant pharmacokinetic aspects, concerns and recommendations

Drug	Main concern	Protein binding (%)	Comments/recommended adjustments in renal and liver disease
Carbamazepine	Hyponatraemia; leukopenia; arrhythmia rash	70–80	No need for adjustment in renal disease; monitor levels in liver disease because of reduction of protein bound fraction; many drug interactions as P450 inducer
Clobazam	Sedation	85	Used for long-term treatment of epilepsy
Clonazepam	Sedation	85	Hepatic metabolism; reduce dose in liver disease; no adjustment needed with renal disease
Gabapentin	Somnolence and dizziness	0	Renally excreted; decrease dose depending on creatinine clearance; supplement after dialysis
Lamotrigine	Rash	55	Must be titrated slowly over 6–8 weeks; 20% dialysable; decreased clearance by >50% in presence of valproate; lower lamotrigine dose
Levetiracetam	Behavioural or psychiatric adverse reactions	<10	Renally excreted; decrease dose depending on creatinine clearance and supplement after dialysis
Oxcarbazepine	Hyponatraemia; rash	38	Active metabolite excreted by the kidneys
Phenobarbital	Cardiovascular depression; sedation	60–90	Up to 25% eliminated renally; supplement after dialysis; many drug interactions as strong P450 inducer
Pregabalin	Dizziness; weight gain	0	Renally excreted; decrease dose depending on creatinine clearance; supplement after dialysis
Phenytoin	Hypotension (i.v.); rash; arrhythmia	90	Adjust according to free levels in renal and liver disease; many drug interactions as strong P450 inducer
Topiramate	Nephrolithiasis; acidosis cognitive changes; glaucoma (rare)	15	Hepatic and renal elimination, with 50–80% unchanged in urine
Valproic acid	Thrombocytopenia; increased bleeding diathesis; increased ammonia	90	Decreased protein binding in uremia; hepatic elimination
Zonisamide	Nephrolithiasis; acidosis	50–60	Renal excretion but extensive metabolism by the liver; long half-life (62 h if healthy and in monotherapy)

i.v., intravenous.

partial seizures in a placebo-controlled study. In study subjects treated with flexible dose regimens of 150–600 mg daily to optimize efficacy and tolerability, discontinuation rates were lower than in subjects treated with 300 mg twice daily starting day 1, due to lower rates of adverse effects, chiefly dizziness, ataxia and weight gain [11]. Topiramate, and to a lesser extent zonisamide, are carbonic anhydrase inhibitors and can exacerbate metabolic acidosis or favour renal calculi formation. Adequate hydration is recommended whenever they are used to promote urinary output and lower the concentration of stone-forming substances.

SEIZURES IN INTENSIVE CARE UNITS

In the ICU setting, seizures are a common neurological manifestation in medical or surgical patients. According to Bleck *et al.*, 12.3% of patients admitted to the medical ICU for non-neurological primary problems had neurological complications, with seizures being the second-leading complication (28.1%, after metabolic encephalopathies, 28.6%). Cerebrovascular insults were the most common cause of seizures, as illustrated in Figure 12.1, indicating aetiologies of seizures and number of patients in each diagnostic category [15]. In a separate series of patients in medical or surgical ICUs who had at least one generalized tonic–clonic seizure, one-third had seizures attributed to abrupt drug withdrawal, usually of a medication given for pain management, such as morphine. One-third had underlying metabolic aetiologies with hyponatraemia and hypocalcaemia being the most frequent [16].

In patients with seizures due to metabolic derangements, correction of these abnormalities may be sufficient to prevent further seizures from occurring. In ICU patients with seizures due to other causes, short-term treatment with an anti-epileptic agent should be considered. The choice of AED, as discussed above, depends on the patient's co-morbidities and potential medication interactions. Treatment in these patients depends largely on the underlying aetiology. For example, for metabolic abnormalities, correction of the underlying disorder will be sufficient and more effective than AEDs. In particular situations, treatment with AEDs will be advisable at least for the short term, especially when the risk of seizures outweighs the risks of treatment and when there is an underlying abnormality that cannot be corrected rapidly. Detailed review of the patient's medications and potential drug interactions should be performed in order to prevent inadvertent changes in efficacy or blood levels and

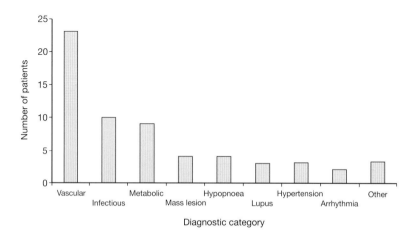

Figure 12.1 Aetiologies of seizures in the medical intensive care unit (number of patients in each diagnostic category) [15].

exacerbation of seizures. For example, there have been several reports of decrease in serum levels of valproic acid by carbapenems, and worsening of seizure control. All described a rapid decline and rapid recovery after discontinuation of the antibiotics. Several mechanisms have been suggested for this interaction, including inhibition of plasma-protein binding and suppression of enterohepatic recirculation [17, 18].

For acute symptomatic seizures, no more than a few weeks of AEDs is recommended (see below). Specific aspects of treatment in different common ICU situations are discussed later.

SEIZURES AND HEPATIC DISEASE

Hepatic failure can either complicate a critical illness or be the main reason for ICU admission. Seizures can arise as a result of increased ammonia levels, abnormal glutamine metabolism, cerebral ischaemia or oedema, accumulation of toxins or associated biochemical abnormalities such as hypoglycaemia, hyponatraemia and hypomagnesaemia [19, 20, 21].

The true incidence of seizures in hepatic encephalopathy is unknown. It has been reported as 2–33% [22]. The most characteristic EEG changes are diffuse background slowing and triphasic waves. Ficker *et al*. reviewed EEGs of 118 patients with hepatic encephalopathy and identified 15% with epileptiform abnormalities. Twelve patients had clinical seizures and most of them died or deteriorated [20]. Status epilepticus can occur but is rare [21]. Ellis *et al.* [19] determined the frequency of subclinical seizures in a cohort of patients with acute liver failure in grade III or grade IV encephalopathy using a bedside cerebral function and activity monitor (two-channel, five-lead EEG). Forty-two patients were enrolled in a controlled clinical trial: 20 patients were given phenytoin and 22 acted as controls. Subclinical seizure activity was recorded in three of the treated patients and 10 of the controls. Autopsy examinations available in 19 patients showed signs of cerebral oedema in 22% of the phenytoin-treated patients compared with 70% of the controls ($P<0.03$). This study supports the important role of continuous EEG monitoring in the critically ill. We recommend performing a complete EEG with a full set of electrodes to rule out subclinical seizures and guide treatment (because these seizures can aggravate cerebral oedema and neurotoxicity) [23]. The full set of electrodes prevents interpretation errors by improving recognition of artefacts and other patterns that could be mistaken for seizures using limited coverage [23, 24]. EEG 'shortcut' techniques such as the cerebral function monitor, designed for assessment of background EEG rather than seizures, should not be used for seizure detection without confirmation by recordings with more electrodes interpreted by a certified electroencephalographer.

When seizures occur in patients with liver disease, the goal should be to rule out an underlying reversible process such as metabolic abnormality, infection or medication toxicity. If AEDs are needed, special considerations should be made in moderate to severe cases of hepatic dysfunction if the drug is metabolized by the liver. Hypoalbuminaemia is often present and leads to increased free (unbound, active portion) blood levels of some AEDs that are highly bound to protein such as phenytoin and valproic acid (VPA). Monitoring free levels of these drugs, particularly free phenytoin, will avoid toxicity and improve seizure control (see Table 12.4).

VPA can cause increased ammonia levels and bleeding dysfunction, even in patients without hepatic disease, which are significant concerns in this patient population. It has been associated with thrombocytopenia, induction of von Willebrand disease (children more than adults), deficiency of vitamin K-dependent coagulation factors and hypofibrinogenaemia [25]. We recommend platelet counts and appropriate laboratory studies whenever bleeding occurs in general when a patient is on VPA, and prior to surgery, particularly neurosurgery. We also consider VPA to be relatively contraindicated in anyone with a coagulopathy.

Anti-seizure drugs favoured in liver disease patients are drugs with low or no protein binding, or those AEDs without hepatic metabolism such as gabapentin, pregabalin and levetiracetam. All these are available orally but an intravenous form of levetiracetam has also become available recently. It has been proven to be well tolerated and has a similar pharmacokinetic profile to the oral form [26]. Doses administered and well tolerated in healthy controls were up to 4000 mg over 15 minutes and 2500 mg over 5 minutes. For all intravenous doses combined, the most frequent adverse effects were CNS related, mostly dizziness. Intravenous levetiracetam is expected to assist in controlling seizures in critically ill patients with liver failure, but no studies have proven this to date.

In a recent study in animal models, Gibbs *et al.* [27] showed that levetiracetam has neuroprotective effect against mitochondrial dysfunction and oxidative stress seen after status epilepticus (SE). Neuroprotective properties have also been reported with topiramate [28, 29]. Further studies in humans are needed to confirm these findings.

SEIZURES AND RENAL DISEASE

Seizures in renal disease are secondary to one or more factors, including hyponatraemia, hypocalcaemia, uraemia itself, hypertensive encephalopathy, medication toxicity or disequilibrium syndrome seen with haemodialysis. In the few studies that looked at occurrence of seizures in patients with renal failure and/or on haemodialysis, seizures occurred in 2–10% of patients [30–32]. Seizures associated with kidney transplants will be discussed later.

Treatment of these patients may be problematic due to hypoalbuminaemia, alteration of AED pharmacokinetics in uraemia and dialysis effect. Drugs chiefly eliminated by the kidneys, especially gabapentin, pregabalin and levetiracetam but also topiramate and phenobarbital, should be used at lower doses in renal failure. It would be wise to avoid carbonic anhydrase inhibitors such as zonisamide or topiramate in patients at risk of nephrolithiasis or when the aetiology of the renal failure is unknown because they increase renal bicarbonate loss (predisposing to acidosis) and stone formation. As far as dialysis effect, drugs that are highly protein bound are not significantly dialysed and do not need to be replaced. Some might be moderately affected (such as lamotrigine, 55% protein bound, 17% dialyzable [33]) and might require pre- and post-dialysis level monitoring to make necessary and individualized adjustments. The AEDs to be replaced following dialysis are gabapentin, pregabalin, ethosuximide, levetiracetam, phenobarbital and topiramate (see Table 12.4). As a rule, if to be used chronically, we check a pre-dialysis level and 2-h post-dialysis level to estimate how much needs to be replaced in a given individual. In general, prior to availability of pre- and post-dialysis levels, one can estimate that concentration post-dialysis will be about half what it was pre-dialysis with these AEDs.

SEIZURES IN PATIENTS WITH CARDIOVASCULAR DISEASE

In patients with cardiovascular disease, mostly if above 60 years of age, new-onset seizures should suggest stroke, either acute or in the past months to years [34]. The reported incidence of post-stroke seizures varies between around 2.5% and 10% depending on the inclusion criteria of the subjects, the underlying type of stroke, age and length of follow up [35–41]. The majority occur within the first 24 h. Early (acute) seizures occur in 4% of strokes [41] and 32% of patients with early seizures have late-onset seizures [42]. The risk of epilepsy in patients with an unprovoked single seizure due to a prior (remote) stroke is often high enough to justify starting AEDs before a second seizure [43]. However, there is no evidence that chronic treatment should be started after acute symptomatic seizures from acute strokes. This situation is probably analogous to acute traumatic brain injury with early seizures (i.e. acute symptomatic seizures): although a risk factor for later development of epilepsy, there is no evidence whatsoever (despite multiple valiant attempts to show this) that AEDs can prevent epileptogenesis [44]. Thus, chronic treatment is not recommended in general, unless there is development of remote symptomatic seizures (i.e. epilepsy).

The electroencephalogram in acute stroke generally shows focal slowing and, less frequently, PLEDs. Once PLEDs are identified, the patient is at high risk (>60%) of having seizures in the acute setting [45]. Owing to this high risk, coupled with the fact that the ischaemic brain is less likely to be able to tolerate the metabolic demand of seizure activity, we recommend treating patients with acute stroke and PLEDs during the acute illness as if they had an acute symptomatic seizure, even if none was noted.

Some AEDs should be used with caution in this population, mainly phenytoin, phenobarbital and carbamazepine. Intravenous phenytoin and phenobarbital are known to cause hypotension. In addition, phenytoin causes cardiac arrhythmias following rapid intravenous infusion. In patients with known atherosclerotic heart disease, maximal infusion rate should be 25 mg/min instead of 50 mg/min, which is the usual recommended rate [46]. Carbamazepine has been shown to cause arrhythmias, even asystole, following overdose, as well as conduction block and Stokes–Adams attacks [47, 48], or severe sick sinus symptoms [49]. Thus, carbamazepine should be used with caution in patients at high risk of cardiac arrhythmias.

SEIZURES IN TRANSPLANT PATIENTS

Seizures in this population are not infrequent and can be secondary to multiple factors: metabolic abnormalities such as hyponatraemia, neurotoxicity from immunosuppressive agents or other medications (see Table 12.3), infectious aetiology, structural lesions of the brain (abscess, brain oedema, infarct) or post-anoxic encephalopathy, including that secondary to septic shock [50].

Besides routine biochemical work-up, brain imaging will be needed. Drug levels of immunosuppressive agents can be useful in certain situations. However, Wijdicks *et al.* looked at FK-506 or tacrolimus neurotoxicity in liver transplant patients. They found that none of their patients had toxic levels and that the levels at the time of the neurotoxicity were similar to the patients without neurotoxicity. They also reported that dose reduction, regardless of the level obtained, resulted in clinical improvement [51]. Sirolimus could also be considered as a substitute immunosuppressant agent for patients with cyclosporine A or tacrolimus neurotoxicity [52].

The incidence of seizures varies depending on the transplanted organ (Table 12.5) but we believe that the reports of seizures are underestimated as none of the studies done so far looked at 24-h continuous EEG in these patients to rule out non-convulsive seizures. Some of the reports include encephalopathy as a neurological complication following transplant, without clarifying EEG findings in these patients; thus, non-convulsive seizures or status epilepticus were not ruled out.

Prophylactic AEDs are not recommended following transplantation. One should recall that prophylactic AEDs are not effective in preventing epilepsy in patients with traumatic

Table 12.5 Seizures after transplantation

Organ transplanted	Incidence of seizures
Liver	5% [76]–25% [77]–33% [78]
Kidney	1% [79]–31% [80]
Heart	2% [81]–6.5% [82]–13% [83]–15% [84]
Lung	22% [85]–27% [86]
Bone marrow	3% [87]–7% [88]–7.5% [89]
Pancreas	13% [90]

brain injury or brain tumours [44, 53]. In fact, there is no situation in which there is good evidence to support the use of prophylactic AEDs for more than 1 week (and only minimal evidence of true clinical benefit when used for 1 week). If acute symptomatic seizures occur in transplant patients, most will not require chronic AEDs as they do not have epilepsy (defined as recurrent unprovoked seizures). Treatment during the acute illness is usually sufficient unless there is a persistent highly epileptogenic brain abnormality or if the patient is unable to tolerate the physiological consequences of seizures, mostly the associated hypersympathetic state. This should be decided on a case-by-case basis depending on the aetiology, as well as the radiological and electrographic findings. If the aetiology is an acute metabolic problem that has been corrected, or any other acute symptomatic cause that is no longer present, there is no indication for prolonged AED use.

Depending on the series, up to a third of liver transplant patients develop seizures (see Table 12.5). In a review of 630 orthotopic liver transplant recipients, Wijdicks *et al.* reported that 28 (4%) had generalized tonic–clonic seizures. None had a history of seizures prior to the transplant. The majority occurred in the perioperative period, mostly post-operative days 4 to 6. Phenytoin was successful in treating all 28 patients and was successfully discontinued in all survivors shortly thereafter [50].

Immunosuppressive drug neurotoxicity is the most common aetiology cited in this population, particularly the calcineurin inhibitors cyclosporine and tacrolimus. These are associated with a wide spectrum of neurotoxic effects, mostly described in liver transplant patients, ranging from tremor and visual hallucinations to more severe symptoms if undiagnosed, including speech difficulties, cortical blindness, posterior leukoencephalopathy and seizures. Factors that may promote the development of serious complications include advanced liver failure, hypertension, hypocholesterolaemia, higher cyclosporine or tacrolimus blood levels and hypomagnesaemia.

In liver transplant patients, intravenous phenytoin or fosphenytoin may be needed for rapid seizure control. Levetiracetam may also be used as discussed earlier and has the advantage of not interacting with other medications and having a favourable side-effect profile (with the exception of some risk of neuropsychiatric/behavioural symptoms). Its oral use has gained popularity within the past few years, particularly for patients with complicated medical issues. Now that it is available intravenously, its use will be even more appealing in this category of critically ill patients. Gabapentin, pregabalin, zonisamide and topiramate can also be advanced relatively rapidly but are only available in oral form. It should be noted that topiramate and zonisamide are carbonic-anhydrase inhibitors and may exacerbate acidosis.

In cardiac transplant patients, phenytoin, phenobarbital and carbamazepine should be used with caution secondary to the risks of arrhythmias (phenytoin, carbamazepine) and cardiovascular depression (phenytoin, phenobarbital). If oxcarbazepine or carbamazepine are used, patients should be closely monitored for hyponatraemia, a common side-effect of these AEDs.

Again, there is no consensus on how long to treat. Decision for long-term treatment is determined after the aetiology has been ascertained, although we usually do not recommend long-term AED use in these patients unless there is a presence of at least one *unprovoked* seizure.

Medication interactions constitute another complicating factor in this population. This issue is discussed in more details in other chapters (see Chapters 1 and 13). Phenytoin, for example, decreases absorption of cyclosporine [54]. All enzyme inducers (phenytoin, phenobarbital, carbamazepine, primidone) can increase the clearance of cyclosporine, steroids, warfarin and many other P450-metabolized medications. On the other hand, cyclosporine and tacrolimus are highly protein bound and could increase levels of unbound AEDs.

HIV

The frequency of seizures in human immunodeficiency virus (HIV) patients has been reported between 3% and 11% [55–57]. A prospective study on HIV patients reported that 3% had new-onset seizures during the study period. The major aetiologies were drug toxicity (47%) and intracranial lesions (35%) [56]. The direct effects of HIV on the brain may be the single most common cause of seizures [55, 58]. Aetiologies are listed in Table 12.6. The majority of seizures were reportedly generalized [55, 56]. Seizure management in HIV-positive patients presents particular problems, especially with respect to drug–disease and drug–drug interactions [59]. HIV-seropositive patients are at higher risk of hypersensitivity reactions. For example, 14–26% of patients who received phenytoin have been reported to develop hypersensitivity reactions [55, 58]. Patients who are hospitalized with HIV may be concomitantly receiving highly active anti-retroviral therapy (HAART). Monitoring of free-phenytoin levels is recommended because of the presence of associated hypoalbuminaemia, especially if the patient is additionally on HAART drugs as some of them are highly protein bound. The protease inhibitors can inhibit or induce the cytochrome P450. Therefore, in this category of patients, AEDs that increase the activity of the relevant P450 isoenzyme should be used with caution (such as phenytoin, phenobarbital or carbamazepine). They may result in insufficient protease-inhibitor drug levels and subsequent increase in viral load. To date, there has been little systematic study of these interactions. Choosing an AED that does not affect the cytochrome P450 system is probably a better choice [59]. We find levetiracetam and gabapentin to be good first choices in this population due to their absence of interactions, rare hypersensitivity and renal clearance, though many other AEDs are also reasonable (see Table 12.4). At the time of choosing which AED to initiate, it is often worth considering co-morbidities: use AEDs that help for neuropathic pain if present, avoid those that promote weight loss (topiramate and zonisamide) if appetite is already suppressed, and so on. Although there were some reports of valproate potentially leading to increased viral replication [60], there is also evidence to the contrary: it has shown potential anti-viral

Table 12.6 Aetiologies of seizures in patients with HIV

Intracranial mass	Toxoplasmosis
	Tuberculoma
	Cryptococcoma
	Lymphoma
	Other abscess
Drug-induced	Zidovudine or foscarnet
Meningitis	Cryptococcus
	Tuberculosis
	Other
Encephalitis	HIV related
	Viral: cytomegalovirus, Epstein–Barr virus
	Other
Vascular	Vasculitis
	Varicella zoster-related stroke
	Infarcts, marantic endocarditis
Progressive multifocal leukoencephalopathy (PML)	
Metabolic	
Illicit drug use	
Alcohol	

activity as an add-on drug in treating latent HIV infection, since it is an inhibitor of an enzyme implicated in maintaining latency of the integrated virus [61] and has been reported to improve HIV-associated neurotoxicity [62].

CANCER

Seizures in cancer patients may be due to several mechanisms: (i) metabolic abnormalities; (ii) chemotherapeutic agents; (iii) vascular events; including embolic events from non-bacterial thrombotic endocarditis; (iv) radiation injury; (v) tumour itself or direct invasion of the brain or leptomeninges; and (vi) central nervous system opportunistic infections [63] and paraneoplastic disease.

The diagnostic measures are the same as explored in the initial section of this chapter. Phenytoin, carbamazepine and phenobarbital are all potent enzyme-inducing AEDs; thus these AEDs can interfere with many chemotherapeutic agents by accelerating their metabolism and reducing their therapeutic effects. This occurs with vinca alkaloids, methotrexate, taxanes and others. Likewise, some chemotherapy drugs can alter the pharmacokinetics of AEDs, resulting in decreased seizure control or toxicity, though this can usually be managed via serum levels and dose adjustments. Other agents, such as valproic acid, are enzyme inhibitors and can potentially increase the serum concentration of some chemotherapeutics. Newer AEDs, such as gabapentin, pregabalin and levetiracetam, are promising in treating seizures in patients with brain tumours as they have no known or expected interactions with chemotherapeutic agents [64, 65].

SEIZURES ON THE OBSTETRICS SERVICE

On consultation of a patient on the maternity floor having a seizure, several specific differential diagnoses come to mind, including:

* Cerebral infarct, haemorrhage or venous sinus thrombosis.
* Vasculitis/vasculopathy. Cerebral angiogram will confirm the diagnosis.
* Tumours (meningioma, choriocarcinoma).
* Eclampsia with RPLS and the associated radiological features of brain oedema (especially posterior white matter), infarcts and haemorrhages. The onset of eclamptic convulsions may be antepartum (38–53%), intrapartum (18–36%) or postpartum (11–44%) [66]. Sibai et al. recorded EEGs in 36 patients with eclampsia and noted that 75% had diffuse or focal slowing, and four patients had 'paroxysmal spike activity' [67]. Besides anti-hypertensive therapy and delivery, magnesium sulphate is the drug of choice in preventing and treating eclampsia; a possible mechanism of action is by stabilizing the endothelium and thus minimizing cerebral oedema. In patients who have prolonged seizures or a seizure while on full dose of magnesium, we recommend loading with an AED as well for the acute setting – phenytoin or fosphenytoin is the usual choice.

UNPROVOKED SEIZURE CLUSTERS

Patients with unprovoked seizures can present to the emergency room with a cluster of seizures and therefore need to be admitted to the hospital for initial work-up and treatment. Single seizures with return to baseline (much more common) do not usually require admission, unless these are new-onset seizures and where it is anticipated that there will be a significant delay in outpatient work-up (depending on the resource setting).

According to the International League Against Epilepsy (ILAE), a first unprovoked seizure is defined as a seizure or flurry of seizures all occurring within 24 h in a person older than 1 month of age with no prior history of unprovoked seizure. Diagnosing epilepsy requires a minimum of two unprovoked seizures [1].

Are clusters of seizures different from single seizures in terms of the management and the recurrence rate? Overall, about 35% of patients with a first seizure are at risk of having a second within the subsequent 3–5 years, although the risks varies from 23% to 71%, depending on the studies, exclusion criteria and the clinical characteristics [68, 69, 70]. Hauser et al. looked at recurrence risk after a first unprovoked seizure, and found that risks were 10%, 24% and 29% at 1, 3 and 5 years respectively for the idiopathic generalized group, contrasting with 26%, 41% and 46% for the remote symptomatic seizure group. Remote symptomatic seizures were defined as seizures in individuals with prior history of CNS insult known to substantially increase the risk for subsequent epilepsy such as head trauma, stroke or CNS infection [68].

Kho et al. studied adult patients presenting with multiple seizures occurring within 24 h (with recovery in between) and compared them with those presenting with single seizures. Patients with status epilepticus were excluded. They found that the recurrence rate at 1 year was almost identical (38% for the single seizure group vs. 40% for the multiple seizures group), regardless of the aetiology or whether or not they were treated [71]. The only variable that independently predicted the seizure recurrence at 1 year was a remote symptomatic aetiology [71, 72].

Patients who have unprovoked status epilepticus or a seizure cluster as their first seizure may have a lower threshold for deciding to begin chronic AEDs. In cryptogenic or idiopathic epilepsy, initial presentation with status epilepticus was not associated with increased risk of subsequent seizures [73] though there may be a greater risk that recurrence will be in the form of another prolonged seizure or cluster (personal communication, W. A. Hauser, 2007). Among remote symptomatic seizure patients, having status epilepticus or post-ictal Todd's paresis increased the risk for recurrence [68]. In patients with status epilepticus or multiple seizures (two or more within 24 h), recurrence risk was 37% at 1 year, 56% at 3 years and 56% at 5 years, compared with 21%, 34% and 43% at 1, 3 and 5 years for those presenting with single seizures. These patients who present with prolonged seizures or clusters should be offered agents for abortive treatment if they have a means of administering it during their seizure (long aura, clusters with recovery between seizures or a care-giver), such as rectal, nasal or buccal benzodiazepines. Rectal diazepam and nasal/buccal midazolam are the most commonly used choices.

CONCLUSION

Hospitalized patients can have seizures of multiple origins, most commonly vascular, infectious or metabolic. These seizures are usually acute symptomatic in nature and the patients do not have epilepsy. Although short-term seizure suppression is often helpful, long-term treatment is usually not required unless unprovoked seizures occur as well. There are multiple choices of AEDs for acute seizures in the hospital, many with few drug interactions, few allergic reactions and no serious adverse effects. This allows rational, individualized choices that are effective and tolerated in most patients.

REFERENCES

1. Guidelines for epidemiologic studies on epilepsy. Commission on Epidemiology and Prognosis, International League Against Epilepsy. *Epilepsia* 1993; 34:592–596.
2. Finocchi V, Bozzao A, Bonamini M et al. Magnetic resonance imaging in posterior reversible encephalopathy syndrome: report of three cases and review of literature. *Arch Gynecol Obstet* 2005; 271:79–85.
3. Servillo G, Bifulco F, De Robertis E et al. Posterior reversible encephalopathy syndrome in intensive care medicine. *Intensive Care Med* 2007; 33:230–236.
4. Aminoff MJ, Simon RP. Status epilepticus. Causes, clinical features and consequences in 98 patients. *Am J Med* 1980; 69:657–666.
5. Claassen J, Mayer SA, Kowalski RG et al. Detection of electrographic seizures with continuous EEG monitoring in critically ill patients. *Neurology* 2004; 62:1743–1748.

6. Pandian JD, Cascino GD, So EL *et al*. Digital video-electroencephalographic monitoring in the neurological–neurosurgical intensive care unit: clinical features and outcome. *Arch Neurol* 2004; 61:1090–1094.

7. Husain AM, Horn GJ, Jacobson MP. Non-convulsive status epilepticus: usefulness of clinical features in selecting patients for urgent EEG. *J Neurol Neurosurg Psychiatry* 2003; 74:189–191.

8. French JA, Kanner AM, Bautista J *et al*. Efficacy and tolerability of the new anti-epileptic drugs I: treatment of new onset epilepsy: report of the Therapeutics and Technology Assessment Subcommittee and Quality Standards Subcommittee of the American Academy of Neurology and the American Epilepsy Society. *Neurology* 2004; 62:1252–1260.

9. Arif H, Buchsbaum R, Weintraub DB *et al*. Comparison and predictors of rash associated with 15 antiepileptic drugs. *Neurology* 2007; 68:1701–1709.

10. French J, Arrigo C. Rapid onset of action of levetiracetam in refractory epilepsy patients. *Epilepsia* 2005; 46:324–326.

11. Elger CE, Brodie MJ, Anhut H *et al*. Pregabalin add-on treatment in patients with partial seizures: a novel evaluation of flexible-dose and fixed-dose treatment in a double-blind, placebo-controlled study. *Epilepsia* 2005; 46:1926–1936.

12. McLean MJ, Gidal BE. Gabapentin dosing in the treatment of epilepsy. *Clin Ther* 2003; 25:1382–1406.

13. Fisher RS, Sachdeo RC, Pellock J *et al*. Rapid initiation of gabapentin: a randomized, controlled trial. *Neurology* 2001; 56:743–748.

14. Bergey GK, Morris HH, Rosenfeld W *et al*. Gabapentin monotherapy: I. An 8-day, double-blind, dose-controlled, multicenter study in hospitalized patients with refractory complex partial or secondarily generalized seizures. The US Gabapentin Study Group 88/89. *Neurology* 1997; 49:739–745.

15. Bleck TP, Smith MC, Pierre-Louis SJ *et al*. Neurologic complications of critical medical illnesses. *Crit Care Med* 1993; 21:98–103.

16. Wijdicks EF, Sharbrough FW. New-onset seizures in critically ill patients. *Neurology* 1993; 43:1042–1044.

17. Sander JW, Perucca E. Epilepsy and comorbidity: infections and antimicrobials usage in relation to epilepsy management. *Acta Neurol Scand Suppl* 2003; 180:16–22.

18. Fudio S, Carcas A, Pinana E *et al*. Epileptic seizures caused by low valproic acid levels from an interaction with meropenem. *J Clin Pharm Ther* 2006; 31:393–396.

19. Ellis AJ, Wendon JA, Williams R. Subclinical seizure activity and prophylactic phenytoin infusion in acute liver failure: a controlled clinical trial. *Hepatology* 2000; 32:536–541.

20. Ficker DM, Westmoreland BF, Sharbrough FW. Epileptiform abnormalities in hepatic encephalopathy. *J Clin Neurophysiol* 1997; 14:230–234.

21. Eleftheriadis N, Fourla E, Eleftheriadis D *et al*. Status epilepticus as a manifestation of hepatic encephalopathy. *Acta Neurol Scand* 2003; 107:142–144.

22. Plum F, Posner J (eds) *Diagnosis of Stupor And Coma*. Philadelphia: TA Davis, 1984.

23. Hirsch LJ, Kull LL. Continuous EEG monitoring in the intensive care unit. *Am J Electroneurodiagnostic Technol* 2004; 44:137–158.

24. Wittman JJ Jr, Hirsch LJ. Continuous electroencephalogram monitoring in the critically ill. *Neurocrit Care* 2005; 2:330–341.

25. Gerstner T, Teich M, Bell N *et al*. Valproate-associated coagulopathies are frequent and variable in children. *Epilepsia* 2006; 47:1136–1143.

26. Ramael S, Daoust A, Otoul C *et al*. Levetiracetam intravenous infusion: a randomized, placebo-controlled safety and pharmacokinetic study. *Epilepsia* 2006; 47:1128–1135.

27. Gibbs JE, Walker MC, Cock HR. Levetiracetam: antiepileptic properties and protective effects on mitochondrial dysfunction in experimental status epilepticus. *Epilepsia* 2006; 47:469–478.

28. Niebauer M, Gruenthal M. Topiramate reduces neuronal injury after experimental status epilepticus. *Brain Res* 1999; 837:263–269.

29. Trojnar MK, Malek R, Chroscinska M *et al*. Neuroprotective effects of antiepileptic drugs. *Pol J Pharmacol* 2002; 54:557–566.

30. Scorza FA, Albuquerque M, Arida RM *et al*. Seizure occurrence in patients with chronic renal insufficiency in regular hemodialysis program. *Arq Neuropsiquiatr* 2005; 63:757–760.

31. Bergen DC, Ristanovic R, Gorelick PB *et al*. Seizures and renal failures. *Int J Artif Organs* 1994; 17:247–251.

32. Glenn CM, Astley SJ, Watkins SL. Dialysis-associated seizures in children and adolescents. *Pediatr Nephrol* 1992; 6:182–186.

33. Fillastre JP, Taburet AM, Fialaire A *et al*. Pharmacokinetics of lamotrigine in patients with renal impairment: influence of haemodialysis. *Drugs Exp Clin Res* 1993; 19:25–32.

34. Hauser WA, Annegers JF, Kurland LT. Incidence of epilepsy and unprovoked seizures in Rochester, Minnesota: 1935–1984. *Epilepsia* 1993; 34:453–468.

35. Giroud M, Gras P, Fayolle H *et al*. Early seizures after acute stroke: a study of 1,640 cases. *Epilepsia* 1994; 35:959–964.

36. Kilpatrick CJ, Davis SM, Tress BM *et al*. Epileptic seizures in acute stroke. *Arch Neurol* 1990; 47:157–160.

37. Lamy C, Domigo V, Semah F *et al*. Early and late seizures after cryptogenic ischemic stroke in young adults. *Neurology* 2003; 60:400–404.

38. Lancman ME, Golimstok A, Norscini J *et al*. Risk factors for developing seizures after a stroke. *Epilepsia* 1993; 34:141–143.

39. Lossius MI, Ronning OM, Slapo GD *et al*. Poststroke epilepsy: occurrence and predictors – a long-term prospective controlled study (Akershus Stroke Study). *Epilepsia* 2005; 46:1246–1251.

40. Bladin CF, Alexandrov AV, Bellavance A *et al*. Seizures after stroke: a prospective multicenter study. *Arch Neurol* 2000; 57:1617–1622.

41. Labovitz DL, Hauser WA, Sacco RL. Prevalence and predictors of early seizure and status epilepticus after first stroke. *Neurology* 2001; 57:200–206.

42. Kilpatrick CJ, Davis SM, Hopper JL *et al*. Early seizures after acute stroke. Risk of late seizures. *Arch Neurol* 1992; 49:509–511.

43. Labovitz DL, Hauser WA. Preventing stroke-related seizures: when should anticonvulsant drugs be started? *Neurology* 2003; 60:365–366.

44. Chang BS, Lowenstein DH. Practice parameter: antiepileptic drug prophylaxis in severe traumatic brain injury: report of the Quality Standards Subcommittee of the American Academy of Neurology. *Neurology* 2003; 60:10–16.

45. Pohlmann-Eden B, Hoch DB, Cochius JI *et al*. Periodic lateralized epileptiform discharges – a critical review. *J Clin Neurophysiol* 1996; 13:519–530.

46. Donovan PJ, Cline D. Phenytoin administration by constant intravenous infusion: selective rates of administration. *Ann Emerg Med* 1991; 20:139–142.

47. Kasarskis EJ, Kuo CS, Berger R, Nelson KR. Carbamazepine-induced cardiac dysfunction. Characterization of two distinct clinical syndromes. *Arch Intern Med* 1992; 152:186–191.

48. Boesen F, Andersen EB, Jensen EK *et al*. Cardiac conduction disturbances during carbamazepine therapy. *Acta Neurol Scand* 1983; 68:49–52.

49. Hewetson KA, Ritch AE, Watson RD. Sick sinus syndrome aggravated by carbamazepine therapy for epilepsy. *Postgrad Med J* 1986; 62:497–498.

50. Wijdicks EF, Plevak DJ, Wiesner RH *et al*. Causes and outcome of seizures in liver transplant recipients. *Neurology*. Dec 1996;47(6):1523–1525.

51. Wijdicks EF, Wiesner RH, Dahlke LJ *et al*. FK506-induced neurotoxicity in liver transplantation. *Ann Neurol* 1994; 35:498–501.

52. Maramattom BV, Wijdicks EF. Sirolimus may not cause neurotoxicity in kidney and liver transplant recipients. *Neurology* 2004; 63:1958–1959.

53. Glantz MJ, Cole BF, Forsyth PA *et al*. Practice parameter: anticonvulsant prophylaxis in patients with newly diagnosed brain tumors. Report of the Quality Standards Subcommittee of the American Academy of Neurology. *Neurology* 2000; 54:1886–1893.

54. Rowland M, Gupta SK. Cyclosporine–phenytoin interaction: re-evaluation using metabolite data. *Br J Clin Pharmacol* 1987; 24:329–334.

55. Wong MC, Suite ND, Labar DR. Seizures in human immunodeficiency virus infection. *Arch Neurol* 1990; 47:640–642.

56. Pascual-Sedano B, Iranzo A, Marti-Fabregas J *et al*. Prospective study of new-onset seizures in patients with human immunodeficiency virus infection: etiologic and clinical aspects. *Arch Neurol* 1999; 56:609–612.

57. Chadha DS, Handa A, Sharma SK *et al*. Seizures in patients with human immunodeficiency virus infection. *J Assoc Physicians India* 2000; 48:573–576.

58. Holtzman DM, Kaku DA, So YT. New-onset seizures associated with human immunodeficiency virus infection: causation and clinical features in 100 cases. *Am J Med* 1989; 87:173–177.

59. Romanelli F, Jennings HR, Nath A *et al*. Therapeutic dilemma: the use of anticonvulsants in HIV-positive individuals. *Neurology* 2000; 54:1404–1407.

60. Romanelli F, Pomeroy C. Concurrent use of antiretrovirals and anticonvulsants in human immunodeficiency virus (HIV) seropositive patients. *Curr Pharm Des* 2003; 9:1433–1439.

61. Lehrman G, Hogue IB, Palmer S *et al*. Depletion of latent HIV-1 infection in vivo: a proof-of-concept study. *Lancet* 2005; 366:549–555.

62. Schifitto G, Peterson DR, Zhong J *et al.* Valproic acid adjunctive therapy for HIV-associated cognitive impairment: a first report. *Neurology* 2006; 66:919–921.

63. Stein DA, Chamberlain MC. Evaluation and management of seizures in the patient with cancer. *Oncology (Williston Park)* 1991; 5:33–39; discussion 40, 47.

64. Vecht CJ, Wagner GL, Wilms EB. Treating seizures in patients with brain tumors: drug interactions between antiepileptic and chemotherapeutic agents. *Semin Oncol* 2003; 30(Suppl 19):49–52.

65. Wagner GL, Wilms EB, Van Donselaar CA *et al.* Levetiracetam: preliminary experience in patients with primary brain tumours. *Seizure* 2003; 12:585–586.

66. Sibai BM. Diagnosis, prevention, and management of eclampsia. *Obstet Gynecol* 2005; 105:402–410.

67. Sibai BM, Spinnato JA, Watson DL *et al.* Effect of magnesium sulfate on electroencephalographic findings in preeclampsia-eclampsia. *Obstet Gynecol* 1984; 64:261–266.

68. Hauser WA, Rich SS, Annegers JF *et al.* Seizure recurrence after a 1st unprovoked seizure: an extended follow-up. *Neurology* 1990; 40:1163–1170.

69. Shinnar S, Berg AT, Moshe SL *et al.* The risk of seizure recurrence after a first unprovoked afebrile seizure in childhood: an extended follow-up. *Pediatrics* 1996; 98:216–225.

70. Berg AT, Shinnar S. The risk of seizure recurrence following a first unprovoked seizure: a quantitative review. *Neurology* 1991; 41:965–972.

71. Kho LK, Lawn ND, Dunne JW *et al.* First seizure presentation: do multiple seizures within 24 h predict recurrence? *Neurology* 2006; 67:1047–1049.

72. Bazil CW, Hauser WA. First seizure: do multiple seizures predict recurrence? *Neurology* 2006; 67:927.

73. Hauser WA, Anderson VE, Loewenson RB *et al.* Seizure recurrence after a first unprovoked seizure. *N Engl J Med* 1982; 307:522–528.

74. Garcia P, Alldredge B. Medication-associated seizures. In: Delanty N (ed.) *Seizures: Medical Causes and Management.* Totowa, NJ: Humana Press Inc., 2001, pp. 145–165.

75. Shuman R, Varelas P. Seizure-inducing drugs used for the critically ill. In: Varelas P (ed.) *Seizures in Critical Care. A guide to diagnosis and therapeutics.* Totowa, NJ: Humana Press Inc., 2005, pp. 261–290.

76. Choi EJ, Kang JK, Lee SA *et al.* New-onset seizures after liver transplantation: clinical implications and prognosis in survivors. *Eur Neurol* 2004; 52:230–236.

77. Adams DH, Ponsford S, Gunson B *et al.* Neurological complications following liver transplantation. *Lancet* 1987; 1:949–951.

78. Martinez AJ, Estol C, Faris AA. Neurologic complications of liver transplantation. *Neurol Clin* 1988; 6:327–348.

79. Jost L, Jost L, Nogues M *et al.* [Neurological complications of renal transplant]. *Medicina (B Aires)* 2000; 60:161–164.

80. McEnery PT, Nathan J, Bates SR *et al.* Convulsions in children undergoing renal transplantation. *J Pediatr* 1989; 115:532–536.

81. Malheiros SM, Almeida DR, Massaro AR *et al.* Neurologic complications after heart transplantation. *Arq Neuropsiquiatr* 2002; 60:192–197.

82. Perez-Miralles F, Sanchez-Manso JC, Almenar-Bonet L *et al.* Incidence of and risk factors for neurologic complications after heart transplantation. *Transplant Proc* 2005; 37:4067–4070.

83. Cemillan CA, Alonso-Pulpon L, Burgos-Lazaro R *et al.* [Neurological complications in a series of 205 orthotopic heart transplant patients]. *Rev Neurol* 2004; 38:906–912.

84. Grigg MM, Costanzo-Nordin MR, Celesia GG *et al.* The etiology of seizures after cardiac transplantation. *Transplant Proc* 1988; 20(Suppl 3):937–944.

85. Vaughn BV, Ali II, Olivier KN *et al.* Seizures in lung transplant recipients. *Epilepsia* 1996; 37:1175–1179.

86. Wong M, Mallory GB Jr, Goldstein J *et al.* Neurologic complications of pediatric lung transplantation. *Neurology* 1999; 53:1542–1549.

87. Snider S, Bashir R, Bierman P. Neurologic complications after high-dose chemotherapy and autologous bone marrow transplantation for Hodgkin's disease. *Neurology* 1994; 44:681–684.

88. Antonini G, Ceschin V, Morino S *et al.* Early neurologic complications following allogeneic bone marrow transplant for leukemia: a prospective study. *Neurology* 1998; 50:1441–1445.

89. Furlong TG, Gallucci BB. Pattern of occurrence and clinical presentation of neurological complications in bone marrow transplant patients. *Cancer Nurs* 1994; 17:27–36.

90. Kiok MC. Neurologic complications of pancreas transplants. *Neurol Clin* 1988; 6:367–376.

13

Treatment of the epilepsy patient with concomitant medical conditions

Sinead M. Murphy, Norman Delanty

INTRODUCTION

Epilepsy is common, affecting up to 2% of the population [1]. Thus, it is inevitable that most doctors, whether neurologists, surgeons, general practitioners or hospital physicians, will at some stage have to manage a patient with epilepsy. People with epilepsy may have an exacerbation in their seizures due to a concomitant medical condition or its treatment, a person without epilepsy may have an acute symptomatic seizure during an acute illness, or a patient may develop epilepsy associated with a medical condition.

Even though a patient's seizures may be well controlled at baseline, an untimely seizure during a systemic disturbance may impact adversely on outcome, predispose the patient to infections and cause metabolic or cerebral dysfunction. Additionally, the situation may be further complicated by the presence of anti-epileptic drugs (AEDs), as pharmacodynamics and pharmacokinetics may be altered during a systemic illness.

Unfortunately, patients with epilepsy who have co-morbid diseases are often excluded from AED trials, which means there are few data about this group of patients. This chapter addresses the difficult topic of managing the patient with epilepsy and a co-morbid medical condition.

CEREBROVASCULAR DISEASE

Stroke may cause acute symptomatic seizures in the initial post-stroke period, as well as epilepsy in the long term [2]. In fact, stroke is the most common cause of epilepsy in older patients [1]. Stroke treatments, such as thrombolysis and revascularization procedures, may also result in seizures. The risk of seizures is highest after intracerebral haemorrhage (ICH) [3, 4], but they may also occur after ischaemic stroke and in the setting of transient ischaemic attack (TIA) due to focal neuronal dysfunction [5, 6]. Animal studies suggest that the risk of seizures is proportional to the volume of damaged tissue [7].

AED prophylaxis is not recommended after stroke or ICH, unless the patient has had a seizure. The risk of seizures is greatest at presentation, and in patients with lobar haemorrhage. However, seizure occurrence does not appear to affect mortality and the

Sinead M. Murphy, MB, BCh, MRCPI, Specialist Registrar in Neurology, Department of Neurology, Beaumont Hospital, Dublin, Ireland

Norman Delanty, FRCPI, ABPN (Dip), Honorary Senior Lecturer Neurology (RCSI); Consultant Neurologist; Director of Epilepsy Services, Department of Neurology, Beaumont Hospital, Dublin, Ireland

risk of developing epilepsy in patients who have not had a seizure at ICH onset is low, suggesting that AED prophylaxis is unnecessary [8]. In the setting of an acute symptomatic seizure following a stroke or ICH, some would advocate the use of an AED for the initial few weeks, followed by gradual weaning if the patient remains seizure free. If, however, a patient has a remote unprovoked seizure in the setting of an underlying structural lesion such as a focal infarct, most epileptologists would commence long-term AED treatment, as the risk of recurrent seizures is high. The choice of AED is important, as many of the older AEDs are sedating, affect coordination and may impact on rehabilitation. Phenytoin was found to impact adversely on functional outcome post subarachnoid haemorrhage (SAH) [9] and phenytoin, phenobarbital and benzodiazepines were all found to be associated with less independence in activities of daily living (ADL) in patients following focal brain injury [10]. In addition, many stroke patients also have cardiac disease, therefore phenytoin may not be ideal.

Fortunately, epilepsy occurring as a result of stroke is usually relatively easily treated, most patients becoming seizure free on monotherapy [11] and most AEDs being effective [12]. AED choice depends on other factors, such as co-morbidities, medications and side-effect profiles. However, gabapentin and lamotrigine have been found to be useful because of lack of interactions, side-effect profile and efficacy [12, 13]. Although there is a lack of specific data on the other newer AEDs, levetiracetam and topiramate would also be expected to be useful in this patient population, although both may have cognitive and behavioural adverse effects.

CARDIAC DISEASE

Atrial fibrillation (AF) occurs in 9% of patients over the age of 80 years, and prevalence is increasing as the population ages [14]. All patients with AF should be anti-coagulated with warfarin for stroke prevention unless there is a clear contraindication. It is therefore particularly important in this patient group that seizures are well controlled, as a minor injury may cause devastating haemorrhage. Epilepsy, however, is not a contraindication to anti-coagulation. One study found that warfarin remained the drug of choice in elderly patients with AF despite a risk of falls [15]. Several AEDs may interact with warfarin, in particular the enzyme inducers (phenytoin, phenobarbital and carbamazepine), which may enhance its metabolism, requiring an increase in warfarin dose to maintain therapeutic anti-coagulation. Importantly, there is a significant risk of over-anticoagulation if the enzyme-inducing AED is withdrawn. Thus, if an AED is added or withdrawn, the international normalized ratio (INR) should be monitored particularly closely. Phenytoin has an unpredictable effect on the INR as it affects both protein binding and enzyme induction (Table 13.1).

Cardiac arrhythmias have been reported frequently during and after seizures. The most common rhythm seen peri-ictally is a sinus tachycardia, which is a normal physiological response to the seizure [16]. However, symptomatic sinus bradycardias, including asystole,

Table 13.1 Effects of anti-epileptic drugs (AEDs) on the international normalized ratio (INR)

AEDs which may reduce INR	AEDs which may increase INR
Carbamazepine	Phenytoin
Phenobarbital	Valproate
Phenytoin	
Primidone	

may occur. Such patients should be considered for pacemaker insertion [17]. S–T-segment abnormailties have also been reported in association with seizures [18]. Patients with epilepsy who have a history of ischaemic heart disease may therefore be at increased risk of cardiac ischaemic events during a seizure.

It is important to consider that not every patient with recurrent unprovoked episodes of loss of consciousness has epilepsy. It is not uncommon for a patient with syncope to have brief convulsive jerks, which may be misinterpreted as seizure activity. Cardiac conditions, such as arrhythmias, are another common cause of recurrent collapses. Confusingly, some AEDs may even help prevent attacks which are not seizures. For example, patients with long Q–T syndrome may have recurrent episodes of loss of consciousness due to a brief asystole. In this situation, phenytoin, which shortens the Q–T interval, may actually prevent the arrhythmia, thereby giving a false impression of 'seizure' control [19].

Cardiac medications, particularly the class I anti-arrhythmics (lidocaine, flecainide, propafenone), which block sodium channels, may lower the seizure threshold even at therapeutic doses. Some cardiac medications, in particular quinidine and flecainide, are also metabolized by the cytochrome P450 system and may interact with certain AEDs (see 'Drugs and drug interactions' later in this chapter).

Some AEDs have cardiovascular side-effects, particularly when administered by intravenous infusion; this may make acute seizure management difficult in patients with cardiac conditions. Phenytoin infusion causes significant hypotension in approximately 5% of patients [20], and may be pro-arrhythmogenic when administered rapidly. For patients with heart disease, the rate of phenytoin infusion should be <25mg/min [21]. Fosphenytoin, a pro-drug of phenytoin, was initially thought to be free of cardiac adverse effects; however, recent literature suggests that cardiac adverse events are not uncommon [22].

Carbamazepine has also been associated with adverse cardiac events. With acute overdose, acute cardiac failure and tachyarrhythmias have been reported; with chronic use and therapeutic drug levels, bradyarrhythmias and refractory hypertension have been reported [23–25]. It has been suggested that sudden unexpected death in epilepsy (SUDEP) may in some cases be attributable to AED-induced cardiac dysfunction [26]; this remains controversial.

For acute seizure treatment in a patient with cardiac disease, intravenous valproate may be preferred to phenytoin or fosphenytoin, while the second-generation AEDs, such as topiramate and lamotrigine, may have fewer cardiac adverse events for patients requiring long-term seizure prophylaxis [27].

RENAL DISEASE

Seizures may occur in uraemic encephalopathy, dialysis disequilibrium syndrome and dialysis encephalopathy. In addition, renal insufficiency and dialysis may both have effects on AED pharmacokinetics. Renal impairment can alter the fraction of AED absorbed, volume of distribution, protein binding and renal drug clearance.

Renal impairment may alter the gastric pH, cause small intestinal bacterial overgrowth, gastrointestimal tract oedema and impaired gastrointestinal motility [28, 29]. These factors may cause reduced ionization of some drugs and reduce drug absorption.

The volume of distribution of drugs may be increased in patients with end-stage renal failure, resulting in lower total plasma levels. However, protein binding of acidic drugs may be significantly reduced in renal impairment [30]; total plasma levels of AEDs may therefore be misleading. A total drug level may appear within the therapeutic range, despite a toxic-free level. For AEDs metabolized by the liver, changes in protein binding will affect the steady-state plasma concentration, but the free concentration will remain unchanged. For these reasons, it is often more useful to measure free concentrations of AEDs which are highly protein bound, such as phenytoin and valproate.

Renal impairment may affect drug clearance depending on the extent of renal clearance, drug filtration and tubular secretion and resorption. Gabapentin, topiramate, pregabalin and levetiracetam are almost exclusively cleared by the kidneys. These drugs have reduced elimination and prolonged half-lives in patients with renal impairment and dosages should be adjusted accordingly [31]. For other AEDs such as phenytoin, carbamazepine and tiagabine, renal excretion is minimal, and unless creatinine clearance is below 25 ml/min there is no need to adjust the dose (Table 13.2).

Table 13.2 Effect of renal disease on specific anti-epileptic drugs (AEDs)

AED	Protein binding (%)	Half-life (h)	Effect of renal disease
Carbamazepine	80	36; 16–24 with repeated doses; 9–10 with enzyme inducers	Anti-diuretic effect, may increase fluid retention
Felbamate	25		Reduced clearance; prolonged half-life
Gabapentin	0	5–9	Reduced clearance; significantly removed by HD; company advises 200–300 mg bolus post HD
Lamotrigine	50	24–34; doubled with valproate; 15 with enzyme inducers	Prolonged half-life; reduce dose; 20% removed by HD
Levetiracetam	<10	6–8	Reduced clearance; 50% removed by HD; company advise giving 250–500 mg bolus post HD
Oxcarbazepine	40 of active metabolite	Parent drug, 2; active metabolite, 9	Reduced clearance; reduce dose
Phenobarbital	40–50	55–118	Removed by HD; reduce dose
Phenytoin	>90	22–36	Reduced total concentration but increased free fraction; only 2–4% removed by HD; monitor free levels
Pregabalin	0	6	Reduced clearance, prolonged half-life; reduce dose; significantly removed by HD; supplement dose post HD
Tiagabine	96	5–8	Minimal effect
Topiramate	<20	21	Reduced clearance; reduce dose; significantly removed by HD; company advise loading before HD to avoid sub-therapeutic levels. Note: risk of renal stones
Valproate	85–95	12–16	Reduced protein binding; reduced total concentration but increased free fraction; 20% removed by HD
Vigabatrin	0	5–8	Reduced clearance; reduce dose
Zonisamide	40	50–70; 30 with enzyme inducers	Reduced clearance; some is removed by HD

HD, haemodialysis;

Several methods have been proposed to calculate AED dose based on creatinine clearance, volume of distribution and other variables [32]. However, these are complex and the actual drug concentration may vary considerably from that calculated. In patients with renal impairment, AEDs should be slowly initiated at low doses and clinical assessment and drug level monitoring are necessary.

Haemodialysis (HD) may clear AEDs from the circulation depending on their molecular size, water solubility, protein binding, volume of distribution and dialysis conditions. Drugs such as ethosuximide, gabapentin, levetiracetam, phenobarbital, pregabalin and topiramate which are highly water soluble, not protein bound and with a small volume of distribution are readily removed by HD. Carbamazepine, clonazepam, phenytoin, tiagibine and valproate have a low risk of removal, although even these will have some removal during HD.

If an AED has been partially removed by HD, the following equation can be used to calculate the loading dose required to restore the desired plasma concentration [32]:

$$LD = C_{change} \times VD$$

where LD = loading dose; C_{change} = desired change in plasma concentration; VD = volume of distribution.

The kidney is the most commonly transplanted organ, usually as a result of hypertensive disease, diabetes or glomerulonephritis, all of which cause uraemia and may be associated with seizures. The immunosuppressant agents most often used in renal transplantation are cyclosporine, tacrolimus, azathioprine and mycophenolate; most patients are also on steroids. Cyclosporine and tacrolimus are well known to be associated with posterior leukoencephalopathy and seizures [33, 34]. Cyclosporine has also been shown to reduce seizure threshold [35]. These immunosuppressants are mainly metabolized by the liver. Enzyme-inducing AEDs such as phenytoin, carbamazepine and phenobarbital may reduce the plasma concentration of cyclosporine; it is therefore particularly important to monitor cyclosporine levels in such patients. It has been reported that phenytoin and phenobarbital reduce renal allograft survival, possibly due to increased metabolism of immunosuppressive agents [36, 37]. Owing to fewer effects on the cytochrome P450 system and fewer drug interactions, some of the second-generation AEDs are preferred in renal transplant patients with epilepsy; however, gabapentin has been reported in association with acute renal dysfunction in an allograft [38].

If transplant patients with epilepsy have breakthrough seizures, it is important to consider aetiologies other than their epilepsy as the cause. In particular, uraemic encephalopathy, metabolic derangement, opportunistic infection or leukoencephalopathy should be considered.

In summary, gabapentin and levetiracetam may accumulate in patients with renal failure. Valproate, carbamazepine, oxcarbazepine and tiagabine are less likely to cause toxicity, although their protein binding will be affected.

HEPATIC DISEASE

The liver is the principal organ of drug metabolism. Some drugs are absorbed from the gut, delivered to the liver and undergo first-pass metabolism prior to reaching the systemic circulation. Metabolism of these drugs is significantly affected by hepatic vascular supply; if hepatic blood flow is reduced, first-pass metabolism is decreased and more drug reaches the systemic circulation. Other drugs reach the systemic circulation before being delivered to the liver for metabolism; hepatocyte function is more important than the blood supply for their metabolism.

Cytochrome P450 enzymes are involved in Phase I metabolism (non-synthetic metabolism which includes oxidation, reduction and hydrolysis). There is substantial genetic polymorphism within these enzymes, and people may be slow or fast metabolizers. These enzymes are also frequently induced or inhibited by drugs, including AEDs. Phenytoin, phenobarbital and carbamazepine are well-known enzyme inducers (Table 13.3).

The liver is also involved in protein production; impaired protein production reduces the amount of drug that is protein bound, increasing the free fraction. This is relevant for phenytoin, valproate, tiagabine and carbamazepine, which are highly protein bound. The

Table 13.3 Effects of liver disease on specific anti-epileptic drugs (AEDs)

AED	Protein bound (%)	Half-life (h)	Liver disease
Carbamazepine	80	36; 16–24 with repeated doses; 9–10 with enzyme inducers	Reduced protein binding; reduced metabolism
Felbamate	25		Potentially hepatotoxic; inadvisable to use in liver disease
Gabapentin	0	5–9	Not affected
Lamotrigine	50	24–34; doubled with valproate; 15 with enzyme inducers	Slight reduction in clearance and prolonged half-life but considered clinically insignificant in trials
Levetiracetam	<10	6–8	Not affected
Oxcarbazepine	40 of active metabolite	Parent drug, 2; active metabolite, 9	No need to alter dose
Phenobarbital	40–50	55–118	Prolonged half-life; reduced metabolism; reduce dose and increase time between doses
Phenytoin	>90	22–36	Reduced metabolism, therefore accumulates and may become toxic quickly; reduced protein binding; increase in free fraction; monitor free levels
Pregabalin	0	6	Not affected
Tiagabine	96	5–8	Prolonged half-life; increased free fraction; reduce dose; increase time between doses
Topiramate	<20	18–23	Reduced clearance; prolonged half-life; felt to be clinically insignificant
Valproate	85–95	12–16	Reduced protein binding; rarely hepatotoxic
Vigabatrin	0	5–8	Not affected; however, some reports of liver damage
Zonisamide	40	50–70; 30 with enzyme inducers	Reduced metabolism; prolonged half-life; increase interval between dose adjustments

true plasma concentration of phenytoin in a patient with low albumin can be calculated by Equation 2 [39].

$$\text{True plasma phenytoin level} = \frac{\text{observed phenytoin level}}{0.9 \times \left[\dfrac{\text{patient's albumin}}{\text{normal albumin}} \right] + 0.1}$$

All AEDs except levetiracetam, gabapentin, pregabalin and vigabatrin have some hepatic metabolism, therefore hepatic disease may affect pharmacokinetics of most of the AEDs (Table 13.4). Additionally, patients with liver disease may be encephalopathic and have altered pharmacodynamics, having a lower seizure threshold as well as being more vulnerable to the central nervous system (CNS) adverse reactions of AEDs.

Seizures occur frequently after liver transplantation. Immunosuppressants are mainly metabolized by the liver, as are most AEDs. In addition, many AEDs may induce or inhibit hepatic metabolism. These factors make management of epilepsy difficult in patients with a liver transplant. Levetiracetam may be a good choice of AED in such patients because of its predominantly renal metabolism and excretion, low protein binding, lack of enzyme induction, lack of drug interactions and broad-spectrum use in different seizure types [40].

A number of AEDs may rarely be hepatotoxic; the most common culprit is valproate, which is contraindicated in patients with hepatic failure. However, other AEDs, including phenytoin, may cause an acute drug-induced hepatitis. These reactions are idiosyncratic and usually occur soon after commencing the drug. Hepatic toxicity should prompt immediate discontinuation of the offending drug and substitution of an alternative AED.

As gabapentin, pregabalin and levetiracetam are not significantly protein bound or metabolized by the liver, these are good choices for long-term AED in patients with hepatic disease. If a patient with liver disease has an acute seizure, benzodiazepines may be used, although there is an increased risk of respiratory depression.

Table 13.4 Drugs that induce or inhibit hepatic enzymes

Enzyme inducers	Enzyme inhibitors	
Anti-epileptic drugs	*Anti-epileptic drugs*	*Antifungals*
Phenytoin	Valproate	Ketaconazole
Carbamazepine	*Antibiotics*	Itraconazole
Phenobarbital	Erythromycin	Fluconazole
Topiramate	Clarithromycin	*Anti-arrhythmics*
Felbamate	Metronidazole	Amiodarone
Tiagabine	Cotrimoxazole	Quinidine
Zonisamide	Isoniazid	Verapamil
Antibiotics	Ciprofloxacin	*Proton pump inhibitors*
Rifampicin	*Protease inhibitors*	Omeprazole
Rifabutin	Ritonavir	*Antidepressants*
	Indinavir	Fluoxetine
	Nelfinavir	Fluvoxamine
	Saquinavir	Nefazodone
	Histamine 2 blockers	Monoamine oxidase inhibitors
	Cimetidine	Lithium

METABOLIC DISORDERS

Metabolic disturbances are a common cause of seizures, even in patients without epilepsy. In most cases, acute metabolic derangements causing seizures are potentially reversible. Seizures due to metabolic derangements are often refractory to anti-convulsant medications; correction of the underlying abnormality is required.

Hyponatraemia is the most common electrolyte disturbance encountered in clinical practice [41]. It is a common side-effect of many drugs, including carbamazepine and oxcarbazepine. Oxcarbazepine seems to be associated with a higher incidence of hyponatraemia than carbamazepine, 30% vs. 14% in one study [42]. Risk factors for the development of hyponatraemia are age >40, female gender, use of drugs associated with hyponatraemia, psychiatric illness and surgery [43]. It may also be due to the syndrome of inappropriate anti-diuretic hormone secretion (SIADH) which may occur in patients with cerebral pathology. Symptoms of hyponatraemia are lethargy, confusion, muscle twitching, seizures and coma. Chronic mild hyponatraemia may be asymptomatic, and may not need specific treatment. However, acute hyponatraemia associated with neurological symptoms may need urgent treatment, in some cases requiring careful administration of hypertonic saline. It is important not to increase the sodium by more than 12 mmol/l/day as there is a risk of central pontine myelinolysis with a rapid change in sodium. In epilepsy patients with pre-existing hyponatraemia, carbamazepine and oxcarbazepine should not be used if possible. If a patient with epilepsy develops hyponatraemia because of their AED, it may be sufficient to reduce the dose, as the severity of hyponatraemia appears to be dose related; if persistent, however, it may be necessary to use an alternative AED.

Hypernatraemia is much less common than hyponatraemia, but may occur transiently following a convulsion. Significant hypernatraemia may cause intracerebral haemorrhage, cerebral vein rupture, seizures, coma and death. Treatment is water replacement, although again it is important not to correct the sodium too quickly, as there is a risk of cerebral oedema.

Symptomatic hypoglycaemia is a common cause of seizures. Hypoglycaemia is often medication related; other causes are sepsis and inborn errors of metabolism. Serum glucose usually needs to be less than 2.2 mmol/l for seizures to occur. Refractory nocturnal seizures should raise the possibility of insulinoma. Patients with diabetes who suffer from recurrent episodes of symptomatic hypoglycaemia and seizures require modification of their hypoglycaemic medication rather than anti-convulsant treatment. Phenytoin has been shown to interfere with carbohydrate metabolism, the usual effect being hyperglycaemia [44]; however, it has also been reported in association with hypoglycaemia [45, 46]. An alternative AED should be used in patients with diabetes.

Non-ketotic hyperglycaemia (NKH) usually occurs in older patients with non-insulin-dependent diabetes. It is associated with significant morbidity and mortality and often causes seizures. It may be precipitated by infection, surgery or other physiological stress. In contrast, ketotic hyperglycaemia rarely causes seizures, as ketosis is thought to have an anti-convulsant effect. Patients with NKH are often also hyponatraemic and may develop areas of potentially reversible focal cerebral damage [47], both of which increase the risk of seizures. Treatment of NKH is with insulin, fluids and correction of the metabolic abnormalities.

Seizures occur in up to one-quarter of patients admitted emergently with acute hypocalcaemia [48]. Rarely, hypocalcaemia has caused seizures in patients on long-term AEDs such as phenytoin and phenobarbital due to their effects on vitamin D metabolism [49]. Acute valproate overdose has also been associated with hypocalcaemia. Treatment of symptomatic hypocalcaemia is with intravenous calcium gluconate; replacement of magnesium may also be required if the patient has co-existing hypomagnesaemia.

Porphyria is a group of disorders caused by inherited deficits of enzymes involved in haem synthesis. Seizures occur in the hepatic porphyrias: acute intermittent porphyria, hereditary co-poporphyria and variegate porphyria. Between 5% and 20% of patients with porphyria have seizures [50, 51]. Unfortunately, many drugs can precipitate an acute attack, including the enzyme-inducing AEDs. This makes treatment of epilepsy and of acute symptomatic seizures very difficult. Gabapentin and vigabatrin have both been used successfully and appear to have a low risk of precipitating a crisis [52, 53]. Lorazepam seems to have the lowest risk of the benzodiazepines, although all cause porphyrin accumulation [54]. Less is known about the second-generation AEDs; tiagabine and topiramate appear to have the potential to cause an acute attack [55], while oxcarbazepine and levetiracetam have both been used safely in case reports [56–58]. Pregabalin is expected to be safe, although to date there are no published data on its use in porphyria.

THE ACUTELY UNWELL OR PERIPROCEDURAL PATIENT

People with epilepsy are often considered to be at higher risk when undergoing procedures. This is mainly due to the possibility of seizures occurring periprocedurally or due to the potential for interactions between drugs used during the procedure and the patient's AEDs.

Factors which may exacerbate seizures, such as sleep deprivation and alcohol, should be avoided prior to a procedure, and patients undergoing surgery should be advised to take their usual AEDs on the morning of surgery, even if fasting, and should continue their usual doses as soon as it is safe to do so.

Seizures are common after neurosurgical procedures, and are also common following cardiac operations [59], possibly due to complex alterations in metabolism, haemodynamic changes, alteration in blood/clotting factors and cerebral perfusion which may occur during cardiopulmonary bypass.

Although most of the local and general anaesthetic agents may have pro- as well as anti-convulsant effects [60], the actual risk of inducing a seizure is small. Enflurane appears to be associated with the highest risk of seizure [61].

Benzodiazepines are often used perioperatively and may prevent acute seizures, but care must be taken when weaning off these agents to avoid withdrawal seizures. Some analgesics such as the opiates – pethidine (meperidine) in particular – are associated with seizures, and should be avoided, where possible, post-operatively.

AED levels may be altered significantly post-operatively due to changes in hydration, volume of distribution, pharmacokinetics, pharmacodynamics, altered protein binding and blood loss. It is useful to have a baseline AED level at which the patient is seizure free to allow comparison and dose alterations post-operatively.

Patients with epilepsy in the intensive care unit (ICU) are at high risk of seizures. Seizures are often precipitated by this environment, even in patients without any history of epilepsy [62]. Organ failure, metabolic changes, electrolyte and fluid imbalance, cerebral oedema, hypoxia, hypotension and hypoglycaemia are all common occurrences, as is the presence of many drugs which may lower the seizure threshold. Most patients in the ICU are also sleep deprived [63]. Pre-existing AED regimens are often disturbed due to altered absorption, metabolism, dosing schedules and because the patient is unable to take drugs orally. In addition, because of the frequent use of sedation and neuromuscular blocking drugs, it may be difficult to know if a patient is actually seizing.

Oral dosing may be limited in patients who are fasting, post-ictal, have a reduced level of consciousness or who are intubated. Most AEDs can be given via an alternative route if the patient cannot swallow tablets:

- Phenytoin may be given intravenously, in suspension form via enteric tubes, or rectally. If given enterally, it should be given separately from feeds as these may reduce absorption.

- Fosphenytoin, a pro-drug of phenytoin, may be substituted. It can be given intramuscularly, which is useful when access is difficult, or intravenously.
- Phenobarbital may be given intravenously, intramuscularly or rectally. It is also available in liquid form which may be given via enteric tubes.
- Valproate may be given intravenously, as a syrup which may be given via enteric tubes, or by rectal suppositories which give good bioavailability.
- Carbamazepine can be given by suppository using the same dose as orally, and is also available in suspension form which can be given via enteric tubes.
- Benzodiazepines are usually used for acute seizure management rather than for chronic epilepsy treatment, but are available in many different forms which may be useful for patients who are acutely unwell. Lorazepam may be given intravenously or sublingually. Rectal diazepam is well absorbed, and is also available intravenously. Midazolam can be given into the buccal cavity or intranasally.

Most of the newer AEDs are still not available in intravenous form. However, most can be given via enteric tubes in the following preparations:

- Oxcarbazepine suspension
- Lamotrigine (tablets may be crushed)
- Topiramate (sprinkles may be injected using water)
- Levetiracetam liquid (intravenous levetiracetam is at an advanced phase of development and is expected to be commercially available in the near future)
- Gabapentin liquid.

ELDERLY PATIENTS

The incidence of epilepsy is highest in patients >75 years [1], with a point prevalence of 1.5%, and as the population ages doctors will treat increasing numbers of older patients with epilepsy. Treatment of epilepsy in older patients is complicated by alterations in pharmacodynamics and pharmacokinetics, metabolic derangements, presence of multiple co-morbid diseases, polypharmacy and psychosocial factors.

The aetiology of epilepsy in older patients differs from that of young people; the most frequent cause being cerebrovascular disease [64]. Seizures are usually partial in onset and may be mistaken for recurrent strokes or TIAs [65, 66], which may lead to unnecessary investigations and inappropriate treatment. In addition, morbidity and mortality are higher in elderly patients with seizures [67]. However, the literature suggests that if the elderly patient can tolerate the AED, the prognosis is usually good, with seizure freedom rates of over 60% at 1 year [68].

Physiological changes occur with increasing age, and these affect AED absorption and metabolism. Gastric emptying, gastrointestinal blood flow and bowel motility are often reduced and gastric pH higher in elderly people [69]. These affect drug solubility and ionization and may reduce the rate and amount of drug absorbed. In addition, the volume of distribution of a drug may be altered by muscle loss and an increase in fat which occurs with age.

Protein binding is altered due to low levels of albumin, which occurs in normal elderly people as well as those with malnutrition, renal or hepatic disease. This affects AEDs which are highly protein bound such as phenytoin, valproate and carbamazepine, meaning that the free drug level may be more useful in these patients.

Hepatic phase I reactions and renal clearance both decrease with advancing age; elderly patients are therefore at higher risk of AED toxicity at lower doses. While there are no specific recommendations with regard to AED dosing in the elderly, they may develop toxic effects at lower levels and may only tolerate lower doses.

Depression is common in the elderly, as it is in epilepsy. Johnson found that interictal psychiatric features impacted more on quality of life in people with epilepsy than did seizure frequency [70]. Depression is frequently under-diagnosed and inadequately treated, and may impact negatively on long-term outcome. Unfortunately, most anti-depressant medications can lower the seizure threshold. Selective serotonin re-uptake inhibitors (SSRIs) have a lower risk of seizures than the tricyclic anti-depressants. The risk of seizures associated with most anti-depressants is <0.4% overall [71] with a dose-dependent relationship; however, the risk is probably higher in patients with epilepsy and in the elderly. If a patient at higher risk of seizures requires an anti-depressant, using a low dose and slower dose escalation may reduce the seizure risk [72].

Many of the AEDs have cognitive adverse effects, which should be considered prior to prescribing them for elderly people who may be more sensitive to these side-effects. Some of the newer AEDs, such as lamotrigine and zonisamide, may have less cognitive adverse effects than some of the first-generation AEDs.

Osteoporosis is frequent in the elderly population, and fractures are a major cause of morbidity and mortality. Patients with epilepsy on AEDs have double the risk of fractures, probably due to a combination of increased risk of falls due to adverse effects of AEDs, seizure-related trauma and reduced bone health. A number of AEDs, predominantly phenytoin, valproate and phenobarbital have been associated with reduced bone mineral density, although more recent studies have also implicated carbamazepine and oxcarbazepine [73, 74]. Patients at risk should be offered dual energy X-ray absorptiometry (DEXA) scanning and may require treatment with bisphosphonates and calcium and vitamin D supplementation.

One study found that the mean number of daily medications for elderly patients in the community was eight, with 40% prescribed more than nine medications daily [75]. Polypharmacy increases the risk of medication non-compliance, which may in turn increase the risk of seizures. In addition, polypharmacy increases the potential for drug–drug interactions. Elderly patients are more likely to have memory problems and visual impairment and these factors make medication errors more likely. Because of the narrow therapeutic index, lower tolerability and higher adverse effect rate of AEDs in older patients, it is preferable to initiate AEDs at lower doses and titrate more slowly than is necessary in younger patients.

Adverse effects of AEDs are one of the most important problems in epilepsy management in elderly people. Older patients are often excluded from drug trials due to co-morbid illnesses and presence of other medications; however, the literature suggests decreased tolerability of the first-generation AEDs with increasing age [76]. In addition, the recent Veterans' Affairs Cooperative Study found that retention rates in elderly people with epilepsy were better for lamotrigine and gabapentin than for carbamazepine, without any significant difference in rates of seizure freedom [45]. Despite this, phenytoin, carbamazepine and valproate remain the most frequently prescribed AEDs in nursing home residents [77]. Elderly patients are more likely to develop adverse effects of drugs at lower doses, as they tend to tolerate a narrower therapeutic range. Adverse effects such as tremor, ataxia, visual disturbances and sedation are common and occur at lower drug levels in elderly people. These adverse effects in turn increase the risk of falls and of non-compliance.

When choosing an AED for an elderly patient with epilepsy, one needs to consider co-morbid conditions and medications. Monotherapy is preferable as they are often on many other medications, and the recent literature would suggest that the second-generation AEDs are preferable as first-line treatment rather than the more established first-generation AEDs (phenytoin, carbamazepine, valproate). If a patient is on other sedating medications, it would be wise to avoid prescribing potentially sedating AEDs such as gabapentin. A patient with tremor or ataxia may be made worse by valproate, phenytoin and carbamazepine. However, even a carefully chosen medication may be less well tolerated and require lower dose and slower titration in this group of patients.

DRUGS AND DRUG INTERACTIONS

The goal of epilepsy treatment is 'no seizures, no side-effects'. Monotherapy is preferred if possible, because of greater patient compliance with medications, better quality of life, more favourable adverse effect profile, lack of drug interactions and cost issues. However, many patients with epilepsy will require more than one AED, and many patients will also be on other medications for co-morbid conditions. This means that a large proportion of people with epilepsy are at risk of drug interactions.

When new AEDs are undergoing trials, they are almost invariably tested as add-on therapy, meaning that they are initially licensed only as add-on treatment rather than as monotherapy.

Drug interactions may be pharmacodynamic or pharmacokinetic. The clinical significance of a drug interaction depends on the drugs involved as well as patient factors such as age and co-morbid conditions. However, drug interactions are not necessarily harmful. There are several combinations of AEDs with synergistic effects on each other, such as lamotrigine and valproate [78], meaning that lower doses of both are required, which may reduce cost. The combination of phenytoin and valproate also appears to have some synergistic activity, so lower drug levels may confer the same anti-convulsant effect [79, 80]. Using an AED which prolongs the half-life or reduces the metabolism of another may mean prolonging the time between doses, which may improve patient compliance.

There are several ways in which AED absorption may be altered. Activated charcoal, antacids and resins reduce drug absorption by adsorbing drugs onto their surface and preventing passage of drug across the stomach wall. As soon as this occurs, serum concentration of the drug begins to decrease, the rate of decrease depending on its half-life. Metoclopramide and other drugs that increase gastric motility may increase the absorption of drugs, while anticholinergics and other drugs that slow gastric emptying may delay absorption. An increase or decrease in the rate of absorption may not alter drug bioavailability, but may be important if a rapid effect is required. Drugs that alter gastric pH, such as histamine receptor blockers, proton pump inhibitors and antacids, may change ionization of acidic or basic drugs, thereby affecting absorption [81]. All of these local factors may be reduced by the patient taking the interacting drugs several hours apart.

Alterations in protein binding may be another mechanism for drug interactions. This is largely important for drugs which are highly protein bound and have a narrow therapeutic index, such as phenytoin. If one drug is commenced when a patient is stable on another, the new drug will displace some of the original drug from plasma proteins, causing an increase in the unbound fraction [82]. However, when the unbound fraction of a drug increases, more is available for metabolism and clearance, so in fact the drug concentration may decrease. These interactions are unpredictable, so it is important to monitor free AED levels as total levels are misleading.

The most common cause of drug interaction, however, is induced alterations in hepatic metabolism (see Table 13.4). Phenytoin, phenobarbital, carbamazepine, topiramate, tiagabine, zonisamide and felbamate are all metabolized by the cytochrome P450 enzyme system. Several drugs can induce or inhibit these enzymes in a dose-dependent fashion. Carbamazepine, for example, is an autoinducer as it induces the isoenzyme which is responsible for its own metabolism. Phenytoin, phenobarbital, carbamazepine and topiramate all induce cytochrome P450 enzymes, while valproate is an inhibitor. Interactions due to enzyme induction occur relatively slowly, as new proteins have to be synthesized. Those resulting from enzyme inhibition depend on the half-life of the affected drug as it takes approximately five half-lives for a drug to reach a steady-state concentration. Gabapentin, levetiracetam and vigabatrin are only minimally metabolized and so have less potential for these type of interactions.

An important interaction occurs in young women who are using the oral contraceptive (OC) pill. Phenytoin, phenobarbital, carbamazepine, oxcarbazepine, felbamate and topiramate increase the metabolism of ethinyl estradiol and progestogens, reducing the effectiveness of the OC pill. With these AEDs, the dose of oestrogen should be increased to at least 50 μg [83], or an alternative form of contraception used.

One should always remember that patients with chronic medical conditions such as epilepsy are more likely to use over-the-counter non-prescription medications [84]. Several of these, in particular St John's Wort and Ginkgo biloba, may have effects on enzyme activity and have the potential for altering AED metabolism [85]. In addition, some may have pharmacodynamic interactions, and may have a clinically significant effect without any effect on drug levels [86]. Most patients using complementary medicine do not inform their doctor, so it is important to ask the patient directly, as self-medication with over-the-counter medications may be a reason for subtherapeutic or toxic drug levels.

Tables 13.5 and 13.6 list the AEDs which act as either inducers or inhibitors. It is not an exhaustive list of interactions, as there are many other non-AEDs which are also inducers or inhibitors and may cause interactions. Consult the British National Formulary (BNF) [87] for more information.

In conclusion, although the potential for drug interactions is high with AEDs, the majority of patients prescribed potentially interacting drugs do not in fact develop any clinical consequences. Patient factors are probably the most important reason behind this. The physician may prevent serious consequences by being aware of the potential interaction, anticipating it, monitoring the patient clinically and using drug levels wisely. As a general rule, the second-generation AEDs have far fewer pharmacokinetic interactions as most do not have any appreciable effect on metabolizing enzymes. If the risk of a serious interaction is high, it may be preferable to use an alternative drug.

OTHER CONDITIONS WHICH MAY BENEFIT FROM AED TREATMENT

There are a number of other neurological conditions in which AEDs are used. These may occur in patients with co-existing epilepsy. It may be useful in these patients to use an AED which has efficacy for both conditions to avoid polypharmacy and drug interactions.

Migraine affects approximately 15% and epilepsy 2% of the population at any one time [88, 89]. As both are so common it is likely that some patients will have both epilepsy and migraine simply by chance; however, the literature suggests a clear association between the two [90]. One theory behind their association is that both conditions are channelopathies. In some cases, the underlying aetiology may be a clear risk factor for headache and seizures, such as arteriovenous malformations or Sturge–Weber syndrome [91]. In addition, there are several neurological syndromes in which epilepsy and migraine co-occur as part of the syndrome, such as cerebral autosomal dominant arteriopathy with subcortical infarcts and leukoencephalopathy (CADASIL) and mitochondrial diseases. Several of the AEDs, such as topiramate, gabapentin, valproate, lamotrigine and carbamazepine, are effective in migraine prophylaxis [92–96]. Pregabalin is also used in migraine, despite a lack of good evidence in the literature to date.

Neuropathic pain is common and occurs in many diseases such as diabetes, paraneoplastic disorders, multiple sclerosis, systemic vasculitides, human immunodeficiency virus (HIV) and as a result of chemotherapy-associated neuropathy. Several of these conditions are also associated with seizures. Gabapentin and pregabalin both appear to be very effective for neuropathic pain [97, 98]. There is also evidence that oxcarbazepine and lamotrigine are effective [99, 100]. In addition, topiramate, levetiracetam and zonisamide are used, although there is less evidence supporting their effectiveness [101–103].

Restless legs syndrome is a common disorder with a prevalence of up to 9% [104]. There does not appear to be any particular association with epilepsy, but the resulting sleep disruption may exacerbate seizure control. Although dopaminergic agents are usually used as first-line treatment, there is also good evidence for gabapentin [105]. The evidence for

Table 13.5 Enzyme-inducing anti-epileptic drugs (AEDs)

Enzyme inducer/ increases elimination	Substrate	Consequences/management
Phenytoin	AEDs: diazepam, CBZ, PHT, TGB, FBM, PB, TPM, VPA, LTG, ETX, OXC, ZNS	Monitor levels and adjust dose as needed
	Analgesics: morphine, methadone	May need increased dose
	Anti-microbials: metronidazole	Monitor for withdrawal
	Anti-fungals: itraconazole, ketaconazole	Therapeutic failure; use fluconazole
	Anti-depressants: citalopram, nefazodone	Monitor clinically
	Anti-psychotics: haloperidol, olanzepine, clozapine, risperidone, quetiapine	Monitor for decreased response
	Cardiac: warfarin, quinidine, fluvastatin	Monitor international normalized ratio
	Immunosuppressants: cyclosporine, tacrolimus	Increase dose
	Protease inhibitors: ritonavir, indinavir, saquinavir	Monitor levels; consider alternative AED
	Others: theophylline, OCP, corticosteroids	Consider alternative AED; monitor levels; increase dose or use alternative contraception
Phenobarbital	Analgesics: morphine, methadone	May need increased dose
	AEDs: CBZ, TGB, FBM, PHT, VPA, ETX, LTG, OXC, ZNS	Monitor for withdrawal
	Anti-depressants: citalopram, nefazodone	Monitor clinically; may need to increase dose
	Anti-fungals: itraconazole, ketaconazole	Monitor for decreased clinical response
	Anti-psychotics: haloperidol, olanzepine, clozapine, risperidone, quetiapine	Therapeutic failure; use Fluconazole
	Cardiac: warfarin, quinidine, nifedipine, verapamil	Monitor for decreased response
	Immunosuppressants: cyclosporine, tacrolimus	Monitor international normalized ratio
	Protease inhibitors: ritonavir, indinavir, saquinavir	Increase dose
	Others: theophylline, OCP, corticosteroids	Monitor levels; consider alternative AED; increase dose or use alternative contraception
Carbamazepine	Analgesics: methadone	Monitor for withdrawal
	Anti-convulsants: TGB, FBM, PHT, TPM, VPA, ETX, LTG, OXC, ZNS, CBZ	Monitor levels; may need to increase dose or consider alternative AED

Continued overleaf

Enzyme inducer/ increases elimination	Substrate	Consequences/management
	Anti-depressants: amitriptylline, imipramine, trazadone, citalopram, nefazodone	Monitor clinical response
	Anti-fungals: itraconazole, ketaconazole	Therapeutic failure; use fluconazole
	Anti-psychotics: haloperidol, olanzapine, clozapine, risperidone, quetiapine	Monitor for decreased effect
	Cardiac: quinidine, warfarin, felodipine	Increase dose; monitor international normalized ratio; consider alternative AED
	Immunosuppressants: cyclosporine, tacrolimus	Monitor levels; consider alternative AED
	Protease inhibitors: indinavir, ritonavir, saquinavir	Consider alternative AED
	Others: theophylline, OCP, corticosteroids	Monitor levels; incerase OCP dose; use alternative method
Topiramate	Anti-depressants: nefazodone	Monitor clinically
	Anti-psychotics: clozapine, quetiapine	Monitor for decreased effect
	Cardiac: digoxin	Monitor levels
	Others: OCP	Increase dose or use alternative contraception
Felbamate	AEDs: CBZ	Active metabolite increases; increased risk of adverse effects
	Anti-depressants: citalopram, nefazodone	Monitor clinically
	Anti-psychotics: clozapine, quetiapine	Monitor for decreased response
	Others: OCP	Increase dose or use alternative method
Zonisamide	AEDs: CBZ	Variable effect; monitor levels
Vigabatrin	AEDs: PHT	Monitor levels
Oxcarbazepine	Anti-depressants: nefazodone	Monitor clinically
	Anti-psychotics: risperidone, quetiapine	Monitor for decreased response

CBZ, carbamazepine; ETX, ethosuximide; FBM, felbamate; LTG, lamotrigine; OCP, oral contraceptive pill; OXC, oxcarbazepine; PB, phenobarbital; PHT, phenytoin; TGB, tiagabine; TPM, topiramate; VPA, valproate; ZNS, zonisamide.

Table 13.6 Enzyme-inhibiting anti-epileptic drugs (AEDs)

Enzyme inhibitor/decreased elimination	Substrate	Consequences/management
Felbamate	AEDs: PHT, PB, VPA	Decrease dose
	Anti-depressants: citalopram	Monitor clinically
	Anti-psychotics: quetiapine	Monitor for increased response
Oxcarbazepine	AEDs: PHT	Decrease dose
	Antidepressants: citalopram	Monitor clinically
	Antipsychotics: quetiapine	Monitor for increased clinical response
Topiramate	AEDs: PHT	Increased levels
Valproate	AEDs: PB, LTG, FBM	Decrease dose
Zonisamide	AEDs: CBZ	Monitor levels

CBZ, carbamazepine; FBM, felbamate; LTG, lamotrigine; PB, phenobarbital; PHT, phenytoin; VPA, valproate.

carbamazepine, valproate and topiramate is less robust but all have been used with some success [105–107].

Mood disorders are much more prevalent in people with epilepsy than in the general population [108]. This may be due partly to psychosocial issues, as well as to the underlying neurobiological reasons. The most common mood disturbance is depression, occurring in approximately one-quarter of patients. Co-morbid depression may be under-diagnosed in patients with epilepsy; it may influence drug compliance and quality of life. As mentioned previously, there are possible drug interactions between some of the AEDs and anti-depressants. In addition, anti-depressants may lower the seizure threshold, although the seizure risk associated with the selective serotonin reuptake inhibitors is <0.4% [109]. Some AEDs may themselves have anti-depressant effects: lamotrigine, carbamazepine, gabapentin and valproate have been shown to improve mood in depressed patients with epilepsy [110]. Many of the AEDs, however, have also been reported in association with adverse effects on mood [111, 112]. When commencing a patient with depression and epilepsy on a new AED, one should be aware that their mood may be improved or affected adversely.

Bipolar affective disorder has been described as occurring in 12% of people with epilepsy, six times that of people without epilepsy [108]. Several of the AEDs, including carbamazepine, valproate, lamotrigine and oxcarbazepine have been used as mood-stabilizing agents in bipolar affective disorder. One study found that monotherapy using these AEDs in children with epilepsy and bipolar affective disorder was effective for the mood disturbance as well as the seizures [113].

CONCLUSION

Epilepsy frequently occurs in association with another medical condition. In such patients, introduction of a new AED should be accompanied by close monitoring for potential adverse effects. Careful selection of an appropriate AED should allow for seizure control in the majority of patients, bearing in mind potential drug interactions and alterations in pharmacodynamics and pharmacokinetics which may occur due to the underlying disease.

REFERENCES

1. Hauser WA, Annegers JF, Kurland LT. Incidence of epilepsy and unprovoked seizures in Rochester, Minnesota: 1935–1984. *Epilepsia* 1993; 34:453–468.
2. Bladin CF, Alexandrov AV, Bellavance A *et al*. Seizures after stroke: a prospective multicenter study. *Arch Neurol* 2000; 57:1617–1622.
3. Vespa PM, O'Phelan K, Shah M *et al*. Acute seizures after intracerebral hemorrhage: a factor in progressive midline shift and outcome. *Neurology* 2003; 60:1441–1446.
4. Arboix A, Garcia-Eroles L, Massons JB *et al*. Predictive factors of early seizures after acute cerebrovascular disease. *Stroke* 1997; 28:1590–1594.
5. Ferracci F, Moretto G, Gentile M *et al*. Can seizures be the only manifestation of transient ischemic attacks? A report of four cases. *Neurol Sci* 2000; 21:303–306.
6. Giroud M, Gras P, Fayolle H *et al*. Early seizures after acute stroke: a study of 1,640 cases. *Epilepsia* 1994; 35:959–964.
7. Williams AJ, Tortella FC, Lu XM *et al*. Antiepileptic drug treatment of nonconvulsive seizures induced by experimental focal brain ischemia. *J Pharmacol Exp Ther* 2004; 311:220–227.
8. Berger AR, Lipton RB, Lesser ML *et al*. Early seizures following intracerebral hemorrhage: implications for therapy. *Neurology* 1988; 38:1363–1365.
9. Naidech AM, Kreiter KT, Janjua N *et al*. Phenytoin exposure is associated with functional and cognitive disability after subarachnoid hemorrhage. *Stroke* 2005; 36:583–587.
10. Goldstein LB. Common drugs may influence motor recovery after stroke. The Sygen In Acute Stroke Study Investigators. *Neurology* 1995; 45:865–871.
11. Gupta SR, Naheedy MH, Elias D *et al*. Postinfarction seizures. A clinical study. *Stroke* 1988; 19:1477–1481.
12. Alvarez-Sabin J, Montaner J, Padro L *et al*. Gabapentin in late-onset poststroke seizures. *Neurology* 2002; 59:1991–1993.
13. Rowan AJ, Ramsay RE, Collins JF *et al*; VA Cooperative Study 428 Group. New onset geriatric epilepsy: a randomized study of gabapentin, lamotrigine, and carbamazepine. *Neurology* 2005; 64:1868–1873.
14. Go AS, Hylek EM, Phillips KA *et al*. Prevalence of diagnosed atrial fibrillation in adults: national implications for rhythm management and stroke prevention: the Anticoagulation and Risk Factors in Atrial Fibrillation (ATRIA) Study. *JAMA* 2001; 285:2370–2375.
15. Man-Son-Hing M, Nichol G, Lau A *et al*. Choosing antithrombotic therapy for elderly patients with atrial fibrillation who are at risk for falls. *Arch Intern Med* 1999; 159:677–685.
16. Galimberti CA, Marchioni E, Barzizza F *et al*. Partial epileptic seizures of different origin variably affect cardiac rhythm. *Epilepsia* 1996; 37:742–747.
17. Rossetti AO, Dworetzky BA, Madsen JR *et al*. Ictal asystole with convulsive syncope mimicking secondary generalisation: a depth electrode study. *J Neurol Neurosurg Psychiatry* 2005; 76:885–887.
18. Tigaran S, Rasmussen V, Dam M *et al*. ECG changes in epilepsy patients. *Acta Neurol Scand* 1997; 96:72–75.
19. Khan JA, Gowda RM. Novel therapeutics for treatment of long-QT syndrome and torsades de pointes. *Int J Cardiol* 2004; 95:1–6.
20. Binder L, Trujillo J, Parker D *et al*. Association of intravenous phenytoin toxicity with demographic, clinical and dosing parameters. *Am J Emer Med* 1996; 14:398–401.
21. Donovan PJ, Cline D. Phenytoin administration by constant intravenous infusion: selective rates of administration. *Ann Emerg Med* 1991; 20:139–142.
22. Adams BD, Buckley NH, Kim JY *et al*. Fosphenytoin may cause hemodynamically unstable bradydysrhythmias. *J Emerg Med* 2006; 30:75–79.
23. Megarbane B, Leprince P, Deye N *et al*. Extracorporeal life support in a case of acute carbamazepine poisoning with life-threatening refractory myocardial failure. *Intensive Care Med* 2006; 32:1409–1413.
24. Faisy C, Guerot E, Diehl JL *et al*. Carbamazepine-associated severe left ventricular dysfunction. *J Toxicol Clin Toxicol* 2000; 38:339–342.
25. Kasarskis EJ, Kuo CS, Berger R *et al*. Carbamazepine-induced cardiac dysfunction. Characterization of two distinct clinical syndromes. *Arch Intern Med* 1992; 152:186–191.

26. Timmings PL. Sudden unexpected death in epilepsy: is carbamazepine implicated? *Seizure* 1998; 7:289–291.
27. Roberts C, French JA. Anticonvulsants in acute medical illness. In: Delanty N (ed.) *Seizures: Medical Causes and Management*. Totowa, NJ: Humana Press, 2002, pp. 333–356.
28. Hubalewska A, Stompor T, Placzkiewicz E *et al.* Evaluation of gastric emptying in patients with chronic renal failure on continuous ambulatory peritoneal dialysis using 99mTc-solid meal. *Nucl Med Rev Cent East Eur* 2004; 7:27–30.
29. Strid H, Simren M, Stotzer PO *et al.* Patients with chronic renal failure have abnormal small intestinal motility and a high prevalence of small intestinal bacterial overgrowth. *Digestion* 2003; 67:129–137.
30. Reidenberg MM, Drayer DE. Alteration of drug-protein binding in renal disease. *Clin Pharmacokinet* 1984; 9:S18–S26.
31. Randinitis EJ, Posvar EL, Alvey CW *et al.* Pharmacokinetics of pregabalin in subjects with various degrees of renal function. *J Clin Pharmacol* 2003; 43:277–283.
32. Browne TR. Renal disorders. In: Ettinger AB, Devinsky O (eds) *Managing Epilepsy and Co-existing Disorders*. Boston: Butterworth-Heinemann, 2002, pp. 49–62.
33. Munoz R, Espinoza M, Espinoza O *et al.* Cyclosporine-associated leukoencephalopathy in organ transplant recipients: experience of three clinical cases. *Transplant Proc* 2006; 38:921–923.
34. Wong R, Beguelin GZ, de Lima M *et al.* Tacrolimus-associated posterior reversible encephalopathy syndrome after allogeneic haematopoietic stem cell transplantation. *Br J Haematol* 2003; 122:128–134.
35. Racusen LC, McCrindle BW, Christenson M *et al.* Cyclosporine lowers seizure threshold in an experimental model of electroshock-induced seizures in Munich-Wistar rats. *Life Sci* 1990; 46:1021–1026.
36. Wassner SJ, Pennisi AJ, Malekzadeh MH *et al.* The adverse effect of anticonvulsant therapy on renal allograft survival. A preliminary report. *J Pediatr* 1976; 88:134–137.
37. Wassner SJ, Malekzadeh MH, Pennisi AJ *et al.* Allograft survival in patients receiving anticonvulsant medications. *Clin Nephrol* 1977; 8:293–297.
38. Gallay BJ, de Mattos AM, Norman DJ. Reversible acute renal allograft dysfunction due to gabapentin. *Transplantation* 2000; 70:208–209.
39. AMNCH Adult Medicines Guide 2006/7: 224–225.
40. Glass GA, Stankiewicz J, Mithoefer A *et al.* Levetiracetam for seizures after liver transplantation. *Neurology* 2005; 64:1084–1085.
41. Upadhyay A, Jaber BL, Madias NE. Incidence and prevalence of hyponatremia. *Am J Med* 2006; 119:S30–S35.
42. Dong X, Leppik IE, White J *et al.* Hyponatremia from oxcarbazepine and carbamazepine. *Neurology* 2005; 65:1976–1978.
43. Kuz GM, Manssourian A. Carbamazepine-induced hyponatremia: assessment of risk factors. *Ann Pharmacother* 2005; 39:1943–1946.
44. Banner W Jr, Johnson DG, Walson PD *et al.* Effects of single large doses of phenytoin on glucose homeostasis – a preliminary report. *J Clin Pharmacol* 1982; 22:79–81.
45. Di Gennaro G, Quarato PP, Colazza GB *et al.* Hypoglycaemia induced by phenytoin treatment for partial status epilepticus. *J Neurol Neurosurg Psychiatry* 2002; 73:349–350.
46. Manto M, Preiser JC, Vincent JL. Hypoglycemia associated with phenytoin intoxication. *J Toxicol Clin Toxicol* 1996; 34:205–208.
47. Lavin PJ. Hyperglycemic hemianopia: a reversible complication of non-ketotic hyperglycemia. *Neurology* 2005; 65:616–619.
48. Gupta MM. Medical emergencies associated with disorders of calcium homeostasis. *J Assoc Physicians India* 1989; 37:629–631.
49. Ali FE, Al-Bustan MA, Al-Busairi WA *et al.* Loss of seizure control due to anticonvulsant-induced hypocalcemia. *Ann Pharmacother* 2004; 38:1002–1005.
50. Crimlisk HL. The little imitator–porphyria: a neuropsychiatric disorder. *J Neurol Neurosurg Psychiatry* 1997; 62:319–328.
51. Bylesjo I, Forsgren L, Lithner F *et al.* Epidemiology and clinical characteristics of seizures in patients with acute intermittent porphyria. *Epilepsia* 1996; 37:230–235.
52. Zadra M, Grandi R, Erli LC *et al.* Treatment of seizures in acute intermittent porphyria: safety and efficacy of gabapentin. *Seizure* 1998; 7:415–416.
53. Tatum WO 4th, Zachariah SB. Gabapentin treatment of seizures in acute intermittent porphyria. *Neurology* 1995; 45:1216–1217.

54. Lambrecht RW, Gildemeister OS, Pepe JA *et al*. Effects of antidepressants and benzodiazepine-type anxiolytic agents on hepatic porphyrin accumulation in primary cultures of chick embryo liver cells. *J Pharmacol Exp Ther* 1999; 291:1150–1155.

55. Krijt J, Krijtova H, Sanitrak J. Effect of tiagabine and topiramate on porphyrin metabolism in an in vivo model of porphyria. *Pharmacol Toxicol* 2001; 89:15–22.

56. Gaida-Hommernick B, Rieck K, Runge U. Oxcarbazepine in focal epilepsy and hepatic porphyria: a case report. *Epilepsia* 2001; 42:793–795.

57. Paul F, Meencke HJ. Levetiracetam in focal epilepsy and hepatic porphyria: a case report. *Epilepsia* 2004; 45:559–560.

58. Zaatreh MM. Levetiracetam in porphyric status epilepticus: a case report. *Clin Neuropharmacol* 2005; 28:243–244.

59. Gaynor JW, Jarvik GP, Bernbaum J *et al*. The relationship of postoperative electrographic seizures to neurodevelopmental outcome at 1 year of age after neonatal and infant cardiac surgery. *J Thorac Cardiovasc Surg* 2006; 131:181–189.

60. Modica PA, Tempelhoff R, White PF. Pro- and anticonvulsant effects of anesthetics (Part II). *Anesth Analg* 1990; 70:433–444.

61. Voss LJ, Ludbrook G, Grant C *et al*. Cerebral cortical effects of desflurane in sheep: comparison with isoflurane, sevoflurane and enflurane. *Acta Anaesthesiol Scand* 2006; 50:313–319.

62. Varelas PN, Mirski MA. Seizures in the adult intensive care unit. *J Neurosurg Anasthesiol* 2001; 13:163–175.

63. Weinhouse GL, Schwab RJ. Sleep in the critically ill patient. *Sleep* 2006; 29:707–716.

64. Forsgren L, Bucht G, Eriksson S *et al*. Incidence and clinical characterization of unprovoked seizures in adults: a prospective population-based study. *Epilepsia* 1996; 37:224–229.

65. Ramsay RE, Rowan AJ, Pryor FM. Special considerations in treating the elderly patient with epilepsy. *Neurology* 2004; 62:S24–S29.

66. AJ Rowan. Epilepsy and seizures in the aged. In: Ettinger AB, Devinsky O (eds) *Managing Epilepsy and Co-existing Disorders*. Boston: Butterworth-Heinemann, 2002, pp. 433–444.

67. Logroscino G, Hesdorffer DC, Cascino G *et al*. Time trends in incidence, mortality, and case-fatality after first episode of status epilepticus. *Epilepsia* 2001; 42:1031–1035.

68. Rowan AJ, Ramsay RE, Collins JF *et al*. VA Cooperative Study 428 Group. New onset geriatric epilepsy: a randomized study of gabapentin, lamotrigine, and carbamazepine. *Neurology* 2005; 64:1868–1873.

69. O'Donovan D, Hausken T, Lei Y *et al*. Effect of aging on transpyloric flow, gastric emptying, and intragastric distribution in healthy humans – impact on glycemia. *Dig Dis Sci* 2005; 50:671–676.

70. Johnson EK, Jones JE, Seidenberg M *et al*. The relative impact of anxiety, depression, and clinical seizure features on health-related quality of life in epilepsy. *Epilepsia* 2004; 45:544–550.

71. Montgomery SA. Antidepressants and seizures: emphasis on newer agents and clinical implications. *Int J Clin Pract* 2005; 59:1435–1440.

72. Pisani F, Oteri G, Costa C *et al*. Effects of psychotropic drugs on seizure threshold. *Drug Saf* 2002; 25:91–110.

73. Chung S, Ahn C. Effects of anti-epileptic drug therapy on bone mineral density in ambulatory epileptic children. *Brain Dev* 1994; 16:382–385.

74. Babayigit A, Dirik E, Bober E *et al*. Adverse effects of antiepileptic drugs on bone mineral density. *Pediatr Neurol* 2006; 35:177–181.

75. Cannon KT, Choi MM, Zuniga MA. Potentially inappropriate medication use in elderly patients receiving home health care: a retrospective data analysis. *Am J Geriatr Pharmacother* 2006; 4:134–143.

76. Brodie MJ, Overstall PW, Giorgi L. Multicentre, double-blind, randomised comparison between lamotrigine and carbamazepine in elderly patients with newly diagnosed epilepsy. The UK Lamotrigine Elderly Study Group. *Epilepsy Res* 1999; 37:81–87.

77. Huying F, Klimpe S, Werhahn KJ. Antiepileptic drug use in nursing home residents: a cross-sectional, regional study. *Seizure* 2006; 15:194–197.

78. Cuadrado A, de las Cuevas I, Valdizan EM *et al*. Synergistic interaction between valproate and lamotrigine against seizures induced by 4-aminopyridine and pentylenetetrazole in mice. *Eur J Pharmacol* 2002; 453:43–52.

79. Della Paschoa OE, Kruk MR, Hamstra R *et al*. Pharmacodynamic interaction between phenytoin and sodium valproate changes seizure thresholds and pattern. *Br J Pharmacol* 1998; 125:997–1004.

80. Della Paschoa OE, Voskuyl RA, Danhof M. Modelling of the pharmacodynamic interaction between phenytoin and sodium valproate. *Br J Pharmacol* 1998; 125:1610–1616.

81. Sorkin EM, Darvey DL. Review of cimetidine drug interactions. *Drug Intell Clin Pharm* 1983; 17:110–120.
82. Suzuki Y, Nagai T, Mano T *et al.* Interaction between valproate formulation and phenytoin concentrations. *Eur J Clin Pharmacol* 1995; 48:61–63.
83. Crawford P. Interactions between antiepileptic drugs and hormaonal contraception. *CNS Drugs* 2002; 16:263–272.
84. Al-Windi A. Predictors of herbal medicine use in a Swedish health practice. *Pharmacoepidemiol Drug Saf* 2004; 13:489–496.
85. Kupiec T, Raj V. Fatal seizures due to potential herb-drug interactions with Ginkgo biloba. *J Anal Toxicol* 2005; 29:755–758.
86. Samuels N. Herbal remedies and anticoagulant therapy. *Thromb Haemost* 2005; 93:3–7.
87. Appendix 1. Interactions. http://bnf.org
88. Bigal ME, Liberman JN, Lipton RB. Age-dependent prevalence and clinical features of migraine. *Neurology* 2006; 67:246–251.
89. Forsgren L, Beghi E, Oun A *et al.* The epidemiology of epilepsy in Europe – a systematic review. *Eur J Neurology* 2005; 12:245–253.
90. Yankovsky AE, Andermann F, Bernasconi A. Characteristics of headache associated with intractable partial epilepsy. *Epilepsia* 2005; 46:1241–1245.
91. Kossoff EH, Hatfield LA, Ball KL *et al.* Comorbidity of epilepsy and headache in patients with Sturge–Weber syndrome. *J Child Neurol* 2005; 20:678–682.
92. Bussone G, Diener HC, Pfeil J *et al.* Topiramate 100 mg/day in migraine prevention: a pooled analysis of double-blind randomised controlled trials. *Int J Clin Pract* 2005; 59:961–968.
93. Mathew NT, Rapoport A, Saper J *et al.* Efficacy of gabapentin in migraine prophylaxis. *Headache* 2001; 41:119–128.
94. Hering R, Kuritzky A. Sodium valproate in the prophylactic treatment of migraine: a double-blind study versus placebo. *Cephalgia* 1992; 12:81–84.
95. Lampl C, Katsarava Z, Diener HC *et al.* Lamotrigine reduces migraine aura and migraine attacks in patients with migraine with aura. *J Neurol Neurosurg Psychiatry* 2005; 76:1730–1732.
96. Chronicle E, Mulleners W. Anticonvulsant drugs for migraine prophylaxis. *Cochrane Database Syst Rev* 2004; (3): CD003226.
97. Backonja M, Glanzman RL. Gabapentin dosing for neuropathic pain: evidence from randomized, placebo-controlled clinical trials. *Clin Ther* 2003; 25:81–104.
98. Frampton JE, Foster RH. Pregabalin: in the treatment of postherpetic neuralgia. *Drugs* 2005; 65:111–118.
99. Magenta P, Arghetti S, Di Palma F *et al.* Oxcarbazepine is effective and safe in the treatment of neuropathic pain: pooled analysis of seven clinical studies. *Neurol Sci* 2005; 26:218–226.
100. Simpson DM, McArthur JC, Olney R *et al*; Lamotrigine HIV Neuropathy Study Team. Lamotrigine for HIV-associated painful sensory neuropathies: a placebo-controlled trial. *Neurology* 2003; 60:1508–1514.
101. Guay DR. Oxcarbazepine, topiramate, zonisamide, and levetiracetam: potential use in neuropathic pain. *Am J Geritr Pharmacolther* 2003; 1:18–37.
102. Atli A, Dogra S. Zonisamide in the treatment of painful diabetic neuropathy: a randomized, double-blind, placebo-controlled pilot study. *Pain Med* 2005; 6:225–234.
103. Thienel U, Neto W, Schwabe SK *et al*; Topiramate Diabetic Neuropathic Pain Study Group. Topiramate in painful diabetic polyneuropathy: findings from three double-blind placebo-controlled trials. *Acta Neurol Scand* 2004; 110:221–231.
104. Trenkwalder C, Paulus W, Walters AS. The restless legs syndrome. *Lancet Neurol* 2005; 4:465–475.
105. Vignatelli L, Billiard M, Clarenbach P *et al.* EFNS guidelines on management of restless legs syndrome and periodic limb movement disorder in sleep. *Eur J Neurol* 2006; 13:1049–1065.
106. Telstad W, Sorensen O, Larsen S *et al.* Treatment of the restless legs syndrome with carbamazepine: a double blind study. *Br Med J (Clin Res Ed)* 1984; 288:444–446.
107. Eisensehr I, Ehrenberg BL, Rogge Solti S *et al.* Treatment of idiopathic restless legs syndrome (RLS) with slow-release valproic acid compared with slow-release levodopa/benserazid. *J Neurol* 2004; 251:579–588.
108. Ettinger AB, Reed ML, Goldberg JF *et al.* Prevalence of bipolar symptoms in epilepsy vs other chronic health disorders. *Neurology* 2005; 65:535–540.
109. Montgomery SA. Antidepressants and seizures: emphasis on newer agents and clinical implications. *Int J Clin Pract* 2005; 59:1435–1440.
110. Edwards KR, Sackellares JC, Vuong A *et al.* Lamotrigine monotherapy improves depressive symptoms in epilepsy: a double-blind comparison with valproate. *Epilepsy Behav* 2001; 2:28–36.

111. Chouinard MJ, Nguyen DK, Clement JF *et al.* Catatonia induced by levetiracetam. *Epilepsy Behav* 2006; 8:303–307.
112. Ciesielski AS, Samson S, Steinhoff BJ. Neuropsychological and psychiatric impact of add-on titration of pregabalin versus levetiracetam: A comparative short-term study. *Epilepsy Behav* 2006; 9:424–431.
113. Salpekar JA, Conry JA, Doss W *et al.* Clinical experience with anticonvulsant medication in pediatric epilepsy and comorbid bipolar spectrum disorder. *Epilepsy Behav* 2006; 9:327–334.

14

A rational approach to the treatment of status epilepticus

Peter Kinirons, Colin P. Doherty

INTRODUCTION

'Based on this retrospective study, the treatment of SE is remarkable for both inadequacy and ineffectiveness. The inappropriate use of therapeutic regimens in the management of SE may be seen as an important cause of ineffective medical treatment.'

When Gregory Cascino wrote these words in 2001 [1], he was referring to the treatment of status epilepticus (SE) between the years 1965 and 1984. He might have reasonably hoped that the treatment of SE would have improved in the succeeding 20 years. However, while the range of medicines available and the technology underpinning emergency life support has undoubtedly improved, the mortality and morbidity associated with acute prolonged seizure activity has hardly changed. Two general problems continue to mitigate against improved outcome in SE. The first is the failure to recognize the wide spectrum of clinical presentation and the potential hazards of misidentification; the second is the failure to treat in an appropriately aggressive and timely manner. In this chapter, as well as describing the basic epidemiology of SE, we will examine the enduring quality of these problems and discuss methods for addressing them in the modern clinical setting, including the potential application of new pharmacological agents and therapeutic strategies to SE. The aim will be to provide a clear understanding of the pathophysiological consequences of prolonged seizures, rather than to simply provide a basic algorithm for treating SE, thus enabling the reader to adopt a rational approach to its management.

While controversy continues over the extent to which the brain is affected by episodes of non-convulsive SE, there is wide agreement that the prediction, onset, course and failure to adequately treat generalized convulsive status epilepticus (GCSE) presents the biggest challenge to the practising physician in the acute setting. For this reason, the emphasis here will be on GCSE.

HISTORICAL CONTEXT

It is widely written that the earliest historical reference to SE appears on a neo-Babylonian clay tablet known as a cuneiform (wedge-shaped), written in the 6th century BC [2]:

Peter Kinirons, MRCPI, PhD, Epilepsy and Neurophysiology Fellow, Massachusetts General Hospital, Boston, Massachusetts, USA

Colin P. Doherty, MD, MRCPI, Consultant Neurologist, Department of Neurology, St James's Hospital, Dublin; Honorary Senior Lecturer, Royal College of Surgeons in Ireland

'... at the time of his possession his hands and feet are cold, he is much darkened, keeps opening and shutting his mouth, is brown and yellow as to the eyes ... it may go on for some time, but he will die.'

In the modern era, the term 'état de mal' was a colloquial phrase used by French patients in the 1820s to describe the condition of continuous seizures and was first noted in the thesis of Louis Calmeil in 1824 [3]. The Latinized term, status epilepticus, was first used in Bazire's translation of Trousseau in 1867 [4]. In 1874, Bourneville [5] gave a now classical description of SE in a 19-year-old hemiplegic woman (see below), and elevated the notion of clinical observation as a means to understanding SE better.

An important contribution was made in the early 20th century by Clark and Prout [6] when they introduced the notion of repetitive seizures without a return to baseline. They also provided the first pathological description of the cell loss seen in brain subjected to prolonged or repeated seizures.

Most of the above descriptions of status refer to convulsive SE. References to other non-convulsive episodes of prolonged seizures are more difficult to find but they do exist. Charcot was the first to recognize that episodes of fugue could be part of a non-convulsive epileptic spectrum [7]. In 1945, after electroencephalography (EEG) became available, Lennox showed that non-convulsive petit mal seizures could be prolonged and alter behaviour [8]. Later, Gastaut described psychomotor status, showing that prolonged motor and behavioural activity can be attributed to epileptic discharges [9].

DEFINITION AND CLASSIFICATION OF STATUS EPILEPTICUS

Status epilepticus is currently defined by the International League Against Epilepsy (ILAE) as 'an abnormally persistent seizure lasting more than 30 minutes or clusters of seizures without a return to baseline for more than 30 minutes' [10]. This is based on research from animal models showing irreversible neuronal damage occurring due to seizures lasting >30 min, as discussed below. However, patients should not be allowed to seize for this period of time before being treated appropriately for SE. The physiological and molecular changes that occur as a result of prolonged seizures, which will be discussed in detail in this chapter, mean that the longer a seizure continues unabated, the more resistant it becomes to therapy and the more profound the potential consequences. This has led to an 'operational' definition of SE that any seizure lasting more than 5 min should be treated as if it were going to last more than 30 min [11].

Although a number of different classifications exist, Table 14.1 provides a scheme that mirrors the accepted classification of all seizures outlined by the ILAE and thus provides a logical approach to describing status types.

Table 14.1 Classification of status epilepticus

Convulsive	Primary generalized
	Symptomatic generalized
	Secondarily generalized
Non-convulsive	Absence status (typical and atypical)
	Complex partial status
	Simple partial status (aura continua and epilepsia partialis continua/ focal motor status)
	Myoclonic status (post-hypoxic brain injury)
	Non-convulsive status epilepticus (NCSE) in comatose patients

EPIDEMIOLOGY OF STATUS EPILEPTICUS

A number of population-based studies on the epidemiology of SE have been published in the last decade [12–19]. These studies are summarized in Table 14.2. The majority have included both convulsive and non-convulsive SE. In general, the reported incidence range is 10–20/100,000, and is higher in studies from the USA than in those from Europe. All studies record the highest incidence in young children and the elderly. The incidence appears to be higher in blacks than whites [12, 16]. A study from the USA reported that the incidence of SE of all types rose from 8.0/100,000 to 18.1/100,000 between 1935 and 1984 in their study cohort, and attributed this to the ageing of the population and to the greater incidence of myoclonic SE after cardiac arrest [20]. Meanwhile, a more recent report noted a fall of 42% in the incidence of convulsive SE from 1991 to 1998 [16].

Although these studies have included both convulsive and non-convulsive SE, it seems likely that, owing to the difficulty with recognition and the necessity of electroencephalography to make the diagnosis, the incidence of non-convulsive status epilepticus (NCSE) without motor features is probably underestimated. One study looking at the presence of NCSE in 236 unselected comatose patients without clinical manifestation of seizure activity found electroencephalogram (EEG) evidence of SE in 8% of patients [21]. Another study that prospectively looked at 198 patients presenting with altered consciousness found that 59 of them had EEG evidence of NCSE, 23 of whom presented with altered consciousness alone [22].

Data from these epidemiological studies [12–19] reveal that SE occurs on a background of epilepsy in 40–50% of patients. Convulsive SE, most often secondarily generalized in nature, and complex partial SE are by far the most commonly reported seizure types, followed by simple partial and absence SE. In adults, SE most often results from an acute or remote brain insult, particularly stroke, tumour, trauma and central nervous system (CNS) infection, while in children the most common aetiologies are prolonged febrile convulsions, acute CNS infection and acute metabolic derangements, such as hypoglycaemia. In those with pre-existing epilepsy, the most common aetiology is medication withdrawal/non-compliance.

MORTALITY

Although a number of case series from tertiary centres looking at the mortality of SE have been published, the most relevant figures come from the population-based studies discussed above, where mortality ranges from 7% to 39%. These figures are presented in Table 14.2, and represent the reported 30-day case fatality. The reported mortality is higher in the US studies, again possibly reflecting the higher degree of post-anoxic myoclonic SE, which carries an inherently poor prognosis, in these cohorts.

In all of these studies, the aetiology of SE is the most important risk factor for mortality, with the majority of deaths occurring in patients with acute symptomatic SE, particularly after anoxic brain injury, stroke, CNS infection and CNS tumour. Whether this is just a reflection of the severity of the underlying aetiology or a representation of the additional physiological burden of prolonged seizures on a severely ill individual remains difficult to tease out due to the lack of comparative studies. However, Waterhouse et al. [23] reported, in a prospective study, that the mortality of patients with acute stroke and SE was three times that of acute stroke alone, both groups being similar for age and lesion size. This suggests that there is a synergistic effect of SE and the underlying aetiology in causing death, emphasizing the importance of effective treatment.

The other variable that appears to be a consistent risk factor for death from SE in these studies is increased age, most showing age >65 years to be an independent risk factor for death. Children with SE have a much lower mortality rate than the elderly. Other variables that have been reported as increasing risk of death include greater duration of SE [24–27],

Table 14.2 Summary of population-based studies of status epilepticus

Origin	Study type	Study population	SE type	Incidence (per 100000)	Mortality (%)	Authors
Virginia, USA	Prospective	Population based, all ages	All types	41	22	DeLorenzo et al., 1995 [12]
Minnesota, USA	Retrospective	Population based, all ages	All types	18.3	21	Hesdorffer et al., 1998 [13]
Switzerland	Prospective	Population based, all ages	All types	10.3	7.6	Coeytaux et al., 2000 [14]
Germany	Prospective	Population based, adults only	All types	17.1	9.3	Knake et al., 2001 [15]
California, USA	Retrospective	Population based, all ages	Convulsive SE only	6.2	10.7	Wu et al., 2002 [16]
North Italy (urban)	Prospective	Population based, all ages	All types	10.7	39	Vignatelli et al., 2003 [17]
North Italy (rural)	Prospective	Population based, all ages	All types	11.6	7	Vignatelli et al., 2005 [18]
England	Prospective	Population based, children only	Convulsive SE only	17–23	3	Chin et al., 2006 [19]

longer time to initiation of treatment [28], greater impairment of consciousness at presentation [29, 30], and continuous SE (as opposed to intermittent seizing) [31]. In terms of clinical type of SE, myoclonic SE and secondarily generalized SE have been associated with a higher mortality [17] but few data are actually available on the correlation between clinical seizure type and risk of death. Similarly, controversy exists regarding the prognosis of NCSE. Some studies suggest it is a relatively benign condition [32, 33] while others have reported significant mortality and morbidity with the condition [30, 34, 35]. Some of this discrepancy is no doubt due to differences in the type of NCSE and differences in the populations under study, for example outpatient EEG setting vs. intensive care unit (ICU) setting. However, it is becoming apparent that patients with acute, severe underlying aetiologies and those with significant impairment of consciousness are at increased risk of death [30, 36].

Post-SE EEG features including burst suppression, periodic lateralized epileptiform discharges (PLEDs) and after-SE ictal discharges have all been shown to predict a poor outcome [32, 33]. On the other hand, idiopathic SE [12–19], SE related to medication or alcohol withdrawal [15, 16, 24, 37] and normalization of the EEG [38,39] have all been associated with a better outcome.

In terms of the long-term effects of an episode of SE on mortality, a study by Logroscino *et al.* [40] reported that 40% of subjects who survived the first 30 days after an incident episode of SE die within the next 10 years. The long-term mortality rate was threefold that of the general population over the same time period and was worse for those with myoclonic SE, for those who presented with SE lasting more than 24 h, and for those with acute symptomatic SE. The long-term mortality rate was not altered in those with idiopathic/cryptogenic SE.

MORBIDITY AND RISK OF SUBSEQUENT EPILEPSY

The profound physiological changes and impairment of consciousness that occur as a result of both SE and the medications used to treat it increase the risk of systemic complications, particularly of the cardio-respiratory system. Hypotension, hypoxia, aspiration pneumonia, metabolic acidosis and rhabdomyolysis with subsequent renal failure are all recognized complications of prolonged seizures which not only contribute to the overall mortality of the condition, but which also contribute to the morbidity and prolonged hospital stay of those who survive.

From a neurological perspective, the main sequelae of concern are, firstly, the impact of SE on cognitive functioning and, secondly, the risk of developing subsequent epilepsy. It is becoming increasingly clear from animal studies that 30–40 min of continuous seizing is enough to produce neuronal death, particularly in vulnerable areas such as the hippocampus. The implications of this on cognitive functioning in humans after an episode of SE have not yet been formally studied but are obvious. The mechanisms involved in producing neuronal death will be discussed in detail below.

There are limited data on the risk of developing epilepsy after an episode of SE. Prospective studies of children presenting with a first unprovoked seizure have consistently shown that, for idiopathic cases, prolonged seizures and SE (i.e. convulsive SE) do not increase the risk of subsequent epilepsy as compared with non-prolonged seizures [36–44]. However, these studies include only unprovoked seizures and are therefore limited in the number of SE cases, many of which are symptomatic in nature. For these cases the data are not so clearcut. Large, long-term, prospective studies comparing the outcome of brief acute symptomatic seizures and acute symptomatic SE are lacking. Studies of the overall outcome of SE in children report the risk of developing epilepsy after an episode of SE as anything from 11% to 82% [45–52]. In adults, a large retrospective study, which compared rates of epilepsy 10 years after first presentation with either SE or a brief seizure in patients with an acute symptomatic aetiology, found that those with SE were 3.3 times more likely to develop unprovoked seizures, after adjusting for age, sex and cause [53]. It is possible that SE may just represent a marker for the severity of the underlying brain injury in this report. In another study, refractory SE was significantly more often followed by symptomatic epilepsy than non-refractory SE [54]. Most of the studies mentioned are based on convulsive SE. For NCSE there are very few data available on long-term risk of epilepsy.

The risk of epilepsy following febrile SE is also controversial. Early childhood prolonged febrile seizures and febrile SE have long been hypothesized to cause mesial temporal sclerosis (MTS) and associated temporal lobe epilepsy (TLE). This is based mainly on retrospective studies from tertiary epilepsy centres which report a history of febrile SE in 35–63% of patients with MTS [55, 56]. However, neither population-based nor prospective hospital-based studies report a significant association between prolonged febrile convulsions and subsequent MTS [57–59]. It must be noted, however, that these prospective studies are based mainly on brief febrile seizures rather than episodes of febrile SE. As a result, the number of febrile SE cases tends to be small and the duration of the seizures poorly characterized. In addition, the length of follow-up is limited. It is possible that the retrospective studies, which are based mainly on refractory TLE patients, are selecting for the more severe cases of childhood febrile SE. However, recent magnetic resonance imaging (MRI) data showing oedema of the hippocampus following prolonged febrile convulsions with subsequent atrophy at 6-month follow-up [60], as well as animal data showing development of hippocampal atrophy and unprovoked seizures after chemical or electrical induced SE, are supportive of a link [61–64]. Ongoing studies using long-term MRI and clinical follow-up should help to clarify the issue.

In conclusion, it is difficult to fully determine the role of prolonged seizures in contributing to epileptogenesis based on the available evidence.

SPECTRUM OF CLINICAL PRESENTATION OF GCSE

There are several important observations that clinicians interested in improving the care and outcome of patients in SE must recognize. Firstly, SE is a term that applies to a polymorphic clinical disorder in which its more subtle manifestations are often missed. It is not widely understood, even among general neurologists, that there is an agreed and applicable classification even if the treatment solutions are not (see Table 14.1). Another poorly understood notion is the fact that SE, no matter what type, has a clinical trajectory, which is referred to as the 'phases' of SE. They run from the pre-monitory phase, through the established phase and then through to either refractory or resolution phases. Every case of SE will have varying clinical features depending on the phase and so the violent convulsive elements of GCSE will often give way eventually to coma with little or no motor activity during late established and refractory phases. This evolution has been well described in the clinical literature [65]. Furthermore, it is now known that such clinical progression is accompanied by predictable EEG changes and increasing difficulty in treatment (refractoriness) [66], as well as increasing pathological damage [67].

Unfortunately, patients coming in from the community who may have been in GCSE for some time may arrive in the emergency room in one of these late phases. The failure to recognize the phase of SE leads to inevitable delays in treatment and arguably avoidable bad outcomes.

Hughlings Jackson advocated clinicians gaining experience and understanding from describing in detail every single seizure [68]. As mentioned above, it was Bourneville's [69] description of the case of Marie Lamb, an epileptic hemiplegic girl of 19 years in the Salpêtrière, 8 June 1874, that represents the pinnacle of classical seizure description. Seizures began to occur in clusters of three but by 10.45 a.m. consciousness was lost and she had 17 seizures in 1.5 h.

'In the first phase – initiation – the legs, more so the left, were flexed slowly over the thighs and the patient uttered a kind of grunt, then several raucous cries in succession. In the second phase, her eyelids were closed; when opened, her eyes were seen to be strongly deviated to the left, and her face

turned to the right; within four or five seconds, her eyes and face turned to the right; her left arm lay flexed and rigid across her body, the fingers tightly flexed across the thumb; her right arm was also stiff, but extended and raised 20 or 30 cm above her body, the fingers flexed but alongside the thumb; the lower limbs remained flexed and rigid. The third phase was marked by very strong and rapid convulsions of the eyelids and of the frontalis; the mouth was deviated to the extreme right, the right nasolabial furrow strongly accentuated, the left obliterated; at the same time, clonic jerks of moderate intensity were observed in the lower limbs, more so the right; breathing was stertorous and there was much frothing at the mouth.'

It is no exaggeration to say that this is a completely lost skill, relying as we now do on a series of stock phrases, which mean little to the consulting neurologist and even less to the treating clinician.

Treiman [70], in our opinion, gives the best definition of GCSE, which includes the non-motor manifestations and an electroclinical correlation emphasizing the importance of EEG in the late stages. He described GCSE as:

'a paroxysmal or continuous tonic and/or clonic convulsive motor activity that may be symmetric or asymmetric, overt or subtle, and is associated with marked impairment of consciousness and with bilateral (although frequently asymmetric) ictal discharges on the EEG.' [70]

Overt GCSE is characterized by recurrent convulsions, each of which evolves in the same manner as a single generalized tonic–clonic seizure. Each discrete convulsion begins with tonic stiffening, either focal or generalized, which is then replaced by clonic jerking, which increases in amplitude and decreases in frequency until abrupt cessation of the clonic jerks. The average duration of the tonic–clonic phases is initially about 90 s but tends to shorten as GCSE progresses. As this process continues, the overt motor activity begins to die away and is replaced by increasingly subtle behavioural manifestations [71].

One difficult but common clinical scenario is that of arriving at a patient's bedside when the seizure has apparently abated. This problem is rarely addressed in published guidelines. According to the accepted definitions of SE, patients should only be considered to have come out of status when they come back to a level of arousal approaching baseline [10]. The need to rule out a late or possibly even refractory phase of SE is not given due attention and may be responsible for a failure to treat. The use of EEG in a patient with reported prolonged seizures who is not back at baseline cannot be emphasized enough. In fact, the EEG changes in GCSE are almost as predictable as the clinical ones. Initial, unambiguous, discrete electrographic seizures give way to waxing and waning of amplitude, frequency and distribution of ictal discharges; this transitional phase gives way to prolonged periods of continuous ictal activity with little variation in the morphology. Finally, continuous ictal discharges are replaced by flat or suppressed periods punctuated by single discharges in a configuration known as periodic epileptiform discharges (PEDs) (Figure 14.1) [71]. While controversy exists about the true physiological nature of PEDs, in our opinion, it is clear that in the clinical setting of ongoing coma one is obliged to treat the pattern as an extension or residual fragment of GCSE. Assuming one has EEG evidence of seizure termination, there is a clear lack of direction on what to do then. Knowledge of the predictors of outcome, as discussed above, would be extremely valuable to the decision analysis at that point and would probably influence the use of rational measures to avoid bad outcomes.

PHYSIOLOGICAL AND ANATOMICAL CONSEQUENCES OF STATUS EPILEPTICUS

A link between epilepsy and brain damage is amongst the oldest known clinical–neuropathological correlates [72]. What is not clear is what particular role SE has in the creation of this damage. While the link between prolonged episodes of febrile seizures in infancy and hippocampal damage in temporal lobe epilepsy has been used as an example of the effect of SE on the brain, it is also clear that such damage can be present without a history

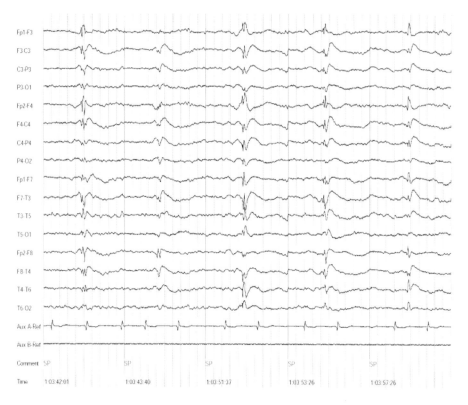

Figure 14.1 Electroencephalogram (EEG) of periodic epileptiform discharges (PEDs) occurring in the late-refractory phase of SE in a patient who has been seizing for more than 5 h. Despite starting as a typical prolonged convulsive seizure, by this time there were no motor manifestations and the EEG and ongoing coma were the only clues to the presence of SE.

of SE. Furthermore, quite why some individuals develop epilepsy after febrile seizures and others do not defies adequate explanation. Research into these phenomena has focused on the presence of genetic susceptibility to damage, which would allow individuals to vary widely in their response to seizure discharges of variable duration. However, until this research, which is in its earliest stages, gives us reproducible biologic markers of both damage and protection, it is incumbent on all physicians to treat prolonged seizures aggressively, not only to avoid brain damage but also to potentially alter the course of epileptogenesis.

While the notion of cell death as a response to seizures is well established both experimentally and clinically, there are in fact a host of physiological changes that occur in the brain, other organs and the circulation, which can influence the extent of central nervous system injury. This section will deal with what we know about the consequences of prolonged seizures and provide tantalizing targets for future protective strategies.

CELL DEATH

The earliest evidence that electrographic seizure discharges alone could kill neurons and that SE-induced neuronal death is not simply the result of secondary complications was obtained by research in animal models in the early 1970s with Meldrum, using the γ-aminobutyric acid A (GABA$_A$) receptor antagonist bicuculline, and Olney using kainic acid, to provoke damage in limbic neurons [73, 74]. Interestingly, Meldrum called this cell loss evidence of 'ischaemic damage' but the usual accompaniments of ischaemic damage such as the reactive changes in microglia, astrocytes and endothelial cells did not appear to be present. In fact, in our experience, the pathology of neuronal damage can appear extremely bland, with neuronal death appearing an almost isolated finding (Figure 14.2).

Nevertheless, these observations led to the excitotoxic hypothesis of cell death in SE. Accordingly, the activation of post synaptic N-methyl-D-aspartate (NMDA) receptors, induced by excessive presynaptic glutamate release, results in excessive calcium influx into neurons which in turn triggers various processes that result in cell death. The remarkable protective effects of NMDA receptor antagonists is a reverse proof of this hypothesis [75]. This theory has stood the test of time but refinements in how we understand the process of cell death have led to new insights into damage susceptibility and possible protection.

There are two principal forms of cell death – necrosis and apoptosis – which at one time were considered totally separate entities but are now considered to be part of a continuum from passive necrotic swelling and lysis to programmed cell death [76]. In seizure-induced damage, the morphology of cell death appears necrotic with calcium influx activating proteases (such as calpain 1 and cathepsin D) and neuronal nitric oxide synthase, which increases nitric oxide production, which in turn generates free radical peroxynitrite that damages DNA. Ultimately, mitochondria swell, and cytoplasmic and lysosomal membranes and essential cytoskeletal proteins are damaged [77].

However, apoptotic pathways have been shown to be active also. Key features of apoptosis are aggregation of chromatin in large masses that abut the nuclear membrane,

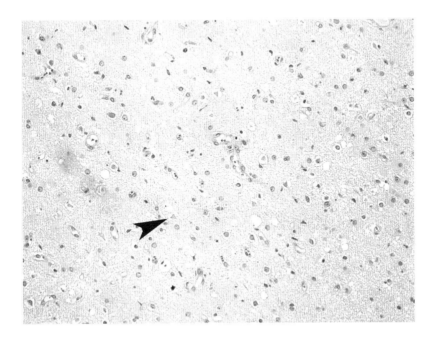

Figure 14.2 Pathology slide of a focal site of epileptic discharge that was surgically extirpated as part of a palliative procedure in a child with refractory focal SE. The slide is remarkable for the blandness of findings showing thickened vessels, eosinophilic atrophied neurons (arrow) and astrocytes with swollen cytoplasm on haematoxylin and eosin (H&E) staining. Only rare lymphocytes and microglia were noted (magnification ×20) [80].

preservation of intracellular organelles, and later dispersion of cell contents in membrane-bound 'apoptotic bodies'. This is considered to be a highly organized process that is controlled by two important families of protein: the caspases (cysteine proteases that cleave proteins at aspartate residues) and Bcl-2 (baculovirus) family of proteins [78].

The exact roles that both necrosis and apoptosis play in regulating cell death and damage is an area of active research. Furthermore, the timing of each phase of the cell death cascade remains unclear. Of extreme practical importance, however, is the fact that this research is leading to the exciting prospect of developing neuroprotective strategies that will seek to attenuate the excitotoxic cascade of events by antagonizing the biochemical necrotic and apoptoic pathways that are active in SE (see below).

BLOOD FLOW

As far back as the 1930s, it has been clear that there is a local increase in blood flow during seizure activity:

'After the attack the cerebral arteries pulsate violently ... Their colour becomes a bright red and arteries which were not seen to pulsate before the seizure may now begin to do so visibly. In fact this recovery may go so far that the veins themselves take on an arterial hue.' [79]

This dramatic 70-year-old description is uncannily similar to the gross operative findings in recent clinical reports [80] (Figure 14.3). In the last 20 years, nuclear imaging studies, such as single photon emission computer tomography (SPECT) and positron emission tomography (PET) using both fluoro-2-deoxy-glucose and oxygen[15] have been used to non-invasively localize seizure foci through the analysis of ictal blood flow and interictal metabolism (see [81] for review). Despite these studies, little is understood about the dynamics of flow in the microcirculation. Some evidence from animal studies suggests that there is uncoupling of metabolism and blood flow in focal seizures with the requirements of metabolism often outstripping the delivery of oxygenated blood [82]. On the other hand, evidence from human studies suggests that, in fact, perfusion outstrips metabolic demand [83].

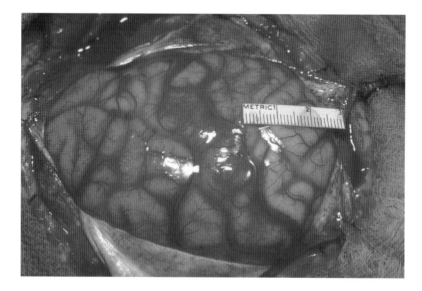

Figure 14.3 Intraoperative image of focal area of refractory discharge. Notice the suffusion of blood on the surface of the brain indicating the arterialization of veins caused by increased blood flow (hyperaemia) to the affected cortex [80].

Advances in structural imaging have further supplemented functional localization after SE. Neuroimaging of the brain directly after prolonged epileptic seizures, either focal or generalized, may reveal focal cerebral abnormalities that are typically transient. Numerous case reports of cerebral hypodensities that enhance with contrast on computerized tomography (CT) have been reported since its first description in 1980 [85]. In most cases, the changes suggested the development of focal cerebral cytotoxic oedema. By the 1990s, a number of reports began appearing in the literature of T2 hyperintensity changes on MRI in similarly focal areas, again associated with SE [85–92]. An example of multi-modal imaging of SE using MRI PET and MRA can be seen in Figure 14.4.

A variety of metabolic events which lead to cytotoxic oedema have been invoked to explain the changes; namely swelling of glial cells, increases in sodium concentration intracellularly secondary to Na/K pump failure [93] and possibly vasogenic oedema caused by excessive glutamate release [94]. While the nature and consequences of such changes in the microcirculation during SE remain a mystery, it is even less clear what connection these changes have to the cell loss alluded to above. It is hoped that the application of new high-field imaging technology, which is increasingly available in the clinical domain, will begin to draw connections between these myriad physiological changes.

OTHER EFFECTS

Hyperthermia

Apart from the model of febrile seizures where temperature elevations are implicated in the genesis of seizures, core body temperature is known to elevate as a result of seizures. The 'fever curve' was a well-known feature of SE reports from the turn of the 20th century, and it was also well known that the temperature elevation was proportional to the duration of SE. It has been shown in recent clinical studies that temperatures exceeding 42 degrees have been recorded in patients in whom status lasted longer than 9 h [25]. Following SE, hyperthermia may persist for some time. It has been shown experimentally that this temperature elevation may well contribute to brain damage and that control of temperature can limit such damage [95]. Furthermore, increased concentrations of glutamate are found in cortical perfusates during hyperthermic induction and during the subsequent seizure [96].

Catecholamines

Marked increases in plasma catecholamine concentrations occur with the initiation of SE and are sustained for a number of hours. These elevations are associated with a parallel and marked elevation in systemic blood pressure and heart rate. Generalized vasoconstriction is a consequence of noradrenaline elevation but these effects are diminished in late SE owing to decreased sensitivity of the vasculature for noradrenaline [97]. Elevations in epinephrine make cardiac arrhythmias and ischaemic changes, as well as elevations in plasma glucose, more likely. Finally, demargination of white blood cells can occur in more than half of patients but the characteristic immature forms (left shift) indicative of infection are absent [98].

Acidosis

A marked rapid acidosis is associated with SE in humans. In baboons with chemically induced status, the pH starts to fall within 1–3 min and reaches its lowest after 15–20 min [97]. In humans studied in the emergency room 84% were acidotic and 32% had a pH <7 [25]. The major cause of acidosis is thought to be peripheral accumulation of lactate from anaerobic metabolism in muscle, although it is also thought that a component of the acidosis is from cerebral venous lactate. Interestingly, SE-induced brain injury does not appear to

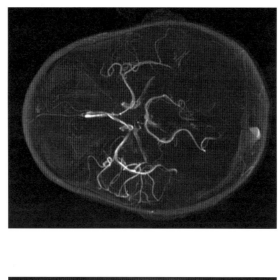

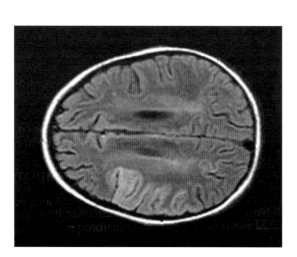

Figure 14.4 Composite figure of imaging in a patient with persistent focal SE lasting 4 weeks. The axial FLAIR image shows signal change in the right frontotemporal area (a), indicating increased brain water. A PET from the same day shows abnormal uptake of radio-labelled glucose co-localized with MR findings in the right frontotemporal regions (b), indicating increased metabolic demand in the region of epileptic discharge. Finally, a magnetic resonance angiogram (MRA) shows increased calibre of MCA territory branches (c), indicating increased blood flow to the area [80].

be exacerbated by acidosis. In fact, modest acidosis has been shown to be protective in excitotoxic injury. The mechanism of protection appears to be that acidosis itself may have an anti-convulsant effect (see the ketogenic diet) which may be mediated by the H^+ inhibition of glutamate acting on the NMDA channel currents [99].

RATIONAL APPROACH TO THERAPY

GENERAL PRINCIPLES

The key to management of SE is to establish the diagnosis quickly, to avoid delay in treatment and to avoid under- or over-use of medications. While GCSE is generally easy to recognize, the possibility of psychogenic seizures always needs to be borne in mind. It is also important to remember that some patients coming in from the community who have been in GCSE for some time may arrive in the emergency room in coma with little or no motor activity. The diagnosis of NCSE, on the other hand, requires a high index of suspicion. It should always be considered in the differential diagnosis of individuals who present with unexplained altered level of consciousness or altered behaviour, particularly those who have a history of epilepsy, a recent change in psychoactive medication or who are unwell for other reasons, both neurological and non-neurological. If EEG is readily available it should be performed to confirm the diagnosis. However, it should not delay treatment if the diagnosis is strongly suspected clinically.

The following section will provide guidelines on the management of SE in the hospital setting. Options are also available for pre-hospital treatment and will be discussed later.

ARRIVING AT THE BEDSIDE – MAKING THE DIAGNOSIS AND ASSESSING RISK OF PROLONGED SEIZURES

According to the operational definition of SE, once a patient is seizing for 5 min or more, they are considered to be in SE. The patient should be commenced on oxygen and vital signs monitored. Intravenous access should be established and blood sent for routine labs and blood culture. Blood glucose should be checked with finger-stick and if low, 50 ml of 50% dextrose should be given. If one suspects malnutrition or alcohol dependence, 100 mg intravenous (i.v.) or intramuscular (i.m.) thiamine should be given prior to the glucose load. The history and exam need to be completed quickly and efficiently, with three key questions in mind:

- What is the likely cause?
- How long has the patient been seizing?
- What is the likely outcome based on the risk factors for mortality?

In terms of determining the likely cause, it is important to remember that approximately 40–50% of cases of GCSE occur in individuals known to have epilepsy and, in the other 50–60%, SE is usually symptomatic in nature. In those with epilepsy, SE is most often related to poor compliance or changes in medication. Simply administering the drug they are withdrawing from can terminate SE even if it requires administration of an oral medicine through a nasogastic tube. These patients typically have a good outcome. As previously mentioned, the main symptomatic causes in adults are stroke, tumour, trauma and CNS infection, while in children febrile SE, CNS infection and acute metabolic derangements are the most common aetiologies. The history and exam should therefore focus on confirming or excluding these. Often the aetiology will not be apparent until the seizures are controlled and further investigations can be carried out. It should be noted that certain clinical findings can be 'normal' in SE, particularly convulsive SE, and do not necessarily point to a localizing pathology. These include hyperthermia, pupillary abnormalities, generalized hyperreflexia and upgoing plantar responses.

The most critical factor to establish is how long the patient has been seizing. This will dictate how aggressive one needs to be with treatment. A patient who arrives in the emergency room after 20–30 min of continuous seizing is at high risk of neurological and systemic complications. Remember, also, that they are less likely to respond to initial benzodiazepine treatment because prolonged seizure activity causes internalization of GABA receptors and the metabolic environment may alter the kinetics and bioavailability of the drug.

In terms of predicting the probable outcome, it is important to assess the patient's risk factors for death, particularly their age and underlying aetiology. Other possible risk factors are discussed above. One should consider early transfer to the intensive care unit for patients with seizures beginning out of hospital and with multiple risks for a poor outcome.

INITIAL TREATMENT

There is no doubt that in terms of the initial pharmacological management of SE, there are few therapeutic options more important in the treatment of potentially damaging *prolonged seizures* of *any type* than the *timely* use of *benzodiazepines*. The rationale for the initial treatment of SE is based on a clinical trial of 384 patients with convulsive SE which compared four different treatment arms [101]: diazepam (0.15 mg/kg), followed by phenytoin (18 mg/kg), lorazepam alone (0.1 mg/kg), phenobarbital alone (15 mg/kg) and phenytoin alone (18 mg/kg). Lorazepam terminated the seizure activity in 64.9%, phenobarbital in 58.2%, diazepam plus phenytoin in 55.8% and phenytoin in 43.6%. An intention-to-treat analysis found no significant difference among treatment groups in patients with overt convulsive SE ($P = 0.12$), except that lorazepam alone was significantly more effective that phenytoin alone. In clinical practice, lorazepam alone is easier and faster to use and hence has become well established as a first agent given to patients in SE of any type. It is preferred to other benzodiazepines because of its longer duration of action. Up to 0.1 mg/kg may be given. As distribution is slow, the rate of injection is not critical. An initial dose of 4 mg is recommended to ensure that adequate plasma levels are achieved quickly. If the patient continues to seize, a second dose may be given after 10 min, and at this stage most physicians would also commence infusion of a second-line agent, typically intravenous phenytoin. Diazepam is an alternative if lorazepam is unavailable (dose 0.5 mg/kg). Both drugs may cause drowsiness, hypotension and respiratory depression. However, because it is relatively lipid insoluble, lorazepam does not tend to accumulate and produce unpredictable respiratory collapse or sudden hypotension, which may occur with diazepam. These drugs are not used for long-term management because of the development of tolerance.

SECOND-LINE TREATMENT

If there is failure to respond to lorazepam, an intravenous infusion of phenytoin or fosphenytoin should be commenced. It is essential to liaise with the anaesthetic services at this stage to make them aware of the situation and the possibility that ICU transfer may be required. Fosphenytoin has the advantage over phenytoin of faster administration and less risk of hypotension. Both should be administered at a dose of 20 mg/kg. There has been a tendency among physicians to use lower doses of phenytoin due to fears of toxicity. However, the risk of phenytoin toxicity at this dose is low and is outweighed by the risks of ongoing SE in those who are under-treated. Epileptic patients who go into SE and who are already taking phenytoin as part of their regimen should be treated with full loading doses initially while the baseline phenytoin level is awaited (if available). If this level is in the medium-to-high range, the succeeding doses of the drug should be reduced.

The rate of infusion should not exceed 50 mg/min, which is equivalent to a 1500-mg infusion given over approximately 30 minutes. It is prudent to reduce this to 30 mg/min in the elderly. For neonates the rate of infusion should not exceed 1 mg/kg/min. The drug should be administered in normal saline to avoid precipitation and other drugs should not be added to the infusion, for the same reason. Owing to its high pH, it may also cause thrombophlebitis (which in severe cases may result in the so-called 'purple glove' syndrome). Phenytoin causes relatively little cerebral or respiratory depression. However, hypotension and cardiac arrhythmia can occur and patients should have their blood pressure and pulse monitored during and after treatment. The risk of severe hypotension or cardiac arrhythmia is low and does not appear to significantly differ from the risks associated with either benzodiazepines or phenobarbital [100]. If there are concerns over the safety of phenytoin use, a good alternative appears to be intravenous valproate. It has the advantage of rapid administration, lower risk of adverse effects and may also offer the benefits of neuroprotection (see below).

It is worth noting that in certain circumstances, it may be reasonable to administer a second-line agent even if the SE is terminated by the initial treatment with lorazepam. This usually arises in the setting of irritative structural lesion, such as a tumour or acute stroke, where the risk of recurrent seizure is high and there is a desire for rapid titration of maintenance AED.

Alternative Second-Line or Third-Line Therapeutic Strategies for Status Epilepticus

These agents should be considered when phenytoin is contraindicated or when the patient continues to seize after its administration (i.e. as a third-line agent). Although there are few data available, it is the authors' opinion that the majority of patients who fail to respond to the combination of benzodiazepine and phenytoin in adequate doses are probably unlikely to respond to a third-line agent and will require intubation and treatment with an anaesthetic agent, as discussed below.

Valproate

Most of the available data on the efficacy of intravenous sodium valproate in treating SE come from non-comparative case series [101–106]. In these studies, the efficacy is reported at between 58% and 100%, as both a first- and second-line agent and in all clinical forms of status, including complex partial SE. However, a recent randomized unblinded study that compared valproate to phenytoin in 68 patients found valproate to be superior at aborting SE as both a first-line (66% vs. 42%) and second-line (79% vs. 25%) agent [107]. There was a suggestion of a synergistic effect with other drugs when valproate was given as the second, third or fourth agent. The drug also has the advantage over phenytoin of better safety, serious side-effects being virtually unheard of in reports. Side-effects that have been reported in occasional patients include respiratory depression, tremor and transient disturbance of liver function tests. It may be given as a rapid intravenous infusion of up to 6 mg/kg/min to a maximum dose of 45 mg/kg, most reports using 20–30 mg/kg at a rate of about 3 mg/kg/min (approximately 2000 mg over 10 min for the average adult). Clearly, large-scale randomized comparative trials are warranted to further clarify the role of the drug in the management of SE.

Levetiracetam

Anecdotal evidence is also beginning to emerge on the use of oral or nasogastric levetiracetam as a treatment for SE [108–111]. Two retrospective case series from the same group have reported that 33–43% of patients with SE of different aetiologies and seizure types responded to levetiracetam, having failed standard SE regimens [109, 111]. The authors noted that although doses between 1000 and 9000 mg/day were given, all responders did so at less than 3000 mg/day and when the drug was commenced within 4 days of the onset of SE. A further case series reported that six patients, refractory to at least two prior AEDs, responded to oral levetiracetam within 96 h at doses up to 3000 mg/day [108]. No significant adverse reactions were reported. Levetiracetam may also be given via nasogastric tube in comatose patients, although absorption may be variable. Levetiracetam can now also be administered intravenously and thus represents an alternative to phenytoin in the acute setting. There are few data currently available on its efficacy. The main advantages of levetiracetam in the setting of SE are ease of administration, rapid titration, easy transition to use as a maintenance anti-epileptic drug (AED) and few drug–drug interactions. Further data are clearly needed before its use can be recommended.

Phenobarbital

Phenobarbital, also known as phenobarbital, is the traditional agent of choice after phenytoin has proven ineffective in the setting of SE. Phenobarbital requires less dilution and can be given as a slow i.v. push over 10 minutes. Phenobarbital is sedating, although not sufficient to induce a burst-suppression EEG pattern when a 20-mg/kg loading dose is administered. Patients need intubation after a loading dose. The drug has a very long half-life of 3–7 days and accumulates in tissues; hence, patients often require a long waking-up period after significant doses are administered. Phenobarbital rarely causes idiosyncratic reactions, but rashes, hepatic dysfunction and aplastic anaemia have been reported.

Topiramate

Evidence supporting the use of topiramate in SE comes from a small number of case series where it has been used in the setting of refractory SE in both children and adults [112–117]. All patients reported thus far appear to have had a favourable response to topiramate in this setting, despite different aetiologies and seizure types, and no serious adverse reactions have been reported. Its multiple mechanisms of action make it a good candidate drug for SE, with the potential for additive effects with other agents. Again, however, prospective clinical trial data are lacking. The drug is typically given in this setting as a suspension, via nasogastric tube in the comatose patient, at doses between 300 and 1600 mg/day. Topiramate is currently not available as an intravenous drug.

REFRACTORY STATUS EPILEPTICUS

SE that is not controlled by the above measures is termed refractory. Refractory SE accounts for between 9% and 31% of all SE and is associated with a mortality rate in the region of 40–50%. Patients should be intubated and ventilated in the ICU. The patient's temperature should be kept below 37°C if possible (see below). The choice of agent to treat the SE lies between continuous intravenous infusions of a barbiturate (such as pentobarbital or thiopentone), midazolam or propofol. As yet, there are no randomized controlled trials comparing the three agents. A meta-analysis of the available data, compiled mainly from case series, suggested that there was no difference in overall mortality between the three agents when continuous infusions were titrated to background EEG suppression [118]. However, pentobarbital appeared to be associated with the lowest rates of short-term treatment failure, breakthrough seizures and need to change to an alternative agent, while midazolam was associated with the highest rates. On the other hand, pentobarbital was associated with a significantly higher rate of hypotension, requiring pressor support than the other two agents. This may well explain why, in a survey of European physicians who treat SE, most prefer the use of propofol or midazolam [119]. It is worth re-emphasizing that continuous infusion therapy simply provides temporary abolition of SE. Optimization of maintenance AED therapy is at least as important as the choice of infusion therapy. Once background suppression of the EEG is achieved, the infusion should be continued for 24 h before tapering. If SE recurs, the AED should be titrated back up and other maintenance AEDs such as levetiracetam, topiramate or valproate added before re-tapering.

Pentobarbital has a rapid onset of action and in adults and older children is given as a loading dose of 5–15 mg/kg at 0.2–0.5 mg/kg/min to suppress epileptiform activity, followed by 1–5 mg/kg/h continuous infusion. The major side-effects are severe hypotension, sedation, respiratory depression and difficulty weaning from the ventilator. Thiopentone is a precursor of phenobarbital that has been commonly used for SE in Europe. The drug has a strong tendency to accumulate and thus blood levels may remain high even after the drug is stopped. Blood level monitoring of both thiopentone and phenobarbital is therefore recommended. Its side-effect profile is similar to that of phenobarbital, although it has a greater tendency to produce severe hypotension, requiring pressor support. It may also cause pancreatitis and hepatic disturbance. It is typically given as a bolus of 100–250 mg over 20 s, followed by 50-mg boluses every 2–3 min until seizures are controlled, followed by an infusion of 3–5 mg/kg/h. After 24 h, the dose should be controlled by blood level monitoring. Blood pressure needs to be monitored via an arterial line and the dose reduced if systolic blood pressure falls below 90 mmHg.

Midazolam is a rapid-onset, short-acting benzodiazepine which is easy to titrate. It is usually given as a 0.2 mg/kg slow i.v. push followed by a continuous infusion of 0.05–0.4 mg/kg/h (may be given up to 3 mg/kg/h). Its rate of elimination is decreased in renal and hepatic failure and by inhibitors of cytochrome CYP 3A, such as verapamil or cimetidine. It appears to be very safe, with little risk of hypotension.

Propofol is given as an initial push of 1–2 mg/kg at 10 mg/min followed by 1–10 mg/kg/h (may be given up to 15 mg/kg/h). Like phenobarbital, prolonged infusions result in slower clearance and accumulation of the drug. The elimination half-life of 2–12 h may be increased up to 3 days after 10-day infusions [120]. However, its duration of clinical effect is much shorter because propofol is rapidly distributed into peripheral tissues, and its effects begin to wear off within half an hour of stopping the infusion. Withdrawal seizures may occur and therefore the drug should be tapered slowly (e.g. 5–10% per hour). During withdrawal, epileptiform-like activity may begin to re-appear on the EEG. In our experience, this is sometimes a transient phenomenon and does not necessarily warrant immediate re-institution of anaesthesia. Studies examining this are lacking, however. Propofol also appears to have neuroexcitatory effects and may produce muscle rigidity and even abnormal movements such as myoclonus. These may be mistaken for seizure activity. The drug is associated with hypotension, often requiring pressor support. High doses (greater than 5 mg/kg/h) over prolonged periods appear to increase the risk of severe side-effects, including hypotension, heart failure, acidosis and rhabdomyolyis – the so-called 'propofol infusion syndrome' – and should be avoided if possible, as should co-treatment with phenobarbital, which appears to increase risk of death [121, 122]. The drug is not recommended for children.

Highly Refractory Status Epilepticus (HRSE)

Despite the therapeutic initiatives outlined above, a small number of patients will remain in SE despite pharmacological suppression of seizures by coma-inducing agents. When confronted with such a scenario, it is vital that a methodical, stepwise review of the case be undertaken before proceeding with further strategies. The following points should be considered:

- Re-evaluate the case and be satisfied that the underlying cause has been identified, particularly metabolic, inflammatory, infectious or iatrogenic causes. In such cases, treatment of the underlying cause may be more beneficial than treatment of the seizures.
- Examine the burst-suppression pattern on EEG and compare the bursts to the seizures evident at the onset of EEG recording, before infusion therapy. Are the bursts in fact

electrographic seizures? If so, further titration of the infusion agent may be warranted. If one infusion therapy does not work, then another should be tried. There is little prospective evidence that one agent is more effective or safer than another. If the initial infusion therapy regimen does not terminate SE after a 24–36-h period, then it should be changed to an alternative.

- Review all imaging studies including MRI, PET and SPECT, if available. Has a structural lesion that might be amenable to surgery been ruled out?
- Check that adequate levels of maintenance AEDs are being used to increase the success of weaning from infusion therapy.
- If the EEG activity is equivocal or difficult to interpret, it is not unreasonable to temporarily discontinue infusion therapies to allow clarification of the current clinical and EEG status. This is sometimes the only way to be sure that the patient is still in SE and may be less risky that prolonged trials of unnecessary treatment.

Therapeutic Options in HRSE

Surgical Intervention

The very high morbidity and mortality rates associated with refractory SE argue for a role for surgical intervention where that SE is focal and particularly where the SE is related to a clearly delineated focal cortical lesion or region. Surgical resection of epileptogenic foci has gained widespread acceptance as a valid therapeutic intervention in chronic epilepsy and the same criteria can be extended to the acute setting of refractory focal SE. In the acute setting, however, consideration of post-operative deficits and the prospect of long-term seizure freedom should be weighed against the risks associated with ongoing focal SE. The likelihood of successful intervention is related to identification of a causative candidate structural lesion or functional epileptogenic region and the timing of surgical resection. Identification of a structural lesion or functional region requires correlation of EEG findings with structural (usually MR) and functional (usually PET or SPECT) imaging. While surgery has been considered as a last-gasp option, it is likely that better outcomes may be obtained with earlier intervention, before the focal SE has evolved into a broader secondarily generalized electroclinical form of SE and without the inherent medical risks following a prolonged ICU admission. There have been a number of reports of successful treatment of refractory focal SE by surgical removal of an underlying structural lesion or brain region [123, 124].

Ketamine

Ketamine is a potent NMDA antagonist that has been used in some institutions in the setting of refractory SE. It is administered as a loading dose of 2 mg/kg, followed by an infusion of 10–50 μg/kg/min. Limited data are available on the use of this infusion therapy in humans. Although its use in refractory SE has theoretic advantages, there is evidence that excessive NMDA excitatory receptor-mediated transmission is an important mechanism of persistent neuronal firing in the setting of downregulation of GABA receptors. The evidence for efficacy of ketamine is largely anecdotal [125]. The reported adverse effects relate to its use as an analgesic, where hallucinations and other transient psychotic sequelae are reported. Ketamine is associated with cardiovascular stimulation and a rise in arterial pressure and heart rate and should be used with caution in patients with systemic or intracranial hypertension. Cerebellar damage has also been reported after longer-term use [126].

Lidocaine Infusion

There are a number of reports of successful use of lidocaine in the setting of refractory SE [127]. This agent should be not be used in patients with co-existing sinoatrial disorders, all grades of atrioventricular block or severe myocardial depression.

Inhalation Anaesthetics

Inhalational anaesthetics are used for the induction and maintenance of anaesthesia. There have been several case reports of successful use of inhalation anaesthetics in the setting of refractory SE including isoflurane and desflurane [128].

Deep Brain Stimulation

Although surface and deep brain stimulation devices are being developed for use in focal and generalized epilepsies, their use has not been reported in humans in the setting of SE.

Transcranial Magnetic Stimulation

Transcranial magnetic stimulation has similarly been evaluated in animal models of focal SE but has not yet been reported to be helpful in human SE.

Electroconvulsive Therapy

While, in theory, it may seem illogical to administer a proconvulsive stimulus in SE, the inhibitory state after a convulsion induced by electroconvulsive therapy has been proposed as possibly beneficial to patients in SE [129]. Electroconvulsive therapy has not been evaluated in a rigorous fashion by clinical trial. In our experience, it has not been helpful in the management of refractory SE.

PRE-HOSPITAL MANAGEMENT

Given that the goal of treatment of SE is to treat early to allow benzodiazepines the best chance to work, pre-hospital treatment is now an essential tool in the management of SE. For patients with known epilepsy, this can be achieved by having a store of buccal midazolam (10 mg in 1-ml syringe) or rectal diazepam (10-mg sachet) available in the home. Relatives and carers should be educated in the use of these products by the local epilepsy service. For other situations, evidence supports the use of i.v. lorazepam or diazepam by the emergency medical services, which are often first at the scene. 2 mg lorazepam or 5 mg diazepam has been shown to be superior to placebo at terminating SE prior to arrival in the emergency room [130]. Again, training of staff is important to avoid under- or over-treatment.

MANAGEMENT OF NCSE

The management of NCSE remains controversial and without clear guidelines. Traditionally, it was felt that this condition followed a more benign course without long-term sequelae. However, there is increasing evidence that NCSE can also result in significant brain damage if allowed to continue unabated [131–133]. In general, we favour a somewhat less aggressive approach than with convulsive SE, following the same initial guidelines outlined above but withholding anaesthetic agents unless the patient is severely obtunded with a depressed level of consciousness, as this recourse is not without its own significant risks. Instead, refractory cases are usually treated with trials of additional second- and third-line agents. Absence SE and simple and complex partial SE in patients known to have epilepsy usually respond well to treatment, whereas acute symptomatic cases are often refractory and only begin to improve with treatment of the underlying cause. For a more detailed discussion of this topic, which is outside the scope of this chapter, the reader is referred Meierkord and Holtkamp's excellent review of this difficult area [134].

NOVEL THERAPEUTIC STRATEGIES FOR STATUS EPILEPTICUS

New approaches to the management of SE fall broadly into the categories of termination of the status itself and, secondly, prevention of the neurological sequelae of SE, commonly termed neuroprotection.

NON-PHARMACOLOGICAL APPROACHES TO SEIZURE TERMINATION

Cooling

It is clear from both animal experiments and the clinical phenomenon of febrile seizures that increases in body temperature have pronounced effects on seizures and epileptic activity. Conversely, it seems that hypothermia may diminish epileptic activity and may become a useful adjunctive strategy in the management of patients with refractory SE. Most of the data are from experimental animals, where cooling has been shown to reduce epileptic activity in both kainic acid and electrical stimulation models of SE in rats [135–137]. In one study, cooling to a maximum of 29°C appeared to have a synergistic effect with diazepam [135]. In humans, moderate hypothermia (30–31°C) combined with thiopental coma was reported to be effective in three paediatric patients with refractory SE [138]. In another study, focal cooling of an epileptogenic focus, performed prior to surgery, appeared to abolish the ictal discharge from the focus [139]. The neurophysiological mechanisms underlying the anti-convulsant effects of cooling are poorly understood, but may include alteration of post-synaptic voltage-gated channels and ion pumps and reduction of presynaptic excitatory neurotransmitter release.

NEUROPROTECTION IN STATUS EPILEPTICUS

As discussed, prolonged seizures may result in neuronal death, which in turn may lead to cognitive decline and epilepsy. As the mechanisms underlying neuronal death in SE become better understood, research has focused on methods of preventing the pathophysiological changes that result in neuronal damage. Thus, most potential neuroprotective agents have targeted excitotoxic pathways, including blockade of glutaminergic NMDA receptors and calcium channels or, alternatively, apoptotic pathways. The data on these agents come from various animal models of SE and are summarized in Table 14.3. No drug is currently approved for use in humans as a neuroprotective agent in SE.

Interpretation of the data on neuroprotection is complicated by the use of different models of SE and administration of the neuroprotective agent at different times before, during and after SE induction, although the trend overall appears to be for better results the earlier the agent is given after SE has commenced. The NMDA receptor antagonists were the first such group to gain recognition in this field but interest in their use has waned due to their potential neurotoxicity. They have been shown to produce neuronal vacuolization and necrosis in animals [140, 141] and some (e.g. phencyclidine) are known to produce psychotic behaviour in humans.

Interestingly, a number of AEDs have been reported to have neuroprotective qualities in addition to their anti-convulsant properties. One of the difficulties in interpreting the data on AEDs is differentiating the neuroprotective effect of reducing seizure activity from an independent effect on the molecular mechanisms underlying neurodegeneration. However, a recent report has suggested that the neuroprotective effect of topiramate may be related to protection of hippocampal mitochondria from high extracellular calcium concentrations, an effect independent of its anti-seizure activity [142]. If these findings can be substantiated in future studies, drugs such as topiramate and valproate may well become the agents of choice for the treatment of SE.

Table 14.3 Summary of neuroprotective agents used in status epilepticus

Class	Agent	Animal model	Initiation of treatment	Effect on cell loss	Effect on epileptogenesis	Reference
NMDA receptor antagonism	Ketamine	(a) Kainic acid; (b) lithium-pilocarpine	(b) 15 min after SE onset	Decreased cell loss in CA1, amygdala, thalamus and piriform cortex	n/a	(a) [143]; (b) [144]
	MK-108	(a–c) Kainic acid; (d) electrical stimulation	(a, b) 90 min after SE onset; (c) ?; (d) 1 h after SE	Decreased cell loss in CA1, CA3 and piriform cortex	(a) No; (d) Yes	(a) [145]; (b) [146]; (c) [143]; (d) [147]
	Phenylcylidine	Kainic acid	?	Decreased cell loss in CA1, amygdala, thalamus and piriform cortex	n/a	[143]
	GCP 40116	Lithium-pilocarpine	15 min after SE onset	Prevents neuronal loss in multiple areas	n/a	[148]
Inhibitors of apoptosis	Caspase inhibitors	(a) Kainic acid; (b) electrical stimulation	(a) 90 min after SE onset	Mild reduction in mossy fibre sprouting	No	(a) [146]; (b) [149]
Anti-epileptic drugs	Gabapentin	Kainic acid	24 h after SE onset	Reduced hippocampal damage	No	[150]
	Levetiracetam	Pilocarpine	30 min after SE onset	No effect	No	[151]
	Phenobarbital	(a–c) Kainic acid	(a) Co-administration; (b, c) 24 h after kainate injection; (d) 1 h after SE	No effect when given at 24 h. Co-administration results in decreased cell loss in dentate gyrus (?anti-convulsant effect)	Reduced susceptibility to kindling when co-administered with kainate	(a) [152]; (b) [153]; (c) [154]; (d) [147]
		(d) Electrical stimulation				
	Valproate	(a) Electrical stimulation	(a) 4 h after SE onset; (b) 24 h after kainate injection	Decreased cell loss in CA1 and CA3	(a) no: (b) prevented spontaneous seizures	(a) [155]; (b) [154]
		(b) Kainic acid				
	Vigabatrin	(a) Electrical stimulation	(a) 2 days after SE onset; (b) 10 min after pilocarpine	Decreased cell loss in CA1, CA3 and dentate gyrus	No	(a) [156]; (b) [157]
		(b) Lithium-pilocarpine				

Continued overleaf

Table 14.3 Continued

Class	Agent	Animal model	Initiation of treatment	Effect on cell loss	Effect on epileptogenesis	Reference
Anti-epileptic drugs	Topiramate	Lithium-pilocarpine	1 h after SE onset	Decreased cell loss in CA1 and CA3	No	[158]
	Pregabalin	Pilocarpine	20 min after pilocarpine injection	Decreased cell loss in enorhinal cortex	Delayed occurrence spontaneous seizures	[159]
Oestrogens	Estradiol benzoate	Kainic acid	48 h before SE onset	Decreased cell loss in CA1 and dentate gyrus	n/a	[160, 161]
Others	Low-dose caffeine	Lithium-pilocarpine	15 days before SE onset	Decreased cell loss in CA1; increased cell loss in piriform cortex	No	[162]

NA, not available.

It must be noted, however, that despite clear, and in some cases pronounced, effects of these agents in reducing cell loss in limbic areas, no agent has been consistently shown to be truly 'anti-epileptogenic'. This suggests that the two processes may in fact be disassociated; that is, that the development of epilepsy is not directly related to the degree of damage to hippocampal structures and that functional alterations in neuronal networking rather than actual neuronal death may be very important in epileptogenesis. It also suggests that extra-hippocampal structures may be more important in the epileptogenic process than previously thought. Clearly, further work will need to be done to better understand this process and it is possible that this may result in a paradigm shift in how we currently understand the process of epileptogenesis following SE.

REFERENCES

1. Cascino GD, Hesdorffer D, Logroscino G et al., Treatment of SE in Rochester, Minnesota, 1965–84. *Mayo Clinic Proc* 2001; 76:39–41.
2. Kinnier Wilson SA, Reynolds EH. Translation and analysis of a cuneiform text forming part of a Babylonian treatise on epilepsy. *Med Hist* 1990; 34:185–198.
3. Calmeil LF. Del'épilepsie, étudiée sous le rapport de son siege et de son influence sur la production de l'aliénation mentale. Thesis, University of Paris, 1824.
4. Trousseau A. *Lectures on clinical medicine delivered at the Hotel Dieu, Paris.* Vol. 1 (trans. P. V. Bazire). London: New Sydenham Society, 1868.
5. Bourneville DM. L'état de mal épileptique. In: Bourneville DM (ed.) *Recherches Cliniques et Thérapeutiques sur l'Épilepsie et l'Hystérie. Compte-rendu des Observations Recueillies à la Salpêtrière.* Paris: Delahaye, 1976.
6. Clark LP, Prout TP. Status epilepticus. A clinical and pathological study in epilepsy. *Am J Insanity* 1903; 60:291–306.
7. Charcot JM. *Clinical lectures on the diseases of the nervous system* (trans. T. Savill). London: New Sydenham Society, 1989.
8. Lennox, W. The petit mal epilepsies. Their treatment with tridone. *JAMA* 1945; 129:1069–1073.
9. Gastaut H, Roger J, Roger A. Sur la signification de certaines fugues épileptiques: Etat de mal temporal. *Rev Neurol* 1956; 94:298–301.
10. Proposal for revised classification of epilepsies and epileptic syndromes. Commission on Classification and Terminology of the International League Against Epilepsy. *Epilepsia* 1989; 30:389–399.
11. Lowenstein DH, Alldredge BK. Status epilepticus. *N Engl J Med* 1998; 338:970–976.
12. DeLorenzo RJ, Pellock JM, Towne AR et al. Epidemiology of status epilepticus. *J Clin Neurophysiol* 1995; 12:316–325.
13. Hesdorffer DC, Logroscino G, Cascino G et al. Incidence of status epilepticus in Rochester, Minnesota, 1965–1984. *Neurology* 1998; 50:735–741.
14. Coeytaux A, Jallon P, Galobardes B et al. Incidence of status epilepticus in French-speaking Switzerland: (EPISTAR). *Neurology* 2000; 55:693–697.
15. Knake S, Rosenow F, Vescovi M et al.; Status Epilepticus Study Group Hessen (SESGH). Incidence of status epilepticus in adults in Germany: a prospective, population-based study. *Epilepsia* 2001; 42:714–718.
16. Wu YW, Shek DW, Garcia PA et al. Incidence and mortality of generalized convulsive status epilepticus in California. *Neurology* 2002; 58:1070–1076.
17. Vignatelli L, Tonon C, D'Alessandro R; Bologna Group for the Study of Status Epilepticus. Incidence and short-term prognosis of status epilepticus in adults in Bologna, Italy. Epilepsia. 2003; 44:964–968.
18. Vignatelli L, Rinaldi R, Galeotti M et al. Epidemiology of status epilepticus in a rural area of northern Italy: a 2-year population-based study. *Eur J Neurol* 2005; 12:897–902.
19. Chin RF, Neville BG, Peckham C et al.; NLSTEPSS Collaborative Group. Incidence, cause, and short-term outcome of convulsive status epilepticus in childhood: prospective population-based study. *Lancet* 2006; 368:222–229.
20. Logroscino G, Hesdorffer DC, Cascino G et al. Time trends in incidence, mortality, and case-fatality after first episode of status epilepticus. *Epilepsia* 2001; 42:1031–1035.
21. Towne AR, Waterhouse EJ, Boggs JG et al. Prevalence of nonconvulsive status epilepticus in comatose patients. *Neurology* 2000; 54:340–345.

22. Privitera M, Hoffman M, Moore JL et al. EEG detection of nontonic–clonic status epilepticus in patients with altered consciousness. *Epilepsy Res* 1994; 18:155–166.
23. Waterhouse EJ, Vaughan JK, Barnes TY et al. Synergistic effect of status epilepticus and ischemic brain injury on mortality. *Epilepsy Res* 1998; 29:175–183.
24. Towne AR, Pellock JM, Ko D et al. Determinants of mortality in status epilepticus. *Epilepsia* 1994; 35:27–34.
25. Aminoff MJ, Simon RP. Status epilepticus. Causes, clinical features and consequences in 98 patients. *Am J Med* 1980; 69:657–666.
26. Sagduyu A, Tarlaci S, Sirin H. Generalized tonic–clonic status epilepticus: causes, treatment, complications and predictors of case fatality. *J Neurol* 1998; 245:640–646.
27. Maegaki Y, Kurozawa Y, Hanaki K et al. Risk factors for fatality and neurological sequelae after status epilepticus in children. *Neuropediatrics* 2005; 36:186–192.
28. Hui AC, Joynt GM, Li H et al. Status epilepticus in Hong Kong Chinese: aetiology, outcome and predictors of death and morbidity. *Seizure* 2003; 12:478–482.
29. Rossetti AO, Hurwitz S, Logroscino G et al. Prognosis of status epilepticus: role of aetiology, age, and consciousness impairment at presentation. *J Neurol Neurosurg Psychiatry* 2006; 77:611–615.
30. Shneker BF, Fountain NB. Assessment of acute morbidity and mortality in nonconvulsive status epilepticus. *Neurology* 2003; 61:1066–1073.
31. Waterhouse EJ, Garnett LK, Towne AR et al. Prospective population-based study of intermittent and continuous convulsive status epilepticus in Richmond, Virginia. *Epilepsia* 1999; 40:752–758.
32. Dunne JW, Summers QA, Stewart-Wyne EG. Nonconvulsive status epilepticus: a prospective study in adult general hospital. *Q J Med* 1987; 23:117–126.
33. Tomson T, Lindbom U, Nilson BY. Nonconvulsive status epilepticus in adults: thirty-two consecutive patients from a general hospital population. *Epilepsia* 1992; 33:829–835.
34. Krumholz A, Sung GY, Fisher RS et al. Complex partial status epilepticus accompanied by serious morbidity and mortality. *Neurology* 1995; 45:1499–1504.
35. Young GB, Jordan KG, Doig GS. An assessment of nonconvulsive seizures in the intensive care unit using continuous EEG monitoring: an investigation of variables associated with mortality. *Neurology* 1996; 47:83–89.
36. Kaplan PW. Prognosis in nonconvulsive status epilepticus. *Epileptic Disord* 2000; 2:185–193.
37. Garzon E, Fernandes RM, Sakamoto AC. Analysis of clinical characteristics and risk factors for mortality in human status epilepticus. *Seizure* 2003; 12:337–345.
38. Jaitly R, Sgro JA, Towne AR et al. Prognostic value of EEG monitoring after status epilepticus: a prospective adult study. *J Clin Neurophysiol* 1997; 14:326–334.
39. Nei M, Lee JM, Shanker VL et al. The EEG and prognosis in status epilepticus. *Epilepsia* 1999; 40:157–163.
40. Logroscino G, Hesdorffer DC, Cascino GD, Anneggers JF, Bagiella E, Hauser WA. Long-term mortality after a first episode of status epilepticus. *Neurology* 2002; 58:537–541.
41. Hauser WA, Anderson VE, Loewenson RB et al. Seizure recurrence after a first unprovoked seizure. *N Engl J Med* 1982; 307:522–528.
42. Shinnar S, Berg AT, Moshe SL et al. Risk of seizure recurrence following a first unprovoked seizure in childhood: a prospective study. *Pediatrics* 1990; 85:1076–1085.
43. Ramos Lizana J, Cassinello Garcia E, Carrasco Marina LL et al. Seizure recurrence after a first unprovoked seizure in childhood: a prospective study. *Epilepsia* 2000; 41:1005–1013.
44. Daoud AS, Ajloni S, El-Salem K et al. Risk of seizure recurrence after a first unprovoked seizure: a prospective study among Jordanian children. *Seizure* 2004; 13:99–103.
45. Maytal J, Shinnar S, Moshe SL et al. Low morbidity and mortality of status epilepticus in children. *Pediatrics* 1989; 83:323–331.
46. Verity CM, Ross EM, Golding J. Outcome of childhood status epilepticus and lengthy febrile convulsions: findings of national cohort study. *BMJ* 1993; 307:225–228.
47. Cavazzuti GB, Ferrari P, Lalla M. Follow-up study of 482 cases with convulsive disorders in the first year of life. *Dev Med Child Neurol* 1984; 26:425–437.
48. Tabarki B, Yacoub M, Selmi H et al. Infantile status epilepticus in Tunisia. Clinical, etiological and prognostic aspects. *Seizure* 2001; 10:365–369.
49. Kwong KL, Chang K, Lam SY. Features predicting adverse outcomes of status epilepticus in childhood. *Hong Kong Med J* 2004; 10:156–159.

50. Kwong KL, Lee SL, Yung A *et al*. Status epilepticus in 37 Chinese children: aetiology and outcome. *J Paediatr Child Health* 1995; 31:395–398.

51. Mah JK, Mah MW. Pediatric status epilepticus: a perspective from Saudi Arabia. *Pediatr Neurol* 1999; 20:364–369.

52. Aicardi J, Chevrie JJ. Convulsive status epilepticus in infants and children. A study of 239 cases. *Epilepsia* 1970; 11:187–197.

53. Hesdorffer DC, Logroscino G, Cascino G *et al*. Risk of unprovoked seizure after acute symptomatic seizure: effect of status epilepticus. *Ann Neurol* 1998; 44:908–912.

54. Holtkamp M, Othman J, Buchheim K *et al*. Predictors and prognosis of refractory status epilepticus treated in a neurological intensive care unit. *J Neurol Neurosurg Psychiatry* 2005; 76:534–539.

55. Cendes F, Andermann F, Gloor P *et al*. Atrophy of mesial structures in patients with temporal lobe epilepsy: cause or consequence of repeated seizures? *Ann Neurol* 1993; 34:795–801.

56. Trinka E, Unterrainer J, Haberlandt E *et al*. Childhood febrile convulsions – which factors determine the subsequent epilepsy syndrome? A retrospective study. *Epilepsy Res* 2002; 50:283–292.

57. Camfield P, Camfield C, Gordon K *et al*. What types of epilepsy are preceded by febrile seizures? A population-based study of children. *Dev Med Child Neurol* 1994; 36:887–892.

58. Tarkka R, Paakko E, Pyhtinen J *et al*. Febrile seizures and mesial temporal sclerosis: no association in a long-term follow-up study. *Neurology* 2003; 60:215–218.

59. Berg AT, Shinnar S, Levy SR *et al*. Childhood-onset epilepsy with and without preceding febrile seizures. *Neurology* 1999; 53:1742–1748.

60. Tasch E, Cendes F, Li LM *et al*. Neuroimaging evidence of progressive neuronal loss and dysfunction in temporal lobe epilepsy. *Ann Neurol* 1999; 45:568–576.

61. Garrido Sanabria ER, Castaneda MT, Banuelos C *et al*. Septal GABAergic neurons are selectively vulnerable to pilocarpine-induced status epilepticus and chronic spontaneous seizures. *Neuroscience* 2006; 142:871–883.

62. Pitkanen A, Nissinen J, Nairismagi J *et al*. Progression of neuronal damage after status epilepticus and during spontaneous seizures in a rat model of temporal lobe epilepsy. *Prog Brain Res* 2002; 135:67–83.

63. Gorter JA, Goncalves Pereira PM, van Vliet EA *et al*. Neuronal cell death in a rat model for mesial temporal lobe epilepsy is induced by the initial status epilepticus and not by later repeated spontaneous seizures. *Epilepsia* 2003; 44:647–658.

64. Nairismagi J, Pitkanen A, Kettunen MI *et al*. Status epilepticus in 12-day-old rats leads to temporal lobe neurodegeneration and volume reduction: a histologic and MRI study. *Epilepsia* 2006; 47:479–488.

65. Treiman DM. Electroclinical features of status epilepticus in the adult. *Epilepsia* 1993; 34(Suppl 1):S2–S11.

66. Handforth A, Cheng JT, Mandelkern MA *et al*. Markedly increased mesiotemporal lobe metabolism in a case with PLEDs: further evidence that PLEDS are a manifestation of partial status epilepticus. *Epilepsia* 1994; 35:876–881.

67. Fujikawa DG. The temporal evolution of neuronal damage from pilocarpine-induced status epilepticus. *Brain Res* 1996; 725:11–22.

68. Critchely M, Critchley E. *John Hughlings Jackson: Father of English Neurology*. New York: Oxford University Press, 1998.

69. Bourneville DM. L'etat de mal epileptique. In: Bourneville DM (ed.) *Recherches Cliniques et Thérapeutiques sur l'Épilepsie et l'Hystérie. Compte-rendu des Observations Recueillies à la Salpêtrière*. Paris: Delahaye, 1976.

70. Treiman DM. Generalized convulsive status in the adult. *Epilepsia* 1993; 34(Suppl 1):S2–S11.

71. Treiman DM. Generalized convulsive status epilepticus. In: Wasterlain CG, Treiman DM (eds) *Status Epilepticus – Mechanisms and Management*. Cambridge, Massachusetts: The MIT Press, 2006, pp. 55–68.

72. DeLorenzo RJ, Hauser WA, Towne AR *et al*. Prospective population based epidemiological study of status epilepticus in Richmond VA. *Neurology* 1996; 46:1029–1032.

73. Meldrum BS, Vigouroux RA, Brierley JB. Systemic factors and epileptic brain damage: prolonged seizures in paralyzed, artificially ventilated baboons. *Arch Neurol* 1973; 29:82–87.

74. Olney JW, Rhee V, Ho OL. Kainic acid: a powerful neurotoxic analogue of glutamate. *Brain Research* 1974; 77:507–512.

75. Fijikawa DG. Prolonged seizures and cellular injury: understanding the connection. *Epilepsy Behav* 2005; 7:S3–S11.

76. Portera-Cailliau C, Price DL, Martin LJ. Excitotoxic neuronal death in the immature brain is an apoptosis–necrosis morphological continuum. *J Comp Neurol* 1997; 378:70–87.

77. Dawson VL, Dawson TM. Nitric oxide neurotoxicity. *J Chem Neuroanat* 1996; 10:179–190.

78. Henshall DC, Simon RP. Epilepsy and apoptosis pathways. *J Cereb Blood Flow Metab* 2005; 25:1557–1572.

79. Penfield W. The evidence of a cerebral vascular mechanism in epilepsy. *Ann Intern Med* 1933; 7:303–310.

80. Doherty CP, Cole AJ, Grant PE *et al*. Multimodal longitudinal imaging of focal status epilepticus. *Can J Neurol Sci* 2004; 31:276–281.

81. Spencer S, Bautista E. Functional neuroimaging in localization of the ictal onset zone. In: Henry T, Duncan J (eds) *Functional Imaging in the Epilepsies*. Philadelphia: Lippincott Williams and Wilkins, 2000, pp. 285–296.

82. Bruehl C, Hagemann G, Witte O. Uncoupling of blood flow and metabolism in focal epilepsy. *Epilepsia* 1998; 39:1235–1242.

83. Franck G, Sadzot B, Salmon E *et al*. Regional cerebral bloodflow and metabolic rates in human focal epilepsy and status epilepticus. *Adv Neurol* 1986; 44:935–948.

84. Henry T, Drury I, Brunberg J *et al*. Focal cerebral magnetic resonance changes associated with partial status epilepticus. *Epilespia* 1994; 35:35–41.

85. Callahan D, Noetzel M. Prolonged absence status epilepticus associated with carbamazepine therapy, increased intracranial pressure and transient MRI abnormalities. *Neurology* 1992; 42:2198–2201.

86. Fazekas F, Kapeller P, Schmidt R *et al*. Magnetic resonance imaging and spectroscopy findings after focal status epilepticus. *Epilepsia* 1995; 36:946–949.

87. Meierkord H, Wieshmann U, Niehaus L *et al*. Structural consequences of status epilepticus demonstrated with serial magnetic resonance imaging. *Acta Neurol Scand* 1997; 96:127–132.

88. Molyneux P, Barker R, Thom M *et al*. Successful treatment of intractable epilepsia partialis continua with multiple subpial transsections. *JNNP* 1998; 65:137–138.

89. Najm I, Wang Y, Shedid D *et al*. MRS metabolic markers of seizures and seizure-induced neuronal damage. *Epilepsia* 1998; 39:244–250.

90. Nohria V, Lee N, Tien R *et al*. Magnetic resonance imaging evidence of hippocampal sclerosis in progression: a case report. *Epilepsia* 1994; 35:1332–1336.

91. Lansberg M, O'Brien M, Norbash A *et al*. MRI abnormalities associated with partial status epilepticus. *Neurology* 1999; 52:1021–1027.

92. Yaffe K, Ferriero D, Barkovich J *et al*. Reversible MRI abnormalities following seizures. *Neurology* 1995; 45:104–108.

93. Zhong J, Petroff O, Prichard J. Barbiturate-reversible reduction of water diffusion coefficient in flurothyl-induced status epilepticus in rats. *Magn Reson Med* 1995; 33:253–256.

94. Lansberg M, O'Brien M, Norbash A *et al*. MRI abnormalities associated with partial status epilepticus. *Neurology* 1999; 52:1021–1027.

95. Liu Z, Gatt A, Mikati M *et al*. Effect of temperature on kainic acid-induced seizures. *Brain Res* 1993; 631:51–58.

96. Morimoto T, Nagao H, Yoshimatsu M *et al*. Pathogenic role of glutamate in hyperthermia-induced seizures. *Epilepsia* 1993; 34:447–452.

97. Meldrum BS, Horton RW. Physiology of status epilepticus in primates. *Arch Neurol* 1973; 28:1–9.

98. Simon RP. Physiologic responses to status epilepticus. In: Wasterlain C, Treiman D (eds) *Status Epilepticus: Mechanisms and Management*. Cambridge, Massachusetts: MIT Press, 2006, pp. 149–161.

99. Tang CM, Dichter, M, Morad M. Modulation of the N-methyl-D-aspartate channel by extracellular H$^+$. *Proc Natl Acad Sci USA* 1990; 87:6445–6449.

100. Treiman DM, Meyers PD, Walton NY *et al*. A comparison of four treatments for generalized convulsive status epilepticus. Veterans Affairs Status Epilepticus Cooperative Study Group. *N Engl J Med* 1998; 339:792–798.

101. Campistol J, Fernandez A, Ortega J. Status epilepticus in children. Experience with intravenous valproate. Update of treatment guidelines. *Rev Neurol* 1999; 29:359–365.

102. Peters CN, Pohlmann-Eden B. Intravenous valproate as an innovative therapy in seizure emergency situations including status epilepticus – experience in 102 adult patients. *Seizure* 2005; 14:164–169.

103. Yu KT, Mills S, Thompson N *et al*. Safety and efficacy of intravenous valproate in pediatric status epilepticus and acute repetitive seizures. *Epilepsia* 2003; 44:724–726.

104. Giroud M, Dumas R. Treatment of status epilepticus by sodium valproate. *Neurophysiol Clin* 1988; 18:21–32.

105. Jha S, Jose M, Patel R. Intravenous sodium valproate in status epilepticus. *Neurol India* 2003; 51:421–422.

106. Uberall MA, Trollmann R, Wunsiedler U *et al*. Intravenous valproate in pediatric epilepsy patients with refractory status epilepticus. *Neurology* 2000; 54:2188–2189.

107. Misra UK, Kalita J, Patel R. Sodium valproate vs phenytoin in status epilepticus: a pilot study. *Neurology* 2006; 67:340–342.

108. Patel NC, Landan IR, Levin J *et al*. The use of levetiracetam in refractory status epilepticus. *Seizure* 2006; 15:137–141.

109. Rossetti AO, Bromfield EB. Determinants of success in the use of oral levetiracetam in status epilepticus. *Epilepsy Behav* 2006; 8:651–654.

110. Mazarati AM, Baldwin R, Klitgaard H *et al*. Anticonvulsant effects of levetiracetam and levetiracetam–diazepam combinations in experimental status epilepticus. *Epilepsy Res* 2004; 58:167–174.

111. Rossetti AO, Bromfield EB. Levetiracetam in the treatment of status epilepticus in adults: a study of 13 episodes. *Eur Neurol* 2005; 54:34–38.

112. Towne AR, Garnett LK, Waterhouse EJ *et al*. The use of topiramate in refractory status epilepticus. *Neurology* 2003; 60:332–334.

113. Perry MS, Holt PJ, Sladky JT. Topiramate loading for refractory status epilepticus in children. *Epilepsia* 2006; 47:1070–1071.

114. Blumkin L, Lerman-Sagie T, Houri T *et al*. Pediatric refractory partial status epilepticus responsive to topiramate. *J Child Neurol* 2005; 20:239–241.

115. Bensalem MK, Fakhoury TA. Topiramate and status epilepticus: report of three cases. *Epilepsy Behav* 2003; 4:757–760.

116. Kahriman M, Minecan D, Kutluay E *et al*. Efficacy of topiramate in children with refractory status epilepticus. *Epilepsia* 2003; 44:1353–1356.

117. Tarulli A, Drislane FW. The use of topiramate in refractory status epilepticus. *Neurology* 2004; 62:837.

118. Claassen J, Hirsch LJ, Emerson RG *et al*. Treatment of refractory status epilepticus with pentobarbital, propofol, or midazolam: a systematic review. *Epilepsia* 2002; 43:146–153.

119. Holtkamp M, Masuhr F, Harms L *et al*. The management of refractory generalised convulsive and complex partial status epilepticus in three European countries: a survey among epileptologists and critical care neurologists. *J Neurol Neurosurg Psychiatry* 2003; 74:1095–1099.

120. Propofol. *Med Lett Drugs Ther* 1990; 32:22.

121. Kumar MA, Urrutia VC, Thomas CE *et al*. The syndrome of irreversible acidosis after prolonged propofol infusion. *Neurocrit Care* 2005; 3:257–259.

122. Cremer OL, Moons KG, Bouman EA *et al*. Long-term propofol infusion and cardiac failure in adult head-injured patients. *Lancet* 2001; 357:117–118.

123. Alexopoulos A, Lachhwani DK, Gupta A *et al*. Resective surgery to treat refractory status epilepticus in children with focal epileptogenesis. *Neurology* 2005; 64:567–570.

124. Costello DJ, Simon MV, Eskandar EN *et al*. Efficacy of surgical treatment of *de novo* adult-onset cryptogenic refractory focal status epilepticus *Arch Neurol* 2006; 63:895–901.

125. Yen W, Williamson J, Bertram EH *et al*. A comparison of three NMDA receptor antagonists in the treatment of prolonged status epilepticus. *Epilepsy Res* 2004; 59:43–50.

126. Ubogu EE, Sagar SM, Lerner AJ *et al*. Ketamine for refractory status epilepticus: a case of possible ketamine-induced neurotoxicity. *Epilepsy Behav* 2003; 4:70–75.

127. Walker IA, Slovis CM. Lidocaine in the treatment of status epilepticus. *Acad Emerg Med* 1997; 4:918–922.

128. Mirsattari SM, Sharpe MD, Young GB. Treatment of refractory status epilepticus with inhalational anesthetic agents isoflurane and desflurane. *Arch Neurol* 2004; 61:1254–1259.

129. Carrasco Gonzalez MD, Palomar M, Rovira R. Electroconvulsive therapy for status epilepticus. *Ann Intern Med* 1997; 127:247–248.

130. Alldredge BK, Gelb AM, Isaacs SM *et al*. A comparison of lorazepam, diazepam, and placebo for the treatment of out-of-hospital status epilepticus. *N Engl J Med* 2001; 345:631–637.

131. Shneker BF, Fountain NB. Assessment of acute morbidity and mortality in nonconvulsive status epilepticus. *Neurology* 2003; 61:1066–1073.

132. Krumholz A, Sung GY, Fisher RS *et al*. Complex partial status epilepticus accompanied by serious morbidity and mortality. *Neurology* 1995; 45:1499–1504.

133. Young GB, Jordan KG, Doig GS. An assessment of nonconvulsive seizures in the intensive care unit using continuous EEG monitoring: an investigation of variables associated with mortality. *Neurology* 1996; 47:83–89.

134. Meierkord H, Holtkamp M. Non-convulsive status epilepticus in adults: clinical forms and treatment. *Lancet Neurol* 2007; 6:329–339.

135. Schmitt FC, Buchheim K, Meierkord H *et al.* Anticonvulsant properties of hypothermia in experimental status epilepticus. *Neurobiol Dis* 2006; 23:689–696.

136. Liu Z, Gatt A, Mikati M *et al.* Effect of temperature on kainic acid-induced seizures. *Brain Res* 1993; 631:51–58.

137. Maeda T, Hashizume K, Tanaka T. Effect of hypothermia on kainic acid-induced limbic seizures: an electroencephalographic and 14C-deoxyglucose autoradiographic study. *Brain Res* 1999; 818:228–235.

138. Orlowski JP, Erenberg G, Lueders H *et al.* Hypothermia and barbiturate coma for refractory status epilepticus. *Crit Care Med* 1984; 12:367–372.

139. Karkar KM, Garcia PA, Bateman LM *et al.* Focal cooling suppresses spontaneous epileptiform activity without changing the cortical motor threshold. *Epilepsia* 2002; 43:932–935.

140. Olney JW, Labruyere J, Price MT. Pathological changes induced in cerebrocortical neurons by phencyclidine and related drugs. *Science* 1989; 244:1360–1362.

141. Olney JW, Labruyere J, Wang G *et al.* NMDA antagonist neurotoxicity: mechanism and prevention. *Science* 1991; 254:1515–1518.

142. Kudin AP, Debska-Vielhaber G, Vielhaber S *et al.* The mechanism of neuroprotection by topiramate in an animal model of epilepsy. *Epilepsia* 2004; 45:1478–1487.

143. Clifford DB, Olney JW, Benz AM *et al.* Ketamine, phencyclidine, and MK-801 protect against kainic acid-induced seizure-related brain damage. *Epilepsia* 1990; 31:382–390.

144. Fujikawa DG. Neuroprotective effect of ketamine administered after status epilepticus onset. *Epilepsia* 1995; 36:186–195.

145. Brandt C, Potschka H, Loscher W *et al.* N-methyl-D-aspartate receptor blockade after status epilepticus protects against limbic brain damage but not against epilepsy in the kainate model of temporal lobe epilepsy. *Neuroscience* 2003; 118:727–740.

146. Ebert U, Brandt C, Loscher W. Delayed sclerosis, neuroprotection, and limbic epileptogenesis after status epilepticus in the rat. *Epilepsia* 2002; 43(Suppl 5):86–95.

147. Prasad A, Williamson JM, Bertram EH. Phenobarbital and MK-801, but not phenytoin, improve the long-term outcome of status epilepticus. *Ann Neurol* 2002; 51:175–181.

148. Fujikawa DG, Daniels AH, Kim JS. The competitive NMDA receptor antagonist CGP 40116 protects against status epilepticus-induced neuronal damage. *Epilepsy Res* 1994; 17:207–219.

149. Narkilahti S, Nissinen J, Pitkanen A. Administration of caspase 3 inhibitor during and after status epilepticus in rat: effect on neuronal damage and epileptogenesis. *Neuropharmacology* 2003; 44:1068–1088.

150. Cilio MR, Bolanos AR, Liu Z *et al.* Anticonvulsant action and long-term effects of gabapentin in the immature brain. *Neuropharmacology* 2001; 40:139–147.

151. Klitgaard HV, Matagne AC, Vanneste-Goemare J *et al.* Effects of prolonged administration of levetiracetam on pilocarpine-induced epileptogenesis. *Epilepsia* 2001; 42(Suppl 7):114–115.

152. Sutula T, Cavazos J, Golarai G. Alteration of long-lasting structural and functional effects of kainic acid in the hippocampus by brief treatment with phenobarbital. *J Neurosci* 1992; 12:4173–4187.

153. Mikati MA, Holmes GL, Chronopoulos A *et al.* Phenobarbital modifies seizure-related brain injury in the developing brain. *Ann Neurol* 1994; 36:425–433.

154. Bolanos AR, Sarkisian M, Yang Y *et al.* Comparison of valproate and phenobarbital treatment after status epilepticus in rats. *Neurology* 1998; 51:41–48.

155. Brandt C, Gastens AM, Sun MZ *et al.* Treatment with valproate after status epilepticus: effect on neuronal damage, epileptogenesis, and behavioral alterations in rats. *Neuropharmacology* 2006; 51:789–804.

156. Halonen T, Nissinen J, Pitkänen A. Chronic elevation of brain GABA levels beginning two days after status epilepticus does not prevent epileptogenesis in rats. *Neuropharmacology* 2001; 40:536–550.

157. André V, Ferrandon A, Marescaux C *et al.* Vigabatrin protects against hippocampal damage but is not antiepileptogenic in the lithium-pilocarpine model of temporal lobe epilepsy. *Epilepsy Res* 2001; 47:99–117.

158. Rigoulot MA, Koning E, Ferrandon A *et al.* Neuroprotective properties of topiramate in the lithium-pilocarpine model of epilepsy. *J Pharmacol Exp Ther* 2004; 308:787–795.

159. Andre V, Rigoulot MA, Koning E *et al.* Long-term pregabalin treatment protects basal cortices and delays the occurrence of spontaneous seizures in the lithium-pilocarpine model in the rat. *Epilepsia* 2003; 44:893–903.

160. Veliskova J, Velisek L, Galanopoulou AS *et al.* Neuroprotective effects of estrogens on hippocampal cells in adult female rats after status epilepticus. *Epilepsia* 2000; 41(Suppl 6):S30–S35.

161. Reibel S, Andre V, Chassagnon S *et al*. Neuroprotective effects of chronic estradiol benzoate treatment on hippocampal cell loss induced by status epilepticus in the female rat. *Neurosci Lett* 2000; 281:79–82.

162. Rigoulot MA, Leroy C, Koning E *et al*. Prolonged low-dose caffeine exposure protects against hippocampal damage but not against the occurrence of epilepsy in the lithium-pilocarpine model in the rat. *Epilepsia* 2003; 44:529–535.

15

Treatment of common co-morbid psychiatric disorders in epilepsy: a review of practical strategies

Andres M. Kanner, Marlis Frey

INTRODUCTION

Psychiatric co-morbidities are relatively frequent in epilepsy [1]. As shown in Table 15.1, the lifetime prevalence rates of the four major psychiatric disorders (mood, anxiety, attention deficit and psychotic disorders) are significantly higher in patients with epilepsy (PWE) than in the general population.

Unfortunately, despite their relatively high prevalence, a timely recognition and treatment of most psychiatric disorders is the exception rather than the rule in this patient population. Other psychiatric disorders have gone unrecognized completely. Such is the case of attention deficit disorders (ADDs) in adults with epilepsy. Indeed, its prevalence in this age group remains unknown. Considering the relatively high prevalence of ADDs in paediatric patients with epilepsy, it is surprising that no attention has been given to these disorders in adults, given that 50–75% of these children are expected to continue to be symptomatic when they enter adult life.

The relatively high co-morbidity of psychiatric disorders in epilepsy is not the expression of psychiatric disorders being only a complication of the seizure disorder. In fact, it reflects a more complex relation between epilepsy and psychiatric disorders and probably the presence of common pathogenic mechanisms shared by these conditions. In fact, a bidirectional relationship has been demonstrated between depression and ADD on the one hand and epilepsy on the other [2]. Thus, not only are PWE at higher risk of experiencing mood disorders, but data from three population-based control studies indicate that people with a history of depression have a four- to seven-fold higher risk of developing epilepsy [3–5]. In one of these studies, a prior history of suicidality was associated with a five-fold increased risk of developing epilepsy [5]. Likewise, the presence of ADDs without hyperactivity was found to be associated with a 2.5-fold higher risk of developing epilepsy [2].

A timely treatment of co-morbid psychiatric disorders is of the essence as they impact negatively on the quality of life of PWE. Furthermore, mood disorders in PWE significantly increase the healthcare costs associated with the management of the seizure disorder. Cramer *et al.* found that patients with untreated depression used significantly more health resources of all types, independent of seizure type or severity [6]. Mild-to-moderate depression was

Andres M. Kanner, MD, Professor of Neurology, Department of Neurological Sciences, Rush Medical College and Rush Epilepsy Center, Rush University Medical Center, Chicago, Illinois, USA

Marlis Frey, MSN, Rush Epilepsy Center, Rush University Medical Center, Chicago, Illinois, USA

Table 15.1 Prevalence rates of psychiatric disorders in epilepsy and the general population

Psychiatric disorder	Prevalence rates	
	Epilepsy	General population
Depression	11–80%	3.3%: dysthymia
		4.9–17%: major depression
Psychosis	2–9.1%	1%: schizophrenia
		0.2%: schizophreniform disorder
Generalized anxiety disorders	15–25%	5.1–7.2%
Panic disorder	4.9–21%	0.5–3%
Attention deficit hyperactivity disorder	12–37%	3–5%

associated with a two-fold increase in medical visits compared with non-depressed controls, while severe depression was associated with a four-fold increase. The presence and severity of depression was a predictor of lower disability scores, irrespective of the duration of the seizure disorder. In this chapter, we review the most relevant aspects of pharmacotherapy of mood, anxiety, ADDs and psychotic disorders in PWE. The treatment of mood and anxiety disorders will be reviewed together, given their frequent co-morbid occurrence and the use of the same class of psychotropic drugs for their management.

TREATMENT OF MOOD DISORDERS

INTERICTAL DEPRESSIVE EPISODES

Interictal depressive episodes/disorders are the most frequent form of depression and, by the same token, the most frequent psychiatric co-morbidity in PWE, with prevalence rates ranging from 11% to 60% [7]. They may mimic major depression, dysthymic, minor depressive and bipolar disorders described in the *Diagnostic and Statistical Manual of Mental Disorders, Fourth Edition* (DSM-IV). In a significant number of patients, however, depression may present with atypical clinical characteristics. In primary depressive disorders, the difference between major depression and dysthymic disorder is based largely on severity, persistence and chronicity. According to DSM-IV criteria, symptoms in both disorders may include combinations of depressed mood, anhedonia, feelings of worthlessness and guilt, decreased ability to concentrate, recurrent thoughts of death and neurovegetative symptoms (i.e. weight loss or gain, insomnia or hypersomnia, psychomotor agitation or retardation and fatigue). The diagnosis of a major depressive episode requires at least 2 weeks of either a depressed mood or anhedonia accompanied by four or more of the additional symptoms cited above occurring *every day* and lasting *the majority* of the day. In contrast, dysthymic disorder is a more chronic but less intense process, with symptoms present more days than not for at least 2 years. Minor depression is similar to major depression in duration but encompasses at least two but fewer than five of the depressive symptoms noted above.

BIPOLAR DISORDERS

Bipolar disorders refer to the mood disorders consisting of manic and/or hypomanic episodes with and/or without depressive episodes. A manic episode consists of a period of at least 1 week's duration with abnormally and persistently elevated or irritable mood, with at least three (or four if there is only irritable mood) of the following associated symptoms: (i) inflated self esteem or grandiosity; (ii) decreased need for sleep; (iii) more talkative than usual or pressured speech; (iv) flight of ideas or racing thoughts; (v) distractibility; and (vi) excessive involvement in pleasurable activities that have a high potential for painful consequences (e.g. unrestricted buying sprees, sexual indiscretions). The difference between manic and hypomanic episodes is also based on severity. A diagnosis of a hypomanic episode is reached after 4 days of a distinct and persistently elevated expansive or irritable mood associated with at least three of the above listed symptoms.

MAJOR DEPRESSION

A diagnosis of major depressive disorder can be made after a single or multiple major depressive episodes. Establishment of whether the depressive episode is the first to occur is of utmost importance as the risk of subsequent major depressive episodes is of 50% after a single episode, 70% after two episodes and almost 100% after more than two episodes [8]. Ten to 15 years after an index major depressive episode, about 80–90% of patients can be expected to have a recurrence.

Patients with dysthymic and minor depressive disorders will often experience one or recurrent major depressive episodes. This is referred to as 'double depression'. Furthermore, recent studies have highlighted the importance of also recognizing sub-syndromal forms of depression, as these are associated with a risk of developing a major depressive episode [9].

ATYPICAL CLINICAL MANIFESTATIONS OF DEPRESSION IN EPILEPSY

As stated above, PWE may often experience depressive disorders that do not meet any *Diagnostic and Statistical Manual of Mental Disorders* diagnostic criteria or may present symptoms of depression intermittently on what is considered today as a sub-syndromal form of depression. In one study that used *Diagnostic and Statistical Manual of Mental Disorders, Third edition Revised* (DSM-III-R) criteria, 50% of depressive disorders had to be classified as atypical depression [10], while this occurred in 25% of depressive disorders in a separate study that used DSM-IV criteria [11]. In a review of the literature, Blumer and Altshuler concluded that the atypical clinical expressions of depression are relatively frequent in PWE [12]. These episodes are more likely to resemble a dysthymic disorder, with respect to the symptom severity; in these forms of depression, symptoms last for periods ranging between several hours and several days that are interrupted by symptom-free periods of similar duration. We have used the term *dysthymic-like disorder of epilepsy* (DLDE) when referring to them [13]. DLDE may consist of anhedonia with or without feelings of hopelessness and helplessness, fatigue, irritability, poor frustration tolerance, and mood liability with recurrent bouts of crying. Some patients also reported changes in appetite and sleep patterns and problems with concentration. Most symptoms exhibited a waxing and waning course, with repeated interspersed symptom-free periods of one to several days' duration. These dysthymic-like disorders also have a negative impact on these patients' quality of life and often can have intermixed episodes of major depression. In open trials, two-thirds of patients with these episodes have been found to experience a complete symptom remission with the use of anti-depressant drugs of the selective serotonin reuptake inhibitor (SSRI) family [13].

It is important for clinicians to recognize whether the symptoms and/or episodes of depression and anxiety are interictal or peri-ictal. Such distinction is significant since interictal symptoms/episodes respond well to pharmacotherapy, while peri-ictal do not.

IDENTIFYING DEPRESSED PATIENTS IN THE NEUROLOGIST'S OFFICE

Inquiry of anhedonia, that is the inability to find pleasure in most activities, is the simplest way of suspecting the existence of a depressive disorder. Second, the use of self-rating screening instruments can be of great assistance. A six-item screening instrument, the neurological disorders depression inventory for epilepsy (NDDI-E), was recently validated to screen for major depressive episodes in patients with epilepsy [14]. This instrument has the advantage of being constructed specifically to minimize confounding factors that plague other instruments, such as adverse events related to anti-epileptic drugs (AEDs) or cognitive problems associated with epilepsy. Completion of the instrument takes less than 3 min. A score of 14 or higher is suggestive of a major depressive episode and indicates that a more in-depth evaluation is necessary. Other self-rating screening instruments developed to identify symptoms of depression in the general population, such as the Beck Depression Inventory-II and the Center for Epidemiologic Studies Depression Scale, are valid instruments to screen symptoms of depression in patients with epilepsy [15]. It should be emphasized that these instruments are *not diagnostic* of major depressive disorders or other mood disorders; follow-up with an in-depth evaluation is necessary. Once the diagnosis of a mood disorder has been established by psychiatric evaluation, the self-rating screening instruments can be given at every visit to measure changes in symptom severity or document symptom remission.

PHARMACOTHERAPY OF DEPRESSION IN EPILEPSY

Before addressing the specific treatment strategies, it is important to review these basic principles:

(i) Did the symptoms of depression appear following the introduction or increase in the dose of an AED known to cause psychiatric adverse events?

(ii) Did the psychiatric symptoms follow the discontinuation of an AED with mood-stabilizing properties (i.e. carbamazepine, oxcarbazepine, valproic acid and lamotrigine)? In such cases, the psychiatric symptoms may be the expression of recurrence of a latent psychiatric disorder that had been in remission (or masked) by the discontinued AED.

(iii) Did the psychiatric symptoms occur after the introduction of an enzyme-inducing AED (carbamazepine, phenytoin, phenobarbital, primidone, high-dose topiramate or oxcarbazepine) in a patient who was already taking a psychotropic drug for a previously recognized depression or anxiety disorder? In such a case, the symptom recurrence may have resulted from a pharmacokinetic interaction between the AED and the psychotropic drug on board that caused a drop in the psychotropic drug's serum concentration. Accordingly, a readjustment in the dose of the psychotropic drug may be sufficient to induce symptom remission.

(iv) Are the psychiatric symptoms temporally related to the seizure occurrence; that is, do they precede (pre-ictal), follow (post-ictal), both, are they the expression of an ictal event, or do they occur interictally with a peri-ictal exacerbation in severity? In the case of pre- or post-ictal without interictal symptoms, pharmacotherapy may fail to yield any benefit. Post-ictal breakthrough symptoms may occur in patients whose interictal symptoms remitted with pharmacotherapy.

(v) Is there a risk factor, other than epilepsy, for the development of the psychiatric disorder, particularly a family history in a first-degree relative?

(vi) Are the psychiatric symptoms related to the remission of seizures following a period of persistent seizures or are they associated with worsening of the patient's seizure disorder? In the former case, the symptoms may be the expression of the phenomenon known as 'forced normalization' or 'alternative psychopathology'.

Today, anti-depressant drugs of the families of the SSRIs and of the selective norepinephrine reuptake inhibitors (SNRIs) have become the first line of pharmacotherapy for primary major, dysthymic and minor depressive disorders. Fortunately, these drugs

Table 15.2 Efficacy of SSRIs and SNRIs in primary depression and anxiety disorders

Anti-depressant drug	Depression	Panic disorder	Generalized anxiety	Starting dose (mg)	Maximal dose (mg)
Paroxetine*	+	+	+	10	60
Sertraline*	+	+		25	200
Fluoxetine*	+	+		10	80
Citalopram*	+			10	60
Escitalopram*	+	+	+	5	30
Venlafaxine[†]	+	+	+	37.5	300

*Selective serotonin reuptake inhibitor (SSRI); [†]selective norepinephrine reuptake inhibitor (SNRI). The SSRI fluvoxamine and the SNRIs mirtazapine and duloxetine were not included in this table due to the absence of any data in patients with epilepsy.

have also been shown to have a therapeutic effect in the treatment of generalized anxiety and panic disorders, which, as stated above, are very frequent co-morbid conditions of mood disorders. Table 15.2 shows the anti-depressant drugs with anti-depressant and anxiolytic and anti-panic properties.

We must keep in mind, however, that the data available for the management of mood disorders in PWE are derived from open trials, based on the experience obtained in the treatment of primary depression disorders. Indeed, to date there has been only one controlled study published in the literature that compared under blind conditions the efficacy of two anti-depressant drugs (amitriptyline and mianserin) with placebo in major depression of PWE [16].

THERAPEUTIC EXPECTATIONS OF PHARMACOTHERAPY OF DEPRESSIVE DISORDERS

A major depressive episode left untreated may last between 6 and 24 months in 90–95% of cases while the remaining 5–10% could last more than 2 years. Two-thirds of patients are expected to 'respond' to anti-depressant medication and in controlled studies, one-third are expected to respond to placebo. Approximately 15–20% of patients will fail to respond to any anti-depressant trial. It is estimated that approximately 50% of patients will reach remission within the first 6 months and about two-thirds within 2 years of the start of therapy.

The variables predictive of relapse include: (i) multiple prior episodes; (ii) severe episodes; (iii) long-lasting episodes; (iv) episodes with psychotic or bipolar features; and (v) incomplete recovery between two consecutive episodes.

The pharmacological treatment of major depressive episodes can be divided into three phases:

1   An *acute phase*, which lasts between 6 and 12 weeks, in which the goal is to achieve a complete symptom remission.
2   A *continuation phase*, which spans the 12th and 52nd weeks, and which aims to prevent the recurrence of a depressive episode. The anti-depressant medication must be maintained at the same dose.
3   A *maintenance phase*, which aims to maintain the patient in a euthymic state indefinitely. Its duration depends on the number of prior major depressive episodes. As stated above, among patients with primary depression, after a first major depressive episode, the probability of future episodes is about 50%; it increases to 70% after a second episode and is more than 90% after a third episode. The decision to keep the patient on anti-depressant drugs beyond the first 12 months and the duration of a maintenance phase should be decided after consultation with a psychiatrist.

CHOICE OF ANTI-DEPRESSANT DRUG

The choice of anti-depressant has to be based on its potential efficacy for the depressive disorder, its safety and tolerability and lack of pharmacokinetic interactions with AEDs. When evaluating the safety and tolerability of anti-depressant drugs in PWE, clinicians must also consider the pharmacokinetic and pharmacodynamic interactions of the AEDs with the anti-depressant drug.

DO ANTI-DEPRESSANT DRUGS WORSEN SEIZURES?

There is a widespread concern among clinicians that anti-depressant drugs can worsen seizures; such a worry is one of the more frequent causes that has limited the prescription of these drugs in PWE who suffer from a depressive disorder. Yet, a careful review of the literature shows that in the general population, an anti-depressant-related increased risk of epileptic seizures has been limited to four anti-depressant drugs: clomipramine, maprotiline, amoxepine and bupropion, and to tricyclic anti-depressant drugs at high plasma serum concentrations resulting from overdoses or encountered in individuals with a genetic predisposition to be a slow metabolizer.

In animal models of epilepsy, anti-depressant drugs that increase the synaptic concentration of serotonin and epinephrine have been found to have anti-convulsant properties. A recent study appears to confirm a 'protective' effect of SSRIs and SNRIs in depressed patients: Alper et al. compared the incidence of seizures between depressed patients randomized to placebo and SSRIs (citalopram, fluoxetine, fluvoxamine), the SNRI venlafaxine and the α_2-antagonist mirtazapine in the course of regulatory studies submitted to the Food and Drug Administration (FDA) [17]. The seizure frequency among patients randomized to placebo was 1501.5 seizures/100 000 years, while that of patients randomized to the anti-depressants was 534.8 seizures/100 000 years. These data clearly indicate the relatively high occurrence of seizures in depressed patients (relative to that of the general population) but it is significantly higher among patients randomized to placebo. These data raise the question of whether the seizure occurrence in depressed patients is an expression of the increased risk of developing epilepsy associated with a history of depression referred to above.

Anti-depressant drugs of the SSRI family are in general safe when used in PWE. Three open trials with SSRIs have found a decrease in seizure frequency in patients with refractory partial epilepsy and one double-blind placebo-controlled study with tricyclic anti-depressants (TCAs) found a significant reduction in absence seizures [18–20]. Finally, in a study of 100 patients with epilepsy, most of whom had pharmacoresistant epilepsy, sertraline was found to *definitely* worsen seizures in only one patient, while in five patients there was a transient increment in seizure frequency which subsided without any changes in dose [13]. We have used the SNRI venlafaxine in more than 100 PWE without identifying any worsening of seizure type or frequency (unpublished data).

PHARMACOKINETIC INTERACTIONS BETWEEN AEDs AND ANTI-DEPRESSANTS

Impact of AEDs on Anti-depressants

Traditional AEDs such as phenytoin, carbamazepine and phenobarbital are potent inducers of the cytochrome P450 (CYP) enzyme system. Oxcarbazepine and topiramate are much less potent inducers of CYP 3A4. AEDs including gabapentin, pregabalin, levetiracetam, tiagabine and lamotrigine do not appear to interfere with CYP activity. The majority of anti-depressant drugs are substrates for one or more or the CYP isozymes [20]. Therefore, co-medication with an enzyme-inducing AED would be expected to increase the systemic clearance of these medications, the result being lower serum concentrations of the psychotropic agent. Specifically, serum concentrations of TCAs such as amitriptyline, nortriptyline, imipramine, desipramine, clomipramine, protriptyline and doxepin, as well as non-TCA agents such as sertraline, paroxetine, mianserin, citalopram and nefazodone, would be expected to be reduced in patients receiving enzyme-inducing AEDs and may require marked increases in dosage in order to maintain a therapeutic anti-depressant response [21].

In contrast to the enzyme-inducing drugs, the AED sodium valproate can inhibit certain CYP (2C9) and uridine 5'-diphosphate-glucuronyltransferase enzymes, and may cause significant increases (50–60%) in serum concentrations of anti-depressants such as amitriptyline or nortriptyline [21].

Impact of Anti-depressant Drugs on AEDs

SSRIs have been found to inhibit the metabolism of some AEDs. For example, several case reports have suggested that SSRIs such as fluoxetine and sertraline have resulted in increased phenytoin and carbamazepine serum concentrations [21, 22]. Fluoxetine has been shown to inhibit several CYP isozymes including CYP 3A4, CYP 2C9, CYP 2C19, CYP 2D6 and CYP 1A2. The active metabolite of fluoxetine, norfluoxetine, has also been shown to inhibit CYP 2D6. Inhibition of CYP 3A4, CYP 2C9 and CYP 2C19 are of the most relevance when considering potential effects on the currently available AEDs.

In vitro experiments examining phenytoin parahydroxylation using human liver microsomes found that among fluoxetine, norfluoxetine, sertraline and paroxetine, fluoxetine was the most potent inhibitor, followed by norfluoxetine, sertraline and to a lesser extent, paroxetine [23]. However, the likelihood of an interaction occurring is relatively low, particularly with paroxetine and sertraline. Indeed, clinical studies did not find an interaction between either sertraline or paroxetine and carbamazepine or phenytoin [24].

The anti-depressant fluvoxamine is not only an inhibitor of CYP 1A2 and 3A4, but is also a potent inhibitor of CYP 2C9 and 2C19. Comedication, therefore, is likely to cause marked increases in phenytoin concentrations [25].

In settings where higher SSRI doses are used, or perhaps in elderly patients who may have reduced clearance of both phenytoin and the SSRI, the potential for a clinically meaningful interaction may be increased. Nefazodone, a CYP 3A4 inhibitor, has been shown to increase carbamazepine serum concentrations [26]. SSRIs with the least potential for causing inhibitory interactions are citalopram and escitalopram. Although definitive studies are lacking, it has also been suggested that venlafaxine and duloxetine are unlikely to cause significant interactions with currently available AEDs.

Pharmacodynamic Interactions between AEDs and Anti-depressants

From a theoretical standpoint, the following potential synergistic adverse events have to be looked for carefully:

- potentiation of weight gain that can be caused by AEDs such as gabapentin, valproic acid, carbamazepine, pregabalin and anti-depressant drugs such as sertraline and paroxetine; and
- potentiation of sexual adverse events. Sexual adverse events, such as decreased libido, anorgasmia and sexual impotence, can be relatively common with AEDs such as the barbiturates (phenobarbital and primidone), but can also be seen with other enzyme-inducing AEDs. Anti-depressant drugs of the SSRIs, monoamino-oxidase inhibitors (MAOIs) and TCAs, as well as the SNRIs are known to cause sexual adverse events. Whether the combination of this type of AEDs and anti-depressants has a 'synergistic adverse effect' on sexual functions has yet to be established. An additional caveat is the direct impact of the seizure disorder on sexual functions which could, in fact, be the variable responsible for the decreased sexual drive independently of the exposure to the AED (or in combination with it).

Single-case reports of various pharmacodynamic interactions have been published in the literature. For example, Dursun *et al.* reported one case of serotonin syndrome resulting from a combination of fluoxetine and carbamazepine [27]. Likewise, Rosenhagen *et al.* recently reported two patients co-medicated with escitalopram, the S-enantiomer of citralopram, and lamotrigine who developed myoclonus, a potential symptom of serotonin syndrome [28]. These authors speculate that lamotrigine may amplify the risk of developing myoclonus in patients receiving SSRIs. Finally, Gernat *et al.* have reported on the development of extrapyramidal syndrome when using fluoxetine in combination with anti-epileptic drugs, but again these were isolated reports [29].

EFFICACY

Table 15.2 summarizes the drugs of the SSRI and SNRI families that have been found to be effective in the treatment of primary depressive disorders, and the recommended starting and maximal doses. From the stand-point of efficacy, the choice of SSRI or SNRI must depend on whether the patient has only a depressive episode or a mixed depression/anxiety (and/or panic) disorder. Furthermore, the elimination of co-morbid anxiety symptoms with a depressive disorder is as important as that of symptoms of depression, as the former have been associated with an increased suicidal risk [30].

Given comparable efficacy among SSRIs and SNRIs, the lack of pharmacokinetic interactions with AEDs and better tolerance, we recommend the use of escitalopram or citalopram first and sertraline as an alternative. If patients have already undergone a trial with an SSRI at optimal doses, clinicians should consider using an SNRI as the next option. In fact, recent studies have suggested that the use of SNRIs can yield symptom remission in patients in whom an SSRI had failed to do so. The suggested advantage of SNRIs is thought to be based on its dual effect on serotonin and norepinephrine neurotransmitters (and at higher doses, on dopaminergic transmission) in contrast to the effect of SSRIs on serotonin alone. It should be noted, however, that venlafaxine yields a noradrenergic effect at moderately high doses, but not at low doses. Such is not the case of the new SNRI duloxetine hydrochloride, which yields noradrenergic effects at lower doses as well as mirtazapine. However, the safety of the latter two drugs in PWE is yet to be established.

There are also data suggesting that SNRIs may be more effective in patients with physical symptoms (pains and aches), fatigue and psychomotor slowing, which can be relatively common complaints in depressed patients. Since a successful treatment of any depressive disorder is one that yields *complete* symptom remission, eradication of these physical symptoms should be always considered, as residual symptoms are associated with a higher risk of recurrence of major depression.

One cautionary note is in order, however: the therapeutic effect of SSRIs and SNRIs may be identified 3–6 weeks after starting the drug. As SSRIs can, at times, cause restlessness and mild anxiety at the start of therapy, a short course of a benzodiazepine such as clonazepam (0.5–1 mg/day) should be considered in patients with co-morbid anxiety and depression. Also, discontinuation of TCAs, SSRIs and SNRIs has to be carried out gradually through a tapering schedule to avert the development of discontinuation emergent symptoms. These include somatic symptoms such as nausea, vomiting, tremors, diaphoresis, ataxia, movement disorders and sleep disturbances. SSRIs and SNRIs with the shorter half-lives are associated with a higher risk of developing these symptoms.

In patients in need of a prompt anxiolytic and sedative effect, the α_2-antagonist mirtazapine may be a good option. The anti-depressant effect of the drug takes up to 4–6 weeks to become apparent, however. Weight gain is a potential problem with this drug and should be closely monitored.

THE USE OF AEDs IN THE TREATMENT OF MOOD DISORDERS IN PWE

The use of an AED with mood-stabilizing properties (if the patient is not taking one already) such as carbamazepine, oxcarbazepine, valproic acid and lamotrigine, can be an alternative strategy to a continuation of the anti-depressant drugs during the maintenance phase. These AEDs are known to have a prophylactic effect against the recurrence of depressive and manic episodes in primary mood disorders, but in mood disorders of PWE, this prophylactic effect has yet to be established. This point is particularly relevant in the management of atypical depressive disorders.

MOOD DISORDERS THAT SHOULD BE MANAGED BY PSYCHIATRISTS FROM THE ONSET

Given their relatively high prevalence in PWE, neurologists should be able to identify the depressive and bipolar disorders described above. They should know how to *initiate* pharmacotherapy for major, dysthymic and minor depressive episodes. Thus, in which type of depressive disorders can a neurologist start pharmacotherapy and when should patients be referred from the start to the care of a psychiatrist? The following are the mood disorders that deserve immediate referral to a psychiatrist.

Any Depressive Episode Associated with Suicidal Ideation

As mentioned above, PWE have a relatively higher suicidal risk than the general population. In the evaluation of any mood (or other psychiatric) disorder, it is essential to investigate the presence of suicidal ideation (active and passive), as well as of any prior history of suicidal attempts, as these patients are the ones at greatest risk.

Any Major Depressive Disorder with Psychotic Features

Approximately 25% of major depressive disorders can present with psychotic features. In such cases, pharmacotherapy has to include anti-psychotic and anti-depressant drugs and at times, the use of electroshock therapy has to be considered. Furthermore, the presence of psychotic symptomatology increases significantly the suicidal risk of these patients. Thus, these patients need to be placed immediately under the care of a psychiatrist.

Any Major Depressive or Dysthymic Episode that has Failed to Respond to Two Prior Trials with SSRI or SNRI at Optimal Doses

The therapeutic expectation of symptom remission with most anti-depressant drugs is of 50–60% of patients. The remaining patients may require a combination of anti-depressant drugs, or the addition of lithium, thyroid drugs or central nervous system stimulants to one or two anti-depressants or electroconvulsive therapy (ECT) to reach a euthymic state. Clearly, these patients require the care of psychiatrists with expertise in refractory mood disorders.

Any Bipolar Disorder

The management of bipolar disorders is fraught with a significantly lower therapeutic success and potential serious complications that go beyond the expected diagnostic and therapeutic skills of neurologists. Thus, patients with bipolar disorders should be referred for psychiatric evaluation and treatment from the start. In patients with 'apparent' stable bipolar disorders, neurologists should at least refer the patient for *one* psychiatric consultation to confirm that optimal treatment options are being considered, but above all to avert a potential worsening of the course of bipolar disease resulting from the inappropriate use of anti-depressant drugs. Indeed, clinicians must keep in mind that the use of anti-depressant medication in a bipolar disorder can facilitate the development of manic and hypomanic episodes and of a rapid cycling bipolar disorder (defined as the presence of four or more depressive, manic or hypomanic episodes in a 12-month period). The American Psychiatric Association guidelines for the treatment of acute depression in bipolar disease advise against an initial use of anti-depressant drugs [31]. Furthermore, a bipolar disorder can begin with recurrent major depressive episodes before the first manic or hypomanic episode occurs. Accordingly, before starting anti-depressant medication for a major depressive episode, or for a dysthymic or minor depressive disorder, neurologists must always inquire about any history of manic or hypomanic episodes as well as any family history of bipolar disease (which is a strong risk factor for the development of this disorder in the patient at hand). Furthermore, a suspicion of potential bipolar illness increases in patients with a first major depressive episode before the age of 20. Indeed, Strober and Carlson followed for a 3- to 4-year period 60 adolescents hospitalized for major depressive episodes. Twenty per cent of these patients went on to develop bipolar illness [32].

TREATMENT OF BIPOLAR DISORDERS IN PWE

Bipolar disorder is an episodic lifelong disease which may begin with a manic, hypomanic or depressive episode. If the bipolar disorder goes untreated, patients may experience 10 or more episodes in the course of their lifetime. While 4–5 years may elapse between the first two episodes, intervals shorten between subsequent episodes. Bipolar patients constitute about 20% of patients with an affective disorder in non-epilepsy patients; the actual prevalence of bipolar disease in PWE remains unknown, however. A population survey carried out in 181 000 households in which 2900 individuals reported a history of epilepsy, found that symptoms of manic depressive illness were identified in 12.2% of PWE, in contrast to 2% of individuals who described themselves as being healthy [33].

The aims of pharmacotherapy in bipolar disorders are to suppress acute major depressive, hypomanic, manic and mixed manic/depressive episodes and reinstate and maintain a euthymic state. Just as in co-morbid depression in epilepsy, the treatment of bipolar disorder in PWE has to be based on data from studies done in non-epilepsy patients. The management of bipolar disorders is fraught with a significantly lower therapeutic success than (unipolar) major depressive and dysthymic disorders and with potential complications, including a higher suicidal risk, co-morbid drug abuse and the development of psychotic episodes. The pharmacologic treatment includes the use of mood stabilizing agents, such as lithium, valproic acid, carbamazepine and lamotrigine. Obviously, in the case of PWE, AEDs with mood-stabilizing properties should be considered before lithium. Furthermore, anti-depressants should be used with great caution in these patients as they increase significantly a risk of triggering manic and hypomanic episodes. Anti-depressant drugs should not be used without a mood-stabilizing drug. Atypical anti-psychotic drugs are also an alternative for these patients. The use of this type of class is reviewed in the section on treatment of psychosis of epilepsy, below.

Lithium is the first 'mood-stabilizing drug' used for the treatment of patients with bipolar disorders. Its use in epileptic patients with affective disorders, however, has been fraught with several problems, including changes in electroencephalogram (EEG) recordings and pro-convulsant effects at therapeutic serum concentrations in non-epileptic patients. Lithium's neurotoxicity and related increase in seizure risk increases with the concurrent use of neuroleptic drugs, in the presence of EEG abnormalities and of a history of central nervous system disorder [34].

Finally, ECT is not contraindicated in depressed PWE. It is a well-tolerated treatment and is worth considering in PWE with very severe depression that fails to respond to anti-depressant drugs [35].

PHARMACOKINETIC AND PHARMACODYNAMIC INTERACTION BETWEEN LITHIUM AND AEDs

There does not appear to be substantial risk for pharmacokinetic interactions between lithium and AEDs. Prior to the discovery of the mood-stabilizing properties of AEDs, lithium was the mood-stabilizing agent *par excellence*. Today, while many AEDs such as valproic acid, carbamazepine and lamotrigine have replaced the use of lithium in the management of bipolar patients, lithium continues to play an important role, above all, in patients with more refractory bipolar disease. It is not infrequent that patients with refractory bipolar illness may be placed on a combination of lithium and valproic acid or lithium and carbamazepine and lamotrigine.

The combination of lithium and carbamazepine has been documented for a long time to cause a synergistic toxicity caused by each individual drug when given alone. Carbamazepine enhances the development of lithium neurotoxicity syndrome, characterized by symptoms of confusion, drowsiness, lethargy, tremor and cerebellar signs, including ataxia [36]. These symptoms occur in the setting of therapeutic serum levels of lithium and carbamazepine. In addition, one can see a decrease in thyroid function tests with lowering of the total and free T4 serum concentrations. Finally, when carbamazepine and lithium are given together, lithium counteracts the hyponatraemic effect of carbamazepine.

The combination of lithium and valproic acid could, in theory, result in an exacerbation of weight gain, as well as tremor, although this interaction has not been documented in systematic studies. Finally, increasing tremor can also be expected when lithium is added to lamotrigine, as both drugs have this potential adverse event, but few data have been published with respect to this potential pharmacodynamic interaction.

ANXIETY DISORDERS

INTERICTAL ANXIETY DISORDERS

As stated above, anxiety disorders are a common co-morbidity in PWE. Panic disorder (PD) and generalized anxiety disorder (GAD) are the most frequent types of anxiety disorders identified in PWE [1]. The DSM-IV classification of anxiety disorders lists six other types: agoraphobia without panic disorder, obsessive compulsive disorder (OCD), social phobia, specific phobia, post-traumatic stress disorder and acute stress disorder. These may also be identified in PWE, but with a much lower frequency. In addition, PWE may often exhibit symptoms of anxiety that fail to meet any DSM-IV diagnostic criteria for a categorical anxiety disorder.

As stated above, PD and GAD are commonly associated with depressive disorders and their presence conveys an increased suicidal risk. Thus, when the primary complaint is that of an anxiety disorder, clinicians must carefully investigate the presence of depressive symptoms or episodes. GAD consists of constant uncontrollable worry on a daily basis of at least 6 months' duration that is associated with at least three of the following six symptoms: restlessness, easy fatiguability, decreased concentration, irritability, muscle tension and sleep disturbances. Given the frequent confusion between *ictal* and *interictal* panic, the differences between the two will be discussed in greater detail in the next section.

To date, there are no screening instruments specifically developed to identify anxiety disorders in PWE. The available screening instruments developed for patients with primary anxiety disorders must be used with caution as they have several items of vegetative symptoms that can easily yield false positive findings and which in reality may be the expression of the seizure disorder or toxicity of the AED.

ICTAL AND PERI-ICTAL SYMPTOMS

Ictal fear or panic is the most frequent ictal psychiatric symptom [37]. It is the sole or predominant clinical expression of a simple partial seizure (aura) or the initial symptom(s) of a complex partial seizure that usually has a mesial temporal lobe origin. Its prevalence has been estimated to harbour around 60% of auras presenting with 'psychiatric' symptoms and 3% of all auras. Frequently, patients fail to recognize and report associated symptoms indicative of an ictal event such as transient confusion or subtle automatisms, which often results in its misdiagnosis and treatment as a PD, and the correct diagnosis is only reached after the patient suffers from a generalized tonic–clonic seizure.

A careful history can help distinguish a PD occurring interictally from ictal panic. Ictal panic is typically brief (less than 30 s in duration), is stereotypical, occurs out of context to concurrent events, and is associated with other ictal phenomena such as periods of confusion of variable duration and subtle or overt automatisms. The intensity of the sensation of fear is mild to moderate and rarely reaches the intensity of a panic attack. On the other hand, interictal panic attacks consist of episodes of 5–20 minutes' duration, which at times may persist for several hours during which the feeling of fear or panic is very intense ('feeling of impending doom') and associated with a variety of autonomic symptoms, including tachycardia, diffuse diaphoresis and shortness of breath. Patients may become completely absorbed by the panic experience to the point where they may not be able to report what is going on around them; however, there is no confusion or loss of consciousness as in complex partial seizures. It is not infrequent for patients to become extremely apprehensive about experiencing another panic attack that may then lead to the development of a full-blown agoraphobia.

The misdiagnosis of ictal fear as a panic disorder may be compounded by the failure to identify an electrographic ictal pattern in simple partial seizures of mesial–temporal origin, above all when the seizure focus is in the amygdala. In such cases, EEG recordings with sphenoidal electrodes placed under fluoroscopic guidance may be necessary to demonstrate the epileptiform activity [38]. Patients with ictal panic may also suffer from interictal panic attacks, which have been identified in up to 25% of PWE.

PHARMACOTHERAPY OF ANXIETY DISORDERS IN PWE

Whether or not the anxiety disorders' response to pharmacotherapy differs between patients with and without epilepsy is yet to be established. To date, the pharmacological treatment of anxiety disorders in PWE is based on the same principles followed in the management of primary anxiety disorders and thus remains empirical. Pharmacological treatment of anxiety disorders depends on the specific type of disorder. Four classes of drugs are typically used: (i) anti-depressant drugs; (ii) benzodiazepines; (iii) AEDs; and (iv) buspirone. In the next section, we will discuss the use of these drugs in the treatment of GAD, PD, social phobia and OCD.

Anti-depressant Drugs

As shown in Table 15.2, several of the SSRIs have shown efficacy in GAD and PD; all SSRIs have also shown efficacy in OCD, but in contrast to the treatment of GAD and PD, a therapeutic effect may not be noticed for 6–12 weeks. However, a cautionary note is in order: patients with PD may be extremely sensitive to adverse events of psychotropic drugs. Accordingly, a lower initial dose should be considered and a slower titration followed than those in the treatment of mood disorders. In the case of GAD and PD, absence of desired therapeutic effect with an SSRI should be followed by a trial with the SNRI venlafaxine or duloxetine. As in the case of mood disorders, the anxiolytic effect of these drugs may not be apparent until the first 4–6 weeks after the start of therapy, for which a temporary use of a benzodiazepine is often an option.

Among the older anti-depressant drugs, the TCA imipramine is the agent of choice in PD with a comparable efficacy to that of SSRIs and has also been found to be as effective as benzodiazepines in the treatment of GAD. MAOIs are also effective in the treatment of PD.

In patients with a GAD or social phobia and a co-morbid or family risk of bipolar disorder, trials with AEDs with anxiolytic properties such as pregabalin and gabapentin should be considered first.

Benzodiazepines

Their efficacy has been demonstrated in GAD and PD and anxiety secondary to life stressors or medical conditions. The risk of physical dependence and subsequent development of tolerance has limited their use to short-term trials. Typically, they are used in GAD and PD at the start of pharmacotherapy with anti-depressants until the latter agents' therapeutic effect takes over. Alprazolam is the benzodiazepine preferred for PD, while clonazepam is used in GAD.

AEDs

In addition to benzodiazepines, tiagabine, gabapentin, pregabalin and valproic acid have been used by psychiatrists in the treatment of anxiety disorders [39–42]. Tiagabine and pregabalin have been found to be effective in the treatment of GAD and gabapentin in social phobia in double-blind placebo-controlled studies. In PWE who suffer from seizures of frontal lobe origin, tiagabine should be used with caution as it can cause absence stupor. Valproic acid, on the other hand, has been found to cause symptom remission in PD in a small study of 13 patients whose panic attacks failed to respond to anti-depressant agents. These findings need to be confirmed in double-blind controlled studies [42].

Other Drugs

Buspirone is a 5-HT$_{1A}$ agonist agent that has been found to be effective for the treatment of GAD [43]. It is favoured over the use of benzodiazepines because it does not cause drug dependence or withdrawal with long-term use and it lacks any significant pharmacokinetic interactions with other agents. Its onset of efficacy is delayed by several weeks, like that of anti-depressant drugs.

ANXIETY DISORDERS TO BE REFERRED TO PSYCHIATRISTS FROM THE START

- Patients with panic and generalized anxiety disorders who failed to respond to a trial with SSRI or SNRIs (see below).
- Any patient with obsessive compulsive disorders, social phobia and chronic phobias, including agoraphobia with or without panic disorder.

WHEN SHOULD PATIENTS BE REFERRED TO A PSYCHOLOGIST FOR PSYCHOTHERAPY?

Often, mood and anxiety disorders may benefit from a combination of pharmacotherapy and psychotherapy. Anti-depressants can be prescribed by the neurologist while neuropsychologists or clinical psychologists can provide the psychotherapy. In fact, there are several studies that have established the efficacy of cognitive behaviour therapy (CBT) for the management of depressive and anxiety disorders, either by themselves or in combination with pharmacotherapy. In general, CBT comprises short-term treatments of 16 to 20 sessions given over 12 weeks on average [44]. They should only be administered by healthcare professionals who have been trained specifically in this technique.

CBT is often an essential concomitant treatment with pharmacotherapy in the management of panic disorder associated with agoraphobia, and may be sufficient on its own to treat specific phobias, social phobias and compulsions in patients with OCD.

ATTENTION DEFICIT DISORDERS

Attention deficit hyperactivity disorder (ADHD) is a clinically complex, heterogeneous psychiatric disorder diagnosed in childhood with approximately 50% of those patients continuing to exhibit symptoms throughout adult life.

Attention deficit disorders and behavioural disturbances are significantly more common among PWE than in the general population (see Table 15.1). In children, the prevalence rates of inattention, hyperactivity or impulsivity may be affected by severity of epilepsy, with increasing rates seen in children with severe epilepsy [45]. Additionally, disruptive behaviour disorder has been reported in 21% of children with complex partial seizures, 23% of children with generalized seizure disorder and 7% of childhood controls [46].

Prevalence rates may also be affected by type of epilepsy. Generalized epilepsies have been associated with impairment of sustained attention, while non-dominant hemispheric foci are also thought to have an affect on attention. Thirty-three per cent of children with complex partial seizures are reported to have ADHD symptoms, while 37.7% are reported to have predominantly inattentive type, and 29.1% have inattentive type in combined child and adolescent samples [47]. The challenge with evaluating these studies is in combining the various measures which have been used to determine the criteria for presence and severity of ADHD.

No information on ADHD and epilepsy in adults can be found.

ADHD IN CHILDREN

Criteria for the diagnosis of ADHD in children have been established in the *Diagnostic and Statistical Manual of Mental Disorders, Fourth Edition Revised* (DSM-IV-R) with three subtypes: ADHD predominantly inattentive type, ADHD predominantly hyperactive–impulsive type and ADHD combined type.

It has been well established that a majority of children diagnosed with ADHD will continue to exhibit symptoms through adolescence into adulthood. Adolescents with epilepsy face numerous challenges which may be magnified in the presence of attentional issues. Academic issues, potential for anti-social personality disorder, substance use disorder and mood disorder have been found to become salient features for this age group. We have found it easier to elicit sensitive information when interviewing adolescents and parents separately and providing confidentiality when appropriate. In addition, obtaining a comprehensive neuropsychological evaluation by a qualified paediatric neuropsychologist will provide much-needed information on academic issues and social developmental issues. It is most helpful if, in addition to providing an evaluation, the neuropsychologist can function as an advocate/liaison for the patient in implementing appropriate modifications for academic settings.

ADHD IN ADULTS

The DSM-IV-R criteria for adult diagnosis of ADHD contain three critical elements: childhood onset, presence of significant symptoms and impairment from these symptoms in at least two domains of school/work, social interaction or home life. Further evaluation of an initial presentation with a co-morbid condition may lead to an eventual diagnosis of

ADHD. Presenting symptoms and history may need to be corroborated with third parties. Psychiatric disorders most commonly associated with ADHD in adults are anxiety, substance abuse, bipolar disorder or major depressive disorder. Lower educational and occupational achievement has been reported.

PHARMACOLOGICAL INTERVENTIONS

As in the case of mood and anxiety disorders, the pharmacological treatment of ADD in PWE remains empirical and is based on the same strategies followed in the management in primary ADD. The pharmacological agents include central nervous system (CNS) stimulants, anti-depressants, alpha-adrenergic agonists and anti-psychotic drugs.

CNS Stimulants

These are the first choice for therapy of ADHD. Methylphenidate and amphetamine compounds remain the most commonly used stimulants. Their safety and efficacy have been well established and they work in a dose-dependent manner. Their effectiveness in controlling symptoms has varied according to different trials from as high as 68–80% in children to 30–50% in children and adults (28% to ~70% in adolescents).

Our preference is to start with methylphenidate in its immediate-release formulation to establish the desired target dose and then convert to one of the extended-release formulations. Methylphenidate has a low bioavailability (20–25%), which may account for occasional erratic responses. If a trial with methylphenidate is not effective, a switch to dextroamphetamine (Dexedrine®, Adderal®) can be considered. These drugs have a high bioavailability (75%) and redundant hepatic metabolism, but no known pharmacokinetic interactions have been identified with AEDs.

There has been a widespread misperception among clinicians that CNS stimulant drugs can lower the seizure threshold. Several studies have shown methylphenidate to be safe and effective without lowering the seizure threshold in children with epilepsy [48–50].

Because of recent deaths associated with the treatment of stimulant therapy, the Pediatric Advisory Committee of the Food and Drug Administration is reviewing approved ADHD medications for possible cardiac adverse effects. A black box warning has not been recommended at this time. However, we have decided to obtain electrocardiograms, with clearance by a cardiologist if necessary, in our patients prior to starting stimulant pharmacotherapy.

Whether to choose a short-acting or an extended-release formulation depends on the severity of the ADD and the needs of the patient. A short-acting formulation may be sufficient in patients with milder forms of ADD, particularly in adults, and their use can be targeted to specific activities. The advantage of an extended-release formulation is its extended coverage for up to 8 h. In paediatric patients, it may eliminate an often stigmatizing trip to the school nurse during the school day.

We follow the general recommendations of starting on a lower dose and titrate weekly to an effective dose without side-effects. Methylphenidate transdermal, currently under review by the FDA, has been shown to be well tolerated with continuous medication release throughout the day. Studies have shown that children treated with stimulants have a lower risk of substance abuse disorder in later life.

The most frequent adverse events of CNS stimulants include decreased appetite, insomnia, abdominal pain, dry mouth, headaches and nervousness. Approximately 10% of children with ADD may not be able to tolerate these drugs as they become more irritable and mood labile from the initial doses, hence the trial must be discontinued at once in these cases.

Noradrenergic Drug – Atomoxetine

In the absence of a therapeutic response with these CNS stimulants, a trial with atomoxetine, a norepinephrine-reuptake inhibitor and non-stimulant agent, should be considered. This drug has been shown to be effective in the treatment of ADD in both adults and children [51, 52]. Its safety in PWE has not been established, as it is a relatively new agent; however, in our experience with using this agent in patients with refractory epilepsy, no worsening of seizure frequency was established. Furthermore, no increased risk of seizures was reported in the regulatory trials. Seizures have been reported only in the presence of overdoses, however. Doses of atomoxetine should be reduced in the presence of agents inhibiting cytochrome P450 microsomal enzyme system, such as valproic acid.

The most frequent adverse events included dry mouth, insomnia, decreased appetite, decreased libido, erectile dysfunction and dizziness. This drug can cause an increase in the systolic and diastolic blood pressure measurements of 1–3 mmHg and an increase in heart rate of 5 beats/min. Reported cases of hepatotoxicity, resolved with discontinuation of the medication, have led to the addition of a bolded warning to the label. A cautionary note is in order, however: as an adrenergic drug, it can facilitate the development of manic and hypomanic episodes in patients with ADD and co-morbid bipolar disorders.

Anti-depressants

Alternative pharmacological options include the use of anti-depressants. The TCAs are effective in children with ADHD and may be particularly useful in those children with co-morbid ADHD and anxiety disorders. The TCAs used in ADHD have included imipramine, desipramine, and nortriptyline. Clinicians must be on the look-out for cardiac conduction disturbances and a baseline ECG should be done and repeated when patients achieve the target dose. Most children treated with TCAs will have an increase in heart rate. Pulse, blood pressure, ECG, and anti-depressant serum levels should be monitored with a goal of keeping the resting heart rate below 130 beats/min, the PR interval less than 200 ms, and the QRS interval less than 120 ms. Although reportedly effective and well tolerated, bupropion is less appropriate due to its documented potential to lower the seizure threshold. SSRIs have also been used in children with aggressive behaviour.

Other Drugs

Other agents used for the treatment of ADHD include the alpha-adrenergic agonists, clonidine and guanfacine, and the anti-psychotic agents; however, these drugs yield a lower therapeutic effect than CNS stimulants. While clonidine and guanfacine may help reduce hyperactivity, they are less effective in improving attention span. The side-effects of these drugs include sedation. Anti-psychotic drugs can be an alternative therapy for severely hyperactive and impulsive children with ADHD, as well as to manage aggressive behaviour.

Psychotherapies

A cognitive–behavioural approach has been shown to be more beneficial than medication alone in patients with verbal IQ scores of 90 or more and without significant psychopathology. The American Academy of Pediatrics' guidelines are recommending stimulant and/or behaviour techniques to meet target behavioural goals for children with ADHD. This combined approach seems especially appropriate for children with attentional problems and epilepsy since family dysfunction has been reported to be associated with ADHD in children. Collaboration between parents, teachers and physicians in setting target goals for behaviour is essential.

PSYCHOTIC DISORDERS

Psychotic disorders are the less frequent psychiatric co-morbidities in PWE, but their prevalence rates are still significantly higher than those of the general population (see Table 15.1). Psychosis of epilepsy (POE) can present as interictal psychosis of epilepsy, peri-ictal, of which post-ictal psychosis is the most frequently recognized, and the psychotic episodes as an expression of the phenomenon of 'forced normalization'.

Interictal psychosis of epilepsy can be indistinguishable from schizophreniform disorders identified in patients without epilepsy and may present with delusions, hallucinations, referential thinking and thought disorders. However, in a significant proportion of PWE, interictal psychosis differs from that of patients with primary schizophreniform disorders. Slater coined the term of interictal psychosis of epilepsy (IPOE) to describe certain clinical characteristics of these psychotic episodes, which consist of an *absence* of negative symptoms, better pre-morbid history, and less common deterioration of the patient's personality [53]. The psychosis is less severe and more responsive to therapy.

POST-ICTAL PSYCHOSIS

Post-ictal psychotic phenomena can present in the form of isolated symptoms or as a cluster of symptoms mimicking psychotic disorders. Post-ictal psychosis (PIP) corresponds to approximately 25% of POE. The prevalence of post-ictal psychiatric disorders in the general population of patients with epilepsy is yet to be established, but has been estimated to range between 6% and 10% [54]. In a study published in 1996, we estimated the yearly incidence of post-ictal psychiatric disorders among patients with partial epilepsy who are undergoing video-EEG to be 7.9% [55]. The majority, or 6.4%, presented as PIP. Common findings among the different case series of PIP include: (i) a symptom-free period of several hours to several days between the onset of psychiatric symptoms and the time of the last seizure; (ii) a relatively short duration, ranging from several hours to a few days, though occasionally can extend to several weeks; (iii) an effect-laden symptomatology; (iv) the clustering of symptoms into delusional and affective-like psychosis; (v) an increase in the frequency of secondarily generalized tonic–clonic seizures preceding the onset of PIP; (vi) the onset of PIP after having seizures for a mean period of more than 10 years; and (vii) a prompt response to low-dose neuroleptic medication or benzodiazepines.

ALTERNATE PSYCHOSIS OR 'FORCED NORMALIZATION'

The concept of alternate psychosis was developed from observations in 1953 by Landoldt, of an inverse relationship between seizure control and psychotic symptom occurrence, in which he observed a 'normalization' of EEG recordings with the appearance of psychiatric symptoms and coined the term 'forced normalization' [56]. This antagonism between psychosis and epilepsy has been considered by some as the explanation for the therapeutic effect of ECT of psychotic disorders. Forced normalization has been reported in patients with temporal lobe epilepsy and generalized epilepsies; this phenomenon is relatively rare.

Forced normalization presents as a pleomorphic clinical disorder with a paranoid psychosis without clouding of consciousness being the most frequent manifestation. As with other POEs, a richness of affective symptoms has been identified.

The phenomenon of forced normalization has been observed following the use of various AEDs, including phenyl-acetylurea, phenytoin and primidone, valproate and carbamazepine and, more recently, vigabatrin and levetiracetam. In these cases, however, the psychotic disorder was thought to result from the suppression of seizures rather than reflecting an adverse event of the AED. An iatrogenic effect of the AED has to be considered in the differential diagnosis of these patients, however.

TREATMENT OF PSYCHOSIS OF EPILEPSY

Clearly, the primary treatment modality of psychotic symptoms and episodes in PWE is based on pharmacotherapy with anti-psychotic drugs (APDs) and in refractory cases, electroshock therapy.

ANTI-PSYCHOTIC DRUG USE IN EPILEPSY

APDs can be separated into two classes: the 'conventional' APD (CAPD) and 'atypical' APD (AAPD). The mechanism of action of CAPDs resides in their ability to block dopamine (DA_2) receptors, at the level of meso-cortical, nigrostriatal and tubero-infundibular DA pathways [57]. Blockade of the DA receptors at the former pathways is responsible for their anti-psychotic effect, but also results in 'emotional blunting' and cognitive symptoms that often lead to confusion with the 'negative' symptoms of schizophrenia. Blockade at the nigrostriatal pathways results in acute and chronic movement disorders, presenting as parkinsonian symptoms, as well as dystonic and dyskinetic movements, while blockade at the tubero-infundibular pathways results in increased secretion of prolactin. In addition to their DA blockade properties, most of these CAPDs have muscarinic anti-cholinergic, alpha-1 and histaminic blocking properties, responsible for anti-cholinergic adverse effects, weight gain, sedation, dizziness and orthostatic hypotension.

AAPDs are dopamine–serotonin antagonists that target DA_2 and $5-HT_{2A}$ receptors [57]. Their main difference compared with CAPD is the absence or mild occurrence of extrapyramidal adverse events and of hyperprolactinaemia. In addition, this class of drugs has a lesser blunting of effect and several of these AAPDs have mood-stabilizing properties. Hence, AAPDs have, in large part, replaced CAPDs. Today, six AAPDs have been introduced in the USA: clozapine (Clozaril®), risperidone (Risperidal®), olanzapine (Zyprexa®), ziprasidone (Geodon®), quetiapine (Seroquel®) and aripiprazole (Abilify®).

The efficacy of the different AAPDs has been found to be comparable in various head-to-head studies in primary psychotic disorders. Hence, the choice of AAPD must be based on the tolerability profile of the drug. The use of all AAPDs has been associated with an increased risk of hyperglycaemia and type II diabetes mellitus (DM), but the risk is greater with clozapine, olanzapine and quietapine. Risperidone carries an intermediate risk and aripiprazole and ziprasidone have the lowest risk. In addition, these drugs have an increased risk of weight gain, including obesity, which in turn increases the risk of type II DM and dyslipidaemias. Patients with a risk factor of DM (i.e. family history of DM) are at greatest risk of developing these complications. Thus, prior to the start of an AAPD, clinicians must establish: (i) personal or family history of obesity, DM, dyslipidaemias, high blood pressure and heart disease; (ii) weight and height (body mass index > 25); (iii) waist circumference (> 40" in men and 35" in women); (iv) blood pressure (> 130/85); (v) fasting blood glucose (> 110 mg/dl); (vi) fasting cholesterol (> 200 mg/dl) and high-density lipoprotein (< 40 mg/dl); and (vii) fasting triglycerides (> 175 mg/dl). These variables need to be monitored every 3 months in the absence of risk factors or as often as once a month in the case of weight gain of more than 5% or a body mass index > 30.

With the exception of aripiprazole, all AAPDs are sedating, with olanzapine and quietapine being the most sedating of all drugs. There has been a question of whether aripiprazole can cause akathisia, but this has yet to be confirmed.

Is the Use of Anti-psychotic Drugs Safe in PWE?

The pro-convulsant properties of CAPDs have been recognized for a long time and range between 0.5% and 1.2% among non-epileptic patients. The risk is higher with certain drugs and in the presence of the following factors: (i) a history of epilepsy; (ii) abnormal EEG recordings; (iii) history of CNS disorder; (iv) rapid titration of the CAPD dose; (v) high doses of CAPD; and (vi) the presence of other drugs that lower the seizure threshold. For example, when chlorpromazine is used at doses above 1000 mg/day, the incidence of seizures was reported to increase to 9%, in contrast to a 0.5% incidence when lower doses are taken [58]. Haloperidol, molindone, fluphenazine, perfenazine and trifluoperazine are among the CAPDs with a lower seizure risk [59].

With the exception of clozapine, AAPD-related seizure incidence has not been higher than expected in the general population. This finding was confirmed by Alper *et al.* in a study comparing the incidence of seizures of psychotic patients without epilepsy randomized to either placebo or one of the AAPDs (risperidone, olanzapine, quetiapine and aripiprazole) in regulatory studies submitted to the FDA [17]. Thus, during pre-marketing studies of non-epilepsy patients taking AAPD, seizures were reported in 0.3% of patients given risperidone, 0.9% given olanzapine, 0.8% given quietapine (vs. 0.5% on placebo) and 0.4% of patients treated with ziprasidone (data in Physicians' Desk Reference®). In contrast, clozapine has been reported to cause seizures in 4.4% when used at doses above 600 mg/day, while at doses lower than 300 mg/day, the incidence of seizures is less than 1% in non-epilepsy patients.

Unfortunately, the impact of AAPD on seizure occurrence among PWE has not been properly studied with the exception of clozapine. In sixteen patients who had epilepsy before the start of this AAPD, all experienced worsening of seizures while on the drug; eight patients at doses lower than 300 mg/day; three patients at doses between 300 mg/day and 600 mg/day and five at doses higher than 600 mg/day. It goes without saying that this AAPD should be avoided or used with extreme caution in exceptional circumstances in patients with epilepsy.

Clozapine followed by chlorpromazine and loxepine are the three APDs with the highest risk of seizure occurrence. Those with a lower seizure risk include haloperidol, molindone fluphenzine, perfenazine and trifluoperazine and risperidone, among the AAPDs. No data are available on olanzapine and quetiapine and ziprasidone. Whether the presence of AEDs at adequate levels protects patients with epilepsy from breakthrough seizures upon the introduction of APD with pro-convulsant properties, is yet to be established.

Most APDs can cause EEG changes consisting of, above all, slowing of the background activity when used at high doses. In addition, some of these drugs, and particularly clozapine, can cause paroxysmal electrographic changes in the form of interictal sharp waves and spikes. This type of epileptiform activity, however, is not predictive of seizure occurrence. There are data suggesting that a severe disorganization of the EEG recordings is a more likely predictor of seizure occurrence. As a rule, any APD should be started at low doses and should undergo slow dose increments to minimize the risk of seizures in PWE.

In addition to the proconvulsant properties of APD, clinicians must also consider the pharmacokinetic and pharmacodynamic interactions between these drugs and AEDs (see below).

PHARMACOKINETIC AND PHARMACODYNAMIC INTERACTIONS BETWEEN APDs AND AEDs

PHARMACOKINETIC INTERACTIONS

Given that the CYP 450 isozymes play a significant role in the metabolism of the anti-psychotic medications, the effects of AED co-medication upon these drugs is similar to that described for the anti-depressant medications. Enzyme-inducing AEDs, such as carbamazepine and phenytoin, have been reported to increase the clearance, and consequently lower the serum concentration of a number of typical as well as atypical anti-psychotic medications including haloperidol, chlorpromazine, clozapine, risperidone, ziprazidone and olanzapine [56]. Reductions in anti-psychotic concentration may be quite marked. For example, co-medication with carbamazepine has been shown to decrease haloperidol concentrations by 50–60% [22]. This may potentially result in recurrence of psychotic symptoms previously controlled at higher serum concentrations of APDs. By the same token, discontinuation of an AED with enzyme-inducing properties may result in a decrease in the clearance of APD, which in turn can lead to extrapyramidal adverse events caused by an increase in their serum concentrations of CAPDs.

In contrast to the enzyme-inducing AEDs, valproate appears to have minimal pharmacokinetic interactions with these drugs. Several studies have suggested that valproate has only minimal effects on serum concentrations of either haloperidol or risperidone. Valproate has been reported to have modest, variable effects on clozapine concentrations. Also, modest increases were seen in haloperidol concentrations in patients co-medicated with topiramate. AEDs that neither substantially induce nor inhibit the CYP isozyme system are unlikely to result in significant pharmacokinetic interactions with anti-psychotic drugs.

Anti-psychotic drugs are less likely to cause pharmacokinetic changes in AEDs. Yet, among the typical anti-psychotic drugs, both chlorpromazine and thioridazine have been reported to result in increases in phenytoin serum concentrations. With regard to atypical anti-psychotics, risperidone has been noted to result in modest decreases in carbamazepine concentrations [22]. Finally, no significant interaction was noted between olanzapine and lamotrigine.

PHARMACODYNAMIC INTERACTIONS

There are few data on the pharmacodynamic interactions between anti-psychotic and anti-epileptic drugs. From a theoretical standpoint, however, the potential for worsening of adverse events caused by both types of drugs, such as increased weight gain and sexual dysfunction, are to be considered, with increased weight gain being a common and significant adverse event for patients taking AAPDs such as quietapine, risperidone, olanzapine and ziprasidone when given in combination with AEDs that are known to also cause weight gain, such as gabapentin, pregabalin, carbamazepine and valproic acid.

By the same token, exacerbation of sexual dysfunction that can be a common adverse event of the older anti-psychotic drugs, such as those in the family of the phenothiazines can be, in theory, accentuated by the use of enzyme-inducing anti-epileptic drugs. The combination of clozapine and carbamazepine has also been known to enhance the neutropenic effect of each drug, and hence should be avoided.

TREATMENT OF PIP

The prompt recognition of PIP *by neurologists* has major diagnostic and therapeutic implications. First, neurologists can avert the recurrence of PIP by introducing low-dose neuroleptic medication at the first sign of PIP. In most cases, insomnia is the initial presenting symptom. In patients with recurrent PIP, families need to be educated in the recognition of these symptoms so that a timely administration of 1–2 mg of risperidone may avert the start of PIP. In these patients there may be no need to wait for the occurrence of insomnia before administering the drug. Low-dose risperidone can be given for 2 to 5 days and then discontinued [60].

Patients who experience a *de novo* cluster of secondarily generalized tonic–clonic seizures in the course of a video-EEG monitoring study, who are found to have bilateral independent ictal foci and who have a past psychiatric history of depression should be carefully watched for the development of PIP. Patients, family members and nursing staff should be on the look-out for insomnia or a mild thought disorder between 12 and 72 h after the last seizure. If these symptoms were to be identified, low-dose risperidone can be administered as outlined above.

TREATMENT OF PSYCHOTIC EPISODES AS AN EXPRESSION OF FORCED NORMALIZATION

In their review of this topic, Reid and Mothersill concluded that the treatment of alternative psychotic episodes (forced normalization) involves the reduction and/or discontinuation of AED, until overt seizure recurrence causes remission of psychotic symptoms. The rapidity with which AED should be tapered is not clear. Following seizure recurrence and remission of psychotic symptoms, AEDs should be re-introduced slowly [61].

CONCLUDING REMARKS

Psychiatric co-morbidities are relatively frequent in PWE and are associated with a very negative impact on their quality of life. Their timely recognition and treatment is of the essence. The concern that the use of psychotropic drugs can worsen seizures is, more often than not, unfounded or exaggerated. The few psychotropic drugs with well-demonstrated pro-convulsant properties (amoxepine, maprotiline, chlomipramine, bupropion among the anti-depressant drugs, and clozapine among the anti-psychotic drugs) should be avoided in PWE. In drugs such as CAPDs and AAPDs, a low initial dose followed by a slow titration can minimize the occurrence of seizures.

REFERENCES

1. Tellez-Zenteno JF, Patten SB, Jetté N *et al*. Psychiatric comorbidity in epilepsy: a population-based analysis. *Epilepsia* 2007 (online early articles). doi:10.1111/j.1528-1167.2007.
2. Hesdorffer DC, Ludvigsson P, Olafsson E *et al*. ADHD as a risk factor for incident unprovoked seizures and epilepsy in children. *Arch Gen Psychiatry* 2004;61:731–736.
3. Forsgren L, Nystrom L. An incident case referent study of epileptic seizures in adults. *Epilepsy Res* 1999; 6:66–81.
4. Hesdorffer DC, Hauser WA, Annegers JF *et al*. Major depression is a risk factor for seizures in older adults. *Ann Neurol* 2000; 47:246–249.
5. Hesdorffer DC, Hauser WA, Olafsson E *et al*. Depression and suicidal attempt as risk factor for incidental unprovoked seizures. *Ann Neurol* 2006; 59:35–41.
6. Cramer JA, Blum D, Fanning K *et al*; Epilepsy Impact Project Group. The impact of comorbid depression on health resource utilization in a community sample of people with epilepsy. *Epilepsy Behav* 2004; 5:337–342.
7. Kanner AM. Depression in epilepsy: prevalence, clinical semiology, pathogenic mechanisms and treatment. *Biol Psychiatry* 2003; 54:388–398.
8. Stahl SM. Depression and bipolar disorders. In: Stahl SM (ed.) *Essential Pharmacology: Neuroscientific Basis and Practical Applications*. 2nd edn. New York: Cambridge University Press, 2000, pp. 135–197.
9. Paykel ES, Ramana R, Cooper Z *et al*. Residual symptoms after partial remission; an important outcome in depression. *Psychol Med* 1995; 25:1171–1180.
10. Mendez MF, Cummings J, Benson D *et al*. Depression in epilepsy. Significance and phenomenology. *Arch Neurol* 1986; 43:766–770.
11. Wiegartz P, Seidenberg M, Woodard A *et al*. Co-morbid psychiatric disorder in chronic epilepsy: recognition and etiology of depression. *Neurology* 1999; 53(Suppl 2):S3–S8.
12. Blumer D, Altshuler LL. Affective disorders. In: Engel J, Pedley TA (eds) *Epilepsy: A Comprehensive Textbook, vol. II*, Philadelphia: Lippincott-Raven, 1998, pp. 2083–2099.
13. Kanner, AM, Kozak AM, Frey M. The use of sertraline in patients with epilepsy: Is it safe? *Epilepsy Behav* 2000; 1:100–105.
14. Gilliam FG, Barry JJ, Meador KJ *et al*. Rapid detection of major depression in epilepsy: a multicenter study. *Lancet Neurology* 2006; 5:399–405.
15. Jones JE, Herman BP, Woodard JL *et al*. Screening for major depression in epilepsy with common self-report depression inventories. *Epilepsia* 2005; 46:731–735.
16. Robertson M. Forced normalization and the aetiology of depression in epilepsy. In: Trimble MR and Schmitz B (eds) *Forced Normalization and Alternative Psychosis of Epilepsy*. Petersfield: Wrightson Biomedical Publishing Ltd, 1998, pp. 143–168.

17. Alper K, Schwartz KA, Kolts RL *et al*. Seizure incidence in psychopharmacological clinical trials: an analysis of Food and Drug Administration (FDA) summary basis of approval reports. *Biol Psychiatry* 2007; 62:345–354.

18. Favale E, Audenino D, Cocito L, *et al*. The anticonvulsant effect of citalopram as an indirect evidence of serotonergic impairment in human epileptogenesis. *Seizure* 2003; 12:316–318.

19. Favale E, Rubino V, Mainardi P *et al*. Anticonvulsant effect of fluoxetine in humans. *Neurology* 1995; 45:1926–1927.

20. Specchio LM, Iudice A, Specchio N *et al*. Citalopram as treatment of depression in patients with epilepsy. *Clin Neuropharmacol* 2004; 27:133–136.

21. Patsalos P, Perucca E. Clinically important drug interactions in epilepsy: interactions between antiepileptic drugs and other drugs. *Lancet Neurology* 2003; 2:473–481.

22. Trimble MR, Mula M. Antiepileptic drug interactions in patients requiring psychiatric drug treatment. In: Majkowski J, Bourgeois B, Patsalos P, Mattson R (eds) *Antiepileptic Drugs. Combination Therapy and Interactions*. Cambridge: Cambridge University Press, 2005, pp. 350–368.

23. Nelson MH, Birnbaum AK, Remmel RP. Inhibition of phenytoin hydroxylation in human liver microsomes by several selective serotonin re-uptake inhibitors. *Epilepsy Res* 2001; 44:71–82.

24. Andersen BB, Mikkelsen M, Vesterager A *et al*. No influence of the antidepressant paroxetine on carbamazepine, valproate, and phenytoin. *Epilepsy Res* 1991; 10:201–204.

25. Mamiya K, Kojima K, Yukawa E *et al*. Phenytoin intoxication induced by fluvoxamine. *Ther Drug Monit* 2001; 23:75–77.

26. Laroudie C, Salazar DE, Cosson JP *et al*. Carbamazepine–nefazodone interaction in healthy subjects. *J Clin Psychpharmacol* 2000; 20:46–53.

27. Dursun SM, Mathew VM, Reveley MA. Toxic serotonin syndrome after fluoxetine plus carbamazepine. *Lancet* 1993; 342:442–443.

28. Rosenhagen M, Schmidt U, Weber F *et al*. Combination therapy of lamotrigine and escitalopram may cause myoclonus. *J Clin Psychpharmacology* 2006; 26:346–347.

29. Gernaat HB, Van de Woude J, Touw DJ. Fluoxetine and parkinsonism in patients taking carbamazepine. *Am J Psychiatry* 1991; 148:1604–1605.

30. Charney DS, Berman RM, Miller HL. Treatment of depression. In: Schatzberg AF, Nemeroff CB (eds) *Textbook of Psychopharmacology*. 2nd edn. Washington DC: American Psychiatric Association Press, 1998, pp. 705–732.

31. Hirschfield RMA, Bowden CL, Gitlin MJ *et al*. Practice guideline for the treatment of patients with bipolar disorder. *Amer J Psychiatry* 2002; 159(Suppl 4):1–15.

32. Strober M, Carlson G. Bipolar illness in adolescents with major depression: clinical, genetic, and psychopharmacologic predictors in a three- to four-year prospective follow-up investigation. *Arch Gen Psychiatry* 1982; 39:549-555.

33. Ettinger AB, Reed ML, Goldberg JF *et al*. Prevalence of bipolar symptoms in epilepsy vs other chronic health disorders. *Neurology* 2005; 65:535–540.

34. Lithium neuroleptic interactions: electroencephalographic studies. *Res Commun Psychol Psychiatr Behav* 1991; 16:35–40.

35. Blackwood DHR, Cull RE, Freeman CP *et al*. A study of the incidence of epilepsy following ECT. *J Neurol Neurosurg Psychiatry* 1980; 43:1098–1102.

36. Bell AJ, Cole A, Eccleston D *et al*. Lithium neurotoxicity at normal therapeutic levels. *Br J Psychiatry* 1993; 162:688–692.

37. Williams D. The structure of emotions reflected in epileptic experiences. *Brain* 1956; 79:29–67.

38. Kanner AM, Ramirez L, Jones JC. The utility of placing sphenoidal electrodes under the foramen ovale with fluoroscopic guidance. *J Clin Neurophysiol* 1995; 12:72–81.

39. Stahl SM. Anticonvulsants as anxiolytics, Part 1. Tiagabine and other anticonvulsants with actions on GABA. *J Clin Psychiatry* 2004; 65:292–293.

40. Schwartz TL. The use of tiagabine augmentation for treatment-resistant anxiety disorders: a case series. *Psychopharmacol Bull* 2002; 36:53–57.

41. Pande AC, Crockatt JG, Feltner DE *et al*. Pregabalin in generalized anxiety disorder: a placebo-controlled trial. *Am J Psychiatry* 2003; 160:533–540.

42. Baetz M, Bowen RC. Efficacy of divalproex sodium in patients with panic disorder and mood instability who have not responded to conventional therapy. *Can J Psychiatry* 1998; 43:73–77.

43. Davidson JRT, DuPont RL, Hedges D *et al*. Efficacy, safety and tolerability of venlafaxine extended release and buspirone in outpatients with generalized anxiety disorder. *J Clin Psychiatry* 1999; 60:528–535.

44. Linden M, Zubraegel D, Baer T *et al*. Efficacy of cognitive behaviour therapy in generalized anxiety disorders. Results of a controlled clinical trial (Berlin CBT-GAD Study). *Psychother Psychosom* 2005; 74:36–42.

45. Dunn DW, Austin JK. Behavioral issues in pediatric epilepsy. *Neurology* 1999; 53(Suppl 2):S96–S100.

46. McDermott S, Mani S, Krishnaswami S. A population-based analysis of specific behavior problems associated with childhood seizures. *J Epilepsy* 1995; 8:110–118.

47. Dunn DW, Austin JK, Harezlak J *et al*. ADHD and epilepsy in childhood. *Dev Med Child Neurol* 2003; 45:50–54.

48. Feldman H, Crumine P, Handen BL *et al*. Methylphenidate in children with seizures and attention-deficit disorder. *Am J Dis Child* 1989; 143:1081–1086.

49. Gross-Tsur V, Manor O, van der Meere J *et al*. Epilepsy and attention deficit hyperactivity disorder: is methylphenidate safe and effective? *J Pediatr* 1997; 130:670–674.

50. Gucuyener K, Erdemogly AK, Senol S *et al*. Use of methylphenidate for attention-deficit hyperactivity disorder in patients with epilepsy or electroencephalographic abnormalities. *J Child Neurol* 2003; 18:109–112.

51. Hernandez AJC, Barragan PEJ. Efficacy of atomoxetine treatment in children with ADHD and epilepsy. *Epilepsia* 2005; 46(Suppl 6):241.

52. Wernicke JF, Chilcott K, McAfee A *et al*. Seizure risk in patients with ADHD treated with atomoxetine (abstract). *AACAP/CACAP Proceedings* 2005; 32:133.

53. Slater E, Beard AW, Glithero E. The schizophrenia-like psychosis of epilepsy. Discussion and conclusions. *Br J Psychiatry* 1963; 109:95–150.

54. Dongier S. Statistical study of clinical and electroencephalographic manifestations of 536 psychotic episodes occurring in 516 epileptics between clinical seizures. *Epilepsia* 1959: 1:117–142.

55. Kanner AM, Stagno S, Kotagal P *et al*. Postictal psychiatric events during prolonged video-electroencephalographic monitoring studies. *Arch Neurol* 1996; 53:258–263.

56. Wolf P, Trimble MR. Biological antagonism and epileptic psychosis. *Br J Psychiatry* 1985; 146:272–276.

57. Stahl SM. Antipsychotic agents. In: Stahl SM (ed.) *Essential Pharmacology: Neuroscientific Basis and Practical Applications*. 2nd edn. New York: Cambridge University Press, 2000, pp. 401–458.

58. Logothetis J. Spontaneous epileptic seizures and EEG changes in the course of phenothiazine therapy. *Neurology* 1967; 17:869–877.

59. Whitworth AB, Fleischhacker WW. Adverse effects of antipsychotic drugs. *Int Clin Psychopharmacol* 1995; 9(Suppl 5):21–27.

60. Kanner N. Psychosis of epilepsy: a neurologist's perspective. *Epilepsy Behav* 2000; 1:219–227.

61. Reid S, Mothersill IW. Forced normalization: the clinical neurologist's view. In: Trimble MR, Schmitz B (eds) *Forced Normalization and Alternative Psychoses of Epilepsy*. Petersfield: Wrightson Biomedical Publishing Ltd, 1998, pp. 77–94.

16

The treatment of epilepsy in individuals with moderate to severe intellectual disability

Mark Scheepers, Mike Kerr

INTRODUCTION

Perhaps uniquely compared with other groups, epilepsy has a pervasive impact across the lives of people with intellectual disabilities (IDs). Studies suggest that as many as one-fifth of the population of people with intellectual disabilities across the lifespan have epilepsy [1]. Higher prevalence figures are quoted in institutional settings and with decreasing intelligence quotient (IQ) [2–4]. This population will often have complex epilepsy; which can be difficult to treat due to its severity but also due to difficulties in diagnosis, assessing treatment response and differentiating side-effects.

The management of epilepsy in people with an intellectual disability provides a special challenge. Key factors in this challenge include the aetiology and severity of the epilepsy, diagnostic overshadowing, a limited evidence base for interventions, and difficulties in investigation and communication. Managing this population will be a core component of any epilepsy service. The combination of severity and associated chronicity of the epilepsy makes it unlikely that patients can be managed adequately by family physicians and thus specialist services will, or should, be providing chronic disease management.

Notwithstanding all the complexities, management, as in the general population with epilepsy, remains focused on accurate diagnosis and the application of appropriate evidence-based treatments. This chapter will explore how the clinician can approach these issues, find a path through complex individual variation, make the appropriate interventions and improve the quality of life of individuals.

THE INDIVIDUAL WITH INTELLECTUAL DISABILITY

In this chapter we will use the internationally recognized term of severe and profound intellectual disability; whilst terminology varies across countries, this population would be recognized by a composite of IQ under 50, have difficulty with adaptive behaviour and these problems would have an onset in the developmental years. As in any branch of epileptology, characteristics of the individual with an intellectual disability will impact on the diagnostic process, assessment and the implementation of management plans. However, this individual variation is arguably more important due to the great heterogeneity of people with intellectual disability.

Mark Scheepers, MBChB, MRCPsych, Consultant Psychiatrist, ²gether NHS Foundation Trust, Gloucestershire, UK

Mike Kerr, MBChB, MRCPsych, MRCGP, MSc, MPhil, Professor of Learning Disability Psychiatry, Welsh Centre for Learning Disabilities, Cardiff, UK

It is worth considering the following factors in individuals as they may impact on management decisions:

- aetiology and severity of the intellectual disability;
- psychiatric and behavioural problems;
- recognized and unrecognized physical health problems, including swallowing and feeding difficulties; and
- communication difficulties and the individual's ability to understand the treatment.

AETIOLOGY AND SEVERITY OF INTELLECTUAL DISABILITY

The aetiology of the intellectual disability may provide several potentially useful management pointers to further understanding of the epilepsy or the behavioural and physical morbidities the individual may experience. An example of useful markers can be seen in some genetically determined conditions associated with intellectual disability. Angelman's syndrome shows a seizure type believed to be of a cryptogenic generalized nature [5] whilst Fragile X syndrome shows features similar to benign epilepsy with centrotemporal spikes [6]. Epilepsy occurs in 5–10% of people with Down syndrome and has a bimodal age distribution for seizure onset. The first peak is during childhood and presents as infantile spasms, myoclonic, atonic and tonic–clonic seizures. Partial seizures are rarely seen [7]. The second peak is in later life, usually as myoclonic or tonic–clonic seizures, and is often associated with Alzheimer's disease.

Our ability to recognize relatively well-defined epilepsy phenotypes in these conditions is an exciting development and is progressing alongside similar advances in understanding the physical and behavioural phenotypes. These, too, may provide clinically useful information – for example, the understanding of autonomic dysfunction in Rett syndrome where knowledge of the prevalence of hyperventilation and breath-holding allows the clinician to recognize potential diagnostic confusion with absence or complex partial seizures. Behavioural phenotypes can also be valuable when distinguishing the relative impact of seizures and their treatment on behaviour – the development of confusion with Alzheimer's disease in Down syndrome or psychosis in velocardiofacial syndrome being examples of conditions that may be attributed to a medication effect rather than to the condition itself.

An assessment of the individual's level of ability can be an important guide to the probable severity and prognosis of the epilepsy and a pointer to other co-morbid health features [3, 8]. As functional ability decreases so the health concerns increase due, in part, to issues of communication, but equally as a result of co-morbid conditions such as cerebral palsy. Up to one-third of people with IDs have problems with their vision, 40% have problems with hearing and 50% problems with communication, and these may get worse with age.

PSYCHIATRIC AND BEHAVIOURAL PROBLEMS

Psychiatric and behavioural problems impact on social and healthcare delivery and, within epilepsy management, can cause diagnostic uncertainty and complicate outcome assessment. About one in five people with IDs has a behaviour disorder and this can account for as much as one-third of referrals to specialist services. Within this group, there are some who will have a psychiatric diagnosis; however, a significant number will have a behavioural problem not immediately attributable to mental illness. It is therefore an important factor to consider when attributing causality of side-effects resulting from anti-epileptic drug (AED) treatment. It is often difficult to ascertain whether behaviour problems or psychiatric episodes that present in people with IDs and epilepsy are in any way related to their epilepsy or the treatment. Studies that have used a control group have generally found no statistically significant increase in the rate of psychopathology (psychiatric illness, behavioural problems or personality disorder) between those with and those without epilepsy [9–12]. In clinical practice, however, there will frequently be concerns that:

- a behavioural disturbance may be a manifestation of epilepsy;
- epilepsy treatment may worsen an existing behavioural problem; or
- a behavioural problem may be caused by the epilepsy treatment.

PHYSICAL HEALTH PROBLEMS

Individuals with an intellectual disability often have unrecognized physical morbidity [13]. Up to one-third of people with an intellectual disability have an associated physical disability, most often cerebral palsy, which may put them at risk of injury during seizures (particularly dislocation). People with ID and epilepsy have more visits to accident and emergency departments than those with ID and no epilepsy. In addition, people with epilepsy have many more fractures than those with ID but no epilepsy [14]. Screening for unrecognized disease may highlight conditions contributing to deterioration in health mistakenly attributed to epilepsy or its treatment.

There is significant evidence of osteoporosis in people with ID [15, 16], with immobility, short stature and, in women, hypogonadism being significant associations. There is increasing evidence of osteoporosis secondary to AEDs [17, 18] with polypharmacy, and enzyme-inducing drugs considered to be the main culprits. Taking this into consideration, it is important to ensure that people with ID and immobility who also have epilepsy are on the drugs least likely to cause osteoporosis, thereby decreasing the risk of fractures.

Swallowing and feeding difficulties are also common and are associated with gastro-oesophageal reflux, an important consideration when choosing the preparation of anti-epileptic medication. Physical disabilities (particularly associations with immobility and incontinence) are an important consideration when formulating a treatment plan as they may act as a marker of potential early mortality [19]. Published standardized mortality rates indicate that in the general ID population this is 1.6 [20], if epilepsy is added this increases to 5 [20, 21] and if cerebral palsy is added this increases to 5.6 [22].

Hypothyroidism is another common condition in people with ID and needs a specific mention as it may be overlooked, particularly when symptoms of cognitive slowing, decreased mobility or drowsiness are attributed to AEDs.

COMMUNICATION AND CAPACITY

Difficulties with communication can lead to difficulties in history-taking and examination [23, 24]. Many individuals with moderate to severe intellectual disability will be handicapped by their communication difficulties and will be unable to take an active part in the decision-making process. It is important to note the capacity each individual has to make decisions about their treatment and about epilepsy-related risks such as bathing and showering. Where they are unable to participate in the decision-making process, appropriate advocacy is needed to ensure access to the most appropriate treatment for their epilepsy.

DIAGNOSIS AND INVESTIGATIONS

The core investigation in the diagnosis of epilepsy in a patient with an intellectual disability is, as in the general population, the clinical history – with an emphasis on witness description of seizure. The hallmark of the epileptic phenomenon is the paroxysmal nature of the disorder – brief, episodic changes should be described. However, the special characteristics of this population make the gathering and interpretation of these data more complex. In particular, the ability of the individual to communicate may make the recognition of aura and post-ictal phenomena difficult. Furthermore, diagnostic overshadowing is common and an expectation for either behaviour or seizure disorder may influence the objectivity of both carers and professionals when reporting events.

A particularly difficult issue arises over the differential diagnosis of behaviour and epilepsy. It is possible that the clinician may be called upon to assess whether behavioural outbursts or repetitive stereotypic movements or mannerisms have an epileptic basis; this is complicated by the high frequency of behaviour problems and mannerisms in this population [25]. The misdiagnosis of epilepsy is common with reports of 20–25% of patients diagnosed as having epilepsy when they have some other cause for the paroxysms they suffer. Syncope, non-epileptic seizures, panic attacks, hallucinations and movement disorders may be mistaken for seizures but may also co-exist in an individual diagnosed with epilepsy in the ID population. When evaluating an individual's epilepsy the possibility of alternative explanations for these events should be considered.

Clear, unbiased reporting is essential and carers may need education in describing their observations. Video recording of events may further aid diagnosis [26]. In cases of behavioural outbursts, a functional analysis of behaviour may also help in differentiating behaviour from a seizure and clinicians should be well versed in ensuring that baseline behavioural assessments are in place before treatment initiation or change takes place.

As in the general population with epilepsy, electroencephalography may aid in seizure and epilepsy syndrome diagnosis. Video-electroencephalography and telemetry remain important diagnostic tools for the individual with intellectual disability; however, these may not be readily available or the individuals may be unable to tolerate the procedure. Some abnormal movements in people with epilepsy may mimic seizures but video-electroencephalography may show them to be non-seizure related [27]. Observed behaviour may be attributed to epilepsy, particularly in the severely or profoundly disabled patient. Staring and abnormal motor activity have often been reported as epileptic activity which, on subsequent video-electroencephalography, has been demonstrated not to be an epilepsy process 60% of the time [28, 29]. The electroencephalogram (EEG) may be of particular value in those with chronic epilepsy, where, despite adequate treatment, individuals are still suffering regular seizure-like movements.

There is a high prevalence of abnormality found on neuroimaging and in particular magnetic resonance imaging (MRI) [30]. Patients with intellectual disabilities may have difficulties co-operating with the technicians in the MRI suite and may, therefore, need sedation or generalized anaesthesia.

While the diagnosis of epilepsy should be based on clear clinical evidence, it is important to note that having ID should not exclude the individual from the appropriate investigations. In most circumstances, sometimes with repeated attempts, investigations can be completed. The diagnosis of epilepsy should be shared with the individual and their carers and, where possible, discussions around prognosis and long-term objectives should be conducted. The incidence of sudden unexpected death in epilepsy (SUDEP) in this population is so high that individuals and their families will need appropriate counselling regarding its risks and potential prevention.

TREATMENT

It is highly likely that medication will be indicated for the majority of individuals with epilepsy and intellectual disability. The process of introducing treatment is a dynamic one supported by family and individual education. Key components of this are:

- establishing the need for treatment;
- identifying and addressing risk factors;
- treatment choice; and
- managing and assessing treatment.

ESTABLISHING THE NEED FOR TREATMENT

The decision to introduce AEDs is always a balance between the effectiveness of the proposed medication for the target symptoms and the impact of the seizures on the individual, their quality of life and the possible side-effects of the medication. Notwithstanding this balance, the evidence of a pervasive effect of seizures across the lifespan is expanding. The single most important factor affecting quality of life remains uncontrolled seizures [31–34]. Seizure freedom is therefore the ultimate aim of epilepsy treatment and this should also be the starting point in managing epilepsy in people with ID. The impact of seizures on quality of life is broad, affecting life expectancy, physical health, social interaction, emotional well-being and cognitive development (Table 16.1). Unfortunately, seizure freedom is not always achievable, and in these circumstances, an aim to reduce the overall burden of seizure, through reducing seizure frequency or severity, is appropriate.

The decision to treat should be made in the patient's best interests, and formed in discussion with informed carers. A number of questions will need to be explored with the carers in order to assess the impact of epilepsy on quality of life:

- Are the carers concerned about seizures?
- Has the person been injured as a result of a seizure?
- Has the person been admitted to hospital for a seizure?
- Has the person ever had status epilepticus?
- Are the carers concerned about behavioural problems?
- Is the person at increased risk of SUDEP?
- Is there a concern over potential cognitive impact?

IDENTIFYING AND ADDRESSING RISK FACTORS

The treatment of epilepsy does not revolve around only the introduction of medication. Baseline monitoring of different seizures, behaviour, psychiatric symptoms and quality of life will inform treatment decisions and help hugely in understanding the treatment effect.

Behaviour is one of the most important factors affecting the decision-making process in epilepsy management for people with ID. Although there is clear evidence for an increased prevalence of emotional disturbance in people with epilepsy who do not have ID [35],

Table 16.1 Impact of epilepsy on health and quality of life in individuals with an intellectual disability

Area	Potential impact
Mortality	Standardized mortality ratio increased
	High risk of sudden unexpected death in epilepsy
Injury	Increased fracture rate
	Increased attendance at accident and emergency departments
Hospitalization	Increased hospitalization and increased cost
	Management of status epilepticus
	Co-morbid healthcare needs (swallow, chest infections)
Emotional well-being	No group effect on challenging behaviour but likely to be increase in anxiety and depression
Cognition	State-dependent learning disability
	Chronic cognitive deterioration
Social integration	Decreased activities
	Reduced living arrangement choice due to risk assessment

the evidence in people with ID is much less certain [36]. Behaviour problems can often impact upon carers more significantly than seizures, particularly when this behaviour is maladaptive. While the clinician may be concerned about the impact of the seizures, the carer may sometimes be concerned about the individual's behaviour or how this may change. It is therefore important to take account of the individual's behaviour and the impact of the seizures on behaviour.

Baseline monitoring of behaviour is a prerequisite to assessing change appropriately. In order to avoid problems with attribution when managing the epilepsy in an individual who also has behaviour problems, it is important to concurrently monitor the behaviour. In a clinical setting, it is difficult to use research-validated tools, but it is equally difficult to make judgements on hearsay or opinion. A simple traffic light system (red/amber/green) describing how the individual behaves/interacts and a recording system completed alongside this, will significantly aid discussion about behavioural change (Appendices 16.1 and 16.2). With data available from a few weeks before and after the change, it becomes possible to interpret the effect the change has had on the individual, whether this be medication, environmental change or a change in social circumstances. When planning change, it is important to control as many variables as possible in order to better understand the data. For example, it is unreasonable to start a new drug when someone is about to move out of the family home into a new care facility, as if there is a change in behaviour, it will be difficult to attribute this to one or another of the variables.

TREATMENT CHOICE

Comprehensive guidelines exist for the management of epilepsy in the general population, in women [37–39] and in people with an ID [40]. Epilepsy management should be directed by evidence-based research and informed by patient choice. Unfortunately, the evidence base for treatment in people with an ID is insufficient to meet this aim for the majority of clinical epilepsy scenarios. In particular, treatment choice decisions based on the relative efficacy/side-effect profiles of AEDs in people with ID are rare. The most glaring evidence gap is in the area of non-seizure-related impact. Such impact on behaviour, quality of life and general health is of paramount importance to carers.

Randomized placebo controlled add-on trials exist for topiramate in adult patients with ID and for lamotrigine, topiramate and felbamate in patients with Lennox–Gastaut syndrome (the majority of whom will have ID). In addition to these studies, numerous case reviews, case series and prospective studies that provide information on real-life usage of most AEDs are published, but are not able to distinguish the placebo impact and bias. Lastly, clinicians are likely to be influenced by individual clinical practice. Clinical choice is thus likely to be multi-axial in terms of this evidence base – Table 16.2 represents this multi-axial approach.

This inverse relationship between the severity of the seizure disorder and the evidence base needed to treat the seizures remains one of the greater inequalities in care experienced by people with an ID. This absence of information should not be a deterrent to treatment advancement and change where seizures continue to impact on an individual's quality of life.

MANAGING AND ASSESSING TREATMENT

Guidelines on the management of epilepsy in people with ID highlight the following good practice principles in the use of AEDs [40]:

- Ensure that the patient has received appropriate first-line treatment for their seizure type and syndrome.

Table 16.2 A multi-axial approach to treatment choice in patients with an intellectual disability (ID)

Axis	Modality	Decision factors/key variance
1	Aetiology of ID	Behavioural phenotypes Physical characteristics Specific seizure type
2	Epilepsy syndrome severity and choice	Main determinant of drug use and likely outcome
3	Published evidence base	Published side-effect profile in non-ID populations Treatment effect Risk assessment May provide specific guidance
4	Patient and carer choice	Patient's capacity Carer knowledge Fear of change Aspirations Presence of behavioural problems or other individual risk such as feeding
5	Clinical experience and practice-based audit	Crucial for communication of knowledge and experience to patients Ability to reflect local outcome side-effects and knowledge of handling risk

- In patients continuing to have seizures despite appropriate first-line anti-epileptic treatment:

    - review diagnosis
    - review treatment adherence
    - ensure that the maximum tolerated dose has been used.

- If the first drug continues to be ineffective at the maximum tolerated dose, an alternative drug should be introduced slowly without tapering the first. If the patient has a good response to the second drug consider withdrawing the first drug gradually.
- If reasonable options for monotherapy have been explored and acceptable symptom control is still not achieved, long-term two-drug therapy should be tried.
- If the first add-on drug is not effective, withdraw slowly and simultaneously replace with a second add-on drug. This process can be repeated for other possible add-on drugs.
- If symptoms are still not controlled on two drugs, some patients may benefit from an additional third drug.
- Intermittent treatment with benzodiazepines such as clobazam or clonazepam may be useful in preventing clustering of seizures, or particularly on days when seizures need to be avoided. Used intermittently, the risk of developing tolerance to the drug is reduced.

Treatment pathways can be developed and should follow a logical progression through the drugs appropriate to the seizure to be treated (Figure 16.1).

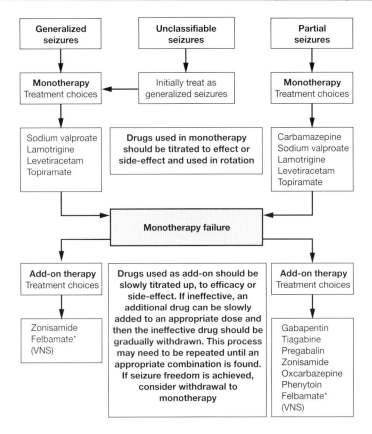

Figure 16.1 Treatment pathway for people with intellectual disabilities. *Licensed in the USA only and has significant side-effects.

RESCUE MEDICATION

Many people with ID and epilepsy have prolonged or clusters of seizures necessitating the use of rescue medication. The decision to use rescue medication should be made by the treating clinician on the basis of the history. Some people may need treatment that can be given to them while they are conscious in order to prevent seizure clusters. The reasons for the clusters need to be understood; some may be predictable, for example excitement at the build-up to a special event, catamenial seizures, or may be a result of the sort of epilepsy they have, where one seizure always leads to another. Others may have prolonged seizures, or may have previously been admitted with status epilepticus and their rescue medication may need to be given to them while they are having a seizure and are unconscious.

Benzodiazepines remain the mainstay of rescue medication, with clobazam, lorazepam and clonazepam all having proven efficacy in the conscious patient, each with differing onset and offset of action. The appropriate drug should be chosen with the desired treatment effect and the half-life of the drug should be taken into consideration. Rectal diazepam has been the gold standard treatment for prolonged seizures, but is often given in an inadequate dose. Recent evidence that the buccal or intranasal route can be safely used to administer midazolam has led to this medication being widely recommended in the UK. Carers are particularly delighted with the use of a treatment that does not require rectal administration, as this has a significant impact on the privacy and dignity of the individual.

Clear guidelines for the administration of rescue medication should be drawn up in order to accompany the individual to the various settings in which they may have care provided (adults may have their day care provided in a separate care facility to where they reside, or their care provider may change suddenly) and in order to minimise the chance for drug errors or inappropriate use of the medication.

Basic principles for the assessment of the use of rescue medication should include:

- Any individual who has epilepsy and intellectual disability should have an assessment of the management of prolonged seizures and/or cluster seizures.
- Where rescue medication is prescribed, a care plan should be completed which must include:

    - drug type and appropriate dose;
    - point at which the drug should be administered;
    - timing before repeat administration;
    - maximum dosage in 24 h; and
    - when to call an ambulance.

- A record of the date, time and who administered the medication should be kept with the individual and this information must be handed over between care teams.
- A review of the use of rescue medication should take place as part of the medication review.

TREATMENT EVALUATION

It is usual, in clinical settings, to assess outcomes in terms of dialogue with the patient over the effectiveness of the treatment, tolerability of the treatment and the lifestyle implications of the diagnosis and treatment. As we have already discussed, in epileptology, the aim is for seizure freedom, tolerable side-effects and a near-normal lifestyle. This is complicated in people with ID who may not be able to explain whether they have side-effects, what the implications are for them, and who may have complex epilepsy that may be difficult to control.

In people with ID, it is therefore important to record and review seizure frequency, seizure severity, quality of life and any significant changes in behaviour.

This package of recording will provide a helpful assessment of the impact of the epilepsy and the treatment prescribed. The assessment of outcome can thus be usefully divided into two groups, the first being the impact on seizures and the second being the impact on behaviour and general health.

IMPACT ON SEIZURES

The recording of seizure change in people with relatively easily recordable seizures is not particularly different to that collected in the general population with epilepsy. Ensuring patient education to gain accurate recording, differentiating seizure types and providing accessible recording tools and charts remains important (Appendices 16.3 and 16.4). Particular challenges are provided by attempts to assess outcome in the individual with severe epilepsy and severe or profound disability. Positive change may need to be evaluated, not through actual frequency of all seizures, but by assessing the change in the most severe seizures, such as atonic seizures, the use of rescue medication such as midazolam, the frequency of hospitalization or the number of seizure-free days. Clinical assessment of global outcome on well-being may guide the clinician; however, such an approach is fraught with pitfalls, in particular the reliability of non-parental care-givers, reporting bias and a tendency to accept the status quo. More objective assessment of outcome through direct computerized assessment of behaviour may offer clearer guidance [41] but its use in clinical care remains limited.

IMPACT ON BEHAVIOUR AND GENERAL HEALTH

Reliable and valid behavioural outcome tools such as the aberrant behaviour checklist [42] are available, but are too complex to administer in a clinical rather than a research setting. Clinical practice is more likely to be driven by carer concerns and these are often influenced by the recent history of behaviour. Having established objective evidence of behavioural change, careful attribution of causation is necessary as this may be the result of numerous other factors including physical health, environmental change or psychological symptoms. While the AEDs, either recently introduced or long term, will frequently be blamed, there is little evidence to support this argument.

A structured clinical assessment is always indicated when behavioural concerns are raised. In some cases, very detailed psychiatric and psychosocial assessment will be needed to identify causative factors. In the clinic setting, a review of the following potential causations may help. Firstly, *seizure change-related behaviour*; where behavioural change is identified in association with major seizure reduction the possibility of forced (paradoxical) normalization [43] is raised. Essentially not provable, the recognition that behaviour may deteriorate as seizure control improves, once recognized, can be communicated to carers and management plans introduced to deal with the behaviour as patients frequently settle over time. *Abnormal illness behaviour* is a challenge in all aspects of epilepsy care and may express itself during treatment change with behaviour abnormalities or non-epileptic attacks. *Seizure-associated behaviours* should be identified through the temporal relationship between seizures and behaviours. This holds true for pre- and post-ictal behaviours. *Ictal behaviour changes* pose a significant diagnostic challenge; these seizures, which present as a behaviour manifestation, are unlikely to arise during treatment change but may do so if the AEDs have modified seizure expression. *Developmental and organic behaviour disturbance* is the most probable cause of behavioural disturbance appearing during treatment change. Such behaviours are the result of the aetiology of the intellectual disability; these should have been present prior to medication change and understandable through either the developmental pattern or the pattern of organic brain damage. *AED-related behaviour change* is a clear possibility. Available evidence suggests that AEDs do not specifically cause aggressive or challenging behaviours. It is likely that behavioural changes are thus linked to intolerance of side-effects with communication difficulties hindering simple expression. Such effects should pass some test of understandability, that is, does the behaviour expressed make sense in terms of a side-effect – this would include agitation, appetite change or irritability. *Concurrent physical illness* can cause similar behavioural manifestations.

CONCLUSION

Epilepsy is a common chronic condition affecting many people with ID. It is important for those managing epilepsy in this population to be aware of the wider impact that the epilepsy and its management have on the individual and their carers. Although the chronic and pervasive impact of epilepsy on the life of individuals with an ID offers many clinical challenges a structured approach, using available evidence and clinical skills, can lead to some real health gains in this population.

REFERENCES

1. Welsh Office. *Welsh Health Survey, 1995.* Cardiff: Welsh Office, 1995.
2. Richardson SA, Katz M, Koller H, McLaren J, Rubenstine B. Some characteristics of a population of mentally retarded young adults in a British city. *Journal of Mental Deficiency Research* 1979; 23:275–287.
3. Corbett J. Epilepsy and mental handicap. In: Laidlaw J, Richens A, Oxley J (eds) *A Textbook of Epilepsy.* 3rd edn. Edinburgh: Churchill Livingstone, 1993, pp. 631–636.
4. Kerr M, Fraser W, Felce D. Primary health care for people with a learning disability; a keynote review. *British Journal of Learning Disabilities* 1996; 24:2–8.
5. Matsumoto A, Kumagai T, Miura K, Miyazaki S, Hayakawa C, Yamanaka T. Epilepsy in Angelman syndrome associated with chromosome 15q deletion. *Epilepsia* 1992; 33:1083–1090.
6. Musumeci SA, Ferri R, Elia M, Colognola R, Bergonzi P, Tassinari C. Epilepsy and Fragile X syndrome: a follow-up study. *Am J Med Genet* 1991; 38:511–513.
7. Appleton R. Aetiology of epilepsy and learning disorders: specific epilepsy syndromes; genetic, chromosomal and sporadic syndromes. In: Trimble MR (ed.) *Learning Disability and Epilepsy: An Integrative Approach.* Guildford: Clarius Press, 2003, pp. 47–64.
8. Welsh Health Planning Forum. *Protocol for Investment in Health Gain: Mental Handicap (Learning Disabilities).* Cardiff: Welsh Office, 1992.
9. Deb S, Hunter D. Psychopathology of people with mental handicap and epilepsy. II: psychiatric illness. *Br J Psychiatry* 1991; 159:826–830.
10. Deb S, Hunter D. Psychopathology of people with mental handicap and epilepsy. I: maladaptive behaviour. *Br J Psychiatry* 1991; 159:822–826.
11. Deb S, Hunter D. Psychopathology of people with mental handicap and epilepsy. III: personality disorder. *Br J Psychiatry* 1991; 159:830–834.
12. Espie CA, Watkins J, Curtice L, Espie A, Duncan R, Ryan JA *et al.* Psychopathology in people with epilepsy and intellectual disability; an investigation of potential explanatory variables. *J Neurol Neurosurg Psychiatry* 2003; 74:1485–1492.
13. Lennox NG, Kerr MP. Primary health care and people with an intellectual disability: the evidence base. *J Intellect Disabil Res* 1997; 41:365–371.
14. Baxter HA. Personal communication, 1999.
15. Center JR, McElduff A, Beange H. Osteoporosis in groups with intellectual disability 1. *J Intellect Dev Disabil* 1994; 19:251–258.
16. Wagemans AMA, Fiolet JFBM, Van der Linden ES, Menheere PPCA. Osteoporosis and intellectual disability: is there any relation? *J Intellect Disabil Res* 1998; 42:370–374.
17. Farhat G, Yamout B, Mikati MA, Demirjian S, Sawaya R, El-Hajj Fuleihan G. Effect of antiepileptic drugs on bone density in ambulatory patients. *Neurology* 2002; 58:1348–1353.
18. Kelso ARC, Cock HR. Advances in epilepsy. *Br Med Bull* 2005; 72:135–148.
19. Hollins S, Attard MT, von Fraunhofer N, McGuigan S, Sedgwick P. Mortality in people with learning disability: risks, causes, and death certification findings in London. *Dev Med Child Neurol* 1998; 40:50–56.
20. Forgren L, Edvinsson S, Nystrom L, Blomquist HK. Influence of epilepsy on mortality in mental retardation: an epidemiological study. *Epilepsia* 1996; 37:956–963.
21. Wieseler NA, Hanson RH, Nord G. Investigation of mortality and morbidity associated with severe self-injurious behaviour. *Am J Ment Retard* 1995; 100:1–5.
22. Morgan CL, Scheepers M, Kerr M. Mortality in patients with intellectual disability and epilepsy. *Curr Opin Psychiatry* 2001; 14:471–475.
23. Duckworth MS, Rhadakrishnan G, Nolan M, Fraser W. Initial encounters between people with a mild mental handicap and psychiatrists: an investigation of a method of evaluating interview skills. *J Intellect Disabil Res* 1993; 37:263–276.
24. Kerr M, Evans S, Nolan M, Fraser W. Assessing clinicians' consultations with people with profound learning disability. *J Intellect Disabil Res* 1995; 39:187–190.
25. Kaufman ME, Levitt HA. A study of three stereotyped behaviours in institutionalised mental defectives. *American Journal of Mental Deficiency* 1965; 69:467–473.
26. Paul A. Epilepsy or stereotypy? Diagnostic issues in people with learning disabilities. *Seizure* 1997; 6:111–120.
27. Donat J, Wright F. Episodic symptoms mistaken for seizures in the neurologically impaired child. *Neurology* 1990; 40:156–157.

28. Desai P, Talwar D. Nonepileptic events in normal and neurologically handicapped children: a video EEG study. *Pediatr Neurol* 1992; 8:127–129.

29. Holmes G, McKeever M, Russman B. Abnormal behaviour or epilepsy? Use of long-term EEG and video monitoring with severely to profoundly mentally retarded patients with seizures. *American Journal of Mental Deficiency* 1983; 87:456–458.

30. Andrews TM, Everitt AD, Sander JW. A descriptive survey of long-term residents with epilepsy and intellectual disability at the Chalfont Centre: is there a relationship between maladaptive behaviour and magnetic resonance imaging findings? *J Intellect Disabil Res* 1999; 43:475–483.

31. Brown S, Betts T, Chadwick D, Hall B, Shorvon S, Wallace S. An epilepsy needs document. *Seizure* 1993; 2:91–103.

32. Hoare P. The development of psychiatric disorder among school children with epilepsy. *Dev Med Child Neurol* 1984; 26:3–13.

33. Vickrey BG. Advances in the measurement of health-related quality of life in epilepsy. *Qual Life Res* 1995; 4:83–85.

34. Espie CA, Paul A, Graham M, Sterrick M, Foley J, McGarvey C. The Epilepsy Outcome Scale: the development of a measure for use with carers of people with epilepsy plus intellectual disability. *J Intellect Disabil Res* 1998; 42:90–96.

35. Scheepers M, Kerr M. Epilepsy and behaviour. *Curr Opin Neurol* 2003; 16:183–187.

36. Krishnamoorthy ES. Neuropsychiatric epidemiology at the interface between learning disability and epilepsy. In: Trimble MR (ed.) *Learning Disability in Epilepsy: An Integrative Approach*. Guildford: Clarius Press, 2003, pp. 17–26.

37. National Institute for Clinical Excellence. *CG20 Epilepsy in adults: Quick reference guide, 2004*. Available at: http://www.nice.org.uk/CG020adultsquickrefguide

38. Scottish Intercollegiate Guidelines Network. *Diagnosis and management of epilepsy in adults Guideline No. 70*. 2003. Available at: http://www.sign.ac.uk/guidelines/fulltext/70/index.html

39. Ben-Menachem E. AAN/AES guidelines on the use of new AEDS. *Epilepsy Currents* 2005; 5:30–32.

40. Working group of the International Association of the Scientific Study of Intellectual Disability. Clinical guidelines for the management of epilepsy in adults with an intellectual disability. *Seizure* 2001; 10:401–409.

41. Smith C, Kerr M, Felce D, Baxter H, Lowe K, Meek A. Exploring the evaluation of anti-epileptic drug change in people with intellectual disabilities and high frequency epileptic seizures: seizure control and sustained responsiveness to the environment. *Epilepsy and Behaviour* 2004; 5:58–66.

42. Aman MG, Singh NN, Stewart AW, Field CJ. The aberrant behavior checklist: a behavior rating scale for the assessment of treatment effects. *American Journal of Mental Deficiency* 1985; 89:485–491.

43. Trimble MR, Schmitz EB. The psychoses of epilepsy/schizophrenia. In: Engel J, Pedley TA (eds) *Epilepsy: A Comprehensive Textbook*. Philadelphia: Lippincott-Raven, 1997, pp. 2071–2082.

Appendix 16.1 Red/Amber/Green (RAG) observation chart

RAG behaviour observation data

Service user name:

Green (Baseline/calm behaviour)	**Amber** (Moved away from baseline, appearing anxious)	**Red** (Appearing anxious/agitated, e.g. shouting or physical aggression, etc.)

Appendix 16.2 Red/Amber/Green (RAG) recording chart

Name:

Date:

Time	08 00	09 00	10 00	11 00	12 00	13 00	14 00	15 00	16 00	17 00	18 00	19 00	20 00	21 00	22 00	23 00	00 00	01 00	02 00	03 00	04 00	05 00	06 00	07 00
Red																								
Amber																								
Green																								
Sleep																								

Reprinted with kind permission from ²gether NHS Foundation Trust, Gloucestershire, UK.

Appendix 16.3 Epileptic seizure record sheet codes

Name:	Date of birth:
Code	**Seizure codes** Describe seizure, including before and after, in detail, without using any jargon.
(A) Generalized tonic–clonic seizure	
(B) Complex partial seizure	
(C) Other	
	Other events that may influence epilepsy Describe event giving detail as required, e.g. behaviour, menstruation, constipation, illness
(1)	
(2)	
(3)	

Reprinted with kind permission from ²gether NHS Foundation Trust, Gloucestershire, UK.

Seizure description sheet (I)

Please use a separate sheet for each seizure type

Name: **Date of birth:**   **Date:**

Complete for each seizure type, e.g. A, B, C – use each letter under YES, NO.

Before

	Yes	No
Aura/unusual sensation, e.g. taste/smell	___	___
Automatisms	___	___
Alteration of appetite	___	___
Change in sleep pattern	___	___
Cold and clammy	___	___
Behaviour change	___	___
Lethargy	___	___
Elation	___	___
Tachycardia	___	___
Scream/cry out	___	___
Undressing	___	___
Other [please state]		

After

	Yes	No
Does the person's body become rigid?	___	___
Does the person's body become floppy?	___	___
Do they experience involuntary/jerky movements?	___	___
If yes, parts of the body affected:		
facial	___	___
whole body	___	___
left arm	___	___
right arm	___	___
left leg	___	___
right leg	___	___
Incontinence:		
urine	___	___
faeces	___	___
Cyanosis	___	___
Cold and clammy	___	___
Froth at mouth	___	___
Change in level of consciousness	___	___
Change in breathing pattern	___	___
Have they a glazed/fixed stare?	___	___
Unusual sounds	___	___
Grind teeth	___	___
Other [please state]		

Reprinted with kind permission from ²gether NHS Foundation Trust, Gloucestershire, UK.

Seizure description sheet (II)

Please use a separate sheet for each seizure type

Name: **Date of birth:** **Date:**

Complete for each seizure type, eg. A, B, C – use each letter under YES, NO.

After	Yes	No
Confusion	____	____
Aggression	____	____
Drowsy	____	____
Headache	____	____
Tearful	____	____
Alteration in appetite	____	____
Thirsty	____	____
Hyperactive	____	____
Partial seizures	____	____
Automatisms	____	____
Other [please state]		

Please state any factors that could precipitate a seizure for this person, e.g. menstrual cycle, flashing lights, stress

Average number of seizures (of this type) per:	A	B	C
Day			
Month			
Year			

	A	B	C
Average duration of seizure (in minutes)			
Average duration of recovery period			

Appendix 16.4 Epilepsy recording chart

Epileptic Seizure Record Chart

Name: Date of Birth: Date completed:

Date (dd/mm/yy)	Time (24h)	Type of Seizure (A, B, C)	During sleep (Y/N)	Specify other events, e.g. menstruation, other illness, constipation, etc.

Reprinted with kind permission from ²gether NHS Foundation Trust, Gloucestershire, UK.

Abbreviations

AAN	American Academy of Neurology
AAPD	atypical anti-psychotic drug
ACTH	adrenocorticotropic hormone
ADD	attention deficit disorder
ADHD	attention deficit hyperactivity disorder
ADL	activities of daily living
AED	anti-epileptic drug
AF	atrial fibrillation
AH	amygdalo-hippocampectomy
ALDH	aldehyde dehydrogenase
AMPA	α-amino-3-hydroxy-5-methyl-4-isoxazeoleproprionic acid
APD	anti-psychotic drug
ATL	anterior temporal lobectomy
AUC	concentration–time curve
BBB	blood–brain barrier
BECTS	benign epilepsy with centrotemporal spikes
CAE	childhood absence epilepsy
CAPD	conventional anti-psychotic drug
CBT	cognitive behaviour therapy
CBZ	carbamazepine
CI	confidence interval
CLB	clobazam
CLZ	clonazepam
CNS	central nervous system
CPR	cardiopulmonary resuscitation
CRH	corticotropin-releasing hormone
CSF	cerebrospinal fluid
CT	computerized tomography
DA	dopamine
DBS	deep brain stimulation
DLDE	dysthymic-like disorder of epilepsy
DM	diabetes mellitus
DMN	dorsal medial nucleus
DWI	diffusion-weighted imaging
ECT	electroconvulsive therapy
EEG	electroencephalogram
EIEE	early infantile epileptic encephalopathy
EME	early myoclonic epileptic encephalopathy
ETX	ethosuximide
EZ	epileptogenic zone

FBM	felbamate
FDA	Food and Drug Administration
FDG	[18F]-fluorodeoxyglucose
FLAIR	fluid-attenuated inversion recovery
fMRI	functional magnetic resonance imaging
FSH	follicle-stimulating hormone
GABA	γ-aminobutyric acid
GAD	generalized anxiety disorder
GBP	gabapentin
GCSE	generalized convulsive status epilepticus
GI	gastrointestinal
GNRH	gonadotrophin-releasing hormone
GTC	generalized-onset tonic–clonic
HAART	highly active anti-retroviral therapy
HD	haemodialysis
HIV	human immunodeficiency virus
HR	hazard ratio
HRSE	highly refractive status epilepticus
HRT	hormone replacement therapy
i.m.	intramuscular
i.v.	intravenous
ICA	internal carotid artery
ICH	intracerebral haemorrhage
ICU	intensive care unit
ID	intellectual disability
iEEG	intracranial electroencephalography
IGE	idiopathic generalized epilepsy
ILAE	International League Against Epilepsy
INR	international normalized ratio
IPOE	interictal psychosis of epilepsy
IQ	intelligence quotient
IS	infantile spasm
IU	international units
JAE	juvenile absence epilepsy
JME	juvenile myoclonic epilepsy
LGS	Lennox–Gastaut syndrome
LH	luteinizing hormone
LTG	lamotrigine
LVT	levetiracetam
MAOI	monoamino-oxidase inhibitor
MCM	major congenital malformation
MDC	multi-disciplinary conference
MEG	magnetoencephalography
MES	maximal electroshock
MR	magnetic resonance
MRI	magnetic resonance imaging
MSI	magnetic source imaging
mTLE	mesial temporal lobe epilepsy
MTS	mesial temporal sclerosis
NAA	N-acetyl aspartate
NCSE	non-convulsive status epilepticus
NKH	non-ketotic hyperglycaemia

NMDA	N-methyl-D-aspartate
NTS	nucleus tractus solitarius
OC	oral contraceptive
OCD	obsessive compulsive disorder
OR	odds ratio
OXC	oxcarbazepine
PCOS	polycystic ovary syndrome
PD	panic disorder
PED	periodic epileptiform discharge
PEMA	phenylethylmalonamide
PET	positron emission tomography
PHB	phenobarbital
PHT	phenytoin
PIP	post-ictal psychosis
PLED	periodic lateralized epileptiform discharge
PLP	pyridoxal 5'-phosphate
PNPO	pyridox(am)ine phosphate oxidase
POE	psychosis of epilepsy
PR	per rectum
PTZ	pentylenetetrazol
PWE	patients with epilepsy
QALY	quality-adjusted life year
QoL	quality of life
RCT	randomized controlled trial
RGB	retigabine
RPLS	reversible posterior leukoencephalopathy syndrome
RR	relative risk
SAH	subarachnoid haemorrhage
SE	status epilepticus
SMEI	severe myoclonic epilepsy in infancy
SNRI	selective norepinephrine reuptake inhibitor
SPECT	single photon emission computer tomography
SREDA	subclinical rhythmic electrical discharges of adulthood
SSRI	selective serotonin reuptake inhibitor
STM	sulthiam
STP	stiripentol
SUDEP	sudden unexpected death in epilepsy
TCA	tricyclic anti-depressant
TGA	transient global amnesia
TGB	tiagabine
TIA	transient ischaemic attack
TLE	temporal lobe epilepsy
TPL	talampanel
TPM	topiramate
TS	tuberous sclerosis
VABS	Vineland Adaptive Behaviour Scale
VGB	vigabatrin
VN	vagus nerve
VNS	vagus nerve stimulation
VPA	valproate
ZNS	zonisamide

Index

A

abortive therapy 225
  in children 97, 108
  in patients with intellectual disability 312–13
absence seizures
  aggravation by AEDs 111
  treatment 8, 15, 142
    in children 89, 95, 109, 193–7
    juvenile AE 198–201
absorption of AEDs, drug interactions 240
acetazolamide, use in catamenial epilepsy 164, 165
acidosis, in status epilepticus 261, 263
acute seizures, management 213–14
  see also abortive therapy
add-on therapy, choice of AED 15, 17
  see also polytherapy
adrenocorticotrophic hormone (ACTH)
  in treatment of EIEE 76
  in treatment of infantile spasms 71–3, 74, 89, 97
aetiology
  in elderly patients 174, 238
  in HIV patients 223
  in hospitalized patients 215, 218
  relationship to long-term seizure control 114
  of status epilepticus 253
ageing population 173
alcohol abuse 136
alpralozam, use in anxiety disorders 293
alternate psychosis 297, 301
alternating hemiplegias of childhood 105
American Academy of Neurology, treatment
    guidelines 194
  for childhood absence seizures 195
  GTC seizures 198
amitryptyline, drug interactions 286–7
ammonia levels, effect of valproate therapy 7
amozepine 301
AMPA (α-amino-3-hydroxy-5-methyl-4-
    isoxazeolepropionic acid) antagonists 145
amphetamine, use in ADHD 295
anaesthetic agents, risk of seizures 237
analgesics
  reduction of seizure threshold 215
  risk of seizures 237
Angelman's syndrome 306

antacids, drug interactions 240
anti-arrhythmic drugs, effect on seizure
    threshold 215, 231
antibiotics, reduction of seizure threshold 215
anticoagulation 230
anti-depressants 239, 244, 284–5
  choice of drug 286
  drug interactions 286–8
  effect on seizures 286
  efficacy 288
  reduction of seizure threshold 215
  use in ADHD 296
  use in anxiety disorders 292–3
  use in bipolar disorders 289–90
anti-epileptic drugs (AEDs) 3
  advantages and disadvantages 91–2
  breastfeeding 161
  as cause of cognitive impairment 113
  choice of agent 14–15, 17, 124, 131, 216–18
    in cancer patients 224
    in cardiac disease 231
    comparative studies 125–6
    in elderly patients 178–82, 238–9
    in hepatic disease 219–20, 233–5
    in HIV patients 223–4
    in intensive care units 218–19
    in obstetric patients 224
    RCTs of new AEDs 126–8
    in renal disease 220
    retrospective outcome studies 128
    in stroke patients 221, 230
    in transplant patients 221–2
  dosing in catamenial epilepsy 164, 165
  dosing during pregnancy 159–60
  dosing in periprocedural patients 237–8
  dosing schedules 19–21
  drug interactions 112–13, 240–1, 242–4
    with anti-depressants 286–8
    with anti-psychotic drugs 299–300
    with lithium 291
    with oral contraceptives 153–5
    pharmacokinetic 5, 143–5
  effects on hepatic enzymes 8, 93–5, 143, 144, 234, 235, 240–4
  after first seizure 121–2

initiation of therapy 16, 120
mechanisms of action 141
monotherapy vs. polytherapy 17–18
neuroprotection in SE 271–2
new molecular targets 145
paediatric dosing ranges 93–5
prophylactic use 221–2
seizure aggravation 111, 204–6
serum levels measurement 18–19
synergistic combinations 142–3
teratogenicity 156–8
timeline of development 124
treatment response 129–31
use in anxiety disorders 293
use in children 90, 93–5
  decision to treat 88
  discontinuation of treatment 98
  treatment of generalized epilepsy 95–6
  treatment of partial epilepsy 89, 95
use in elderly patients 178–82
use in infants 70, 75–6
  for infantile spasms 71, 72–4
  in severe myoclonic epilepsy in infancy 74–5
use in patients with intellectual disability 310–12
  need for treatment 309
  rescue medication 312–13
  treatment choice 310
  treatment evaluation 313–14
use in renal disease 232–3
anti-psychotic drugs 298–9
interactions with AEDs 299–300
antiquitin 67
anxiety disorders 130, 291–2
indications for psychiatric referral 293
prevalence 282
psychotherapy 293–4
aplastic anaemia
  as side-effect of felbamate 9
  as side-effect of valproate therapy 8
apoptosis 259–60
appetite suppression, AEDs 17
aripiprazole 298
arrhythmias 230–1
AEDs as cause 221, 222
asthenia, as side-effect of tiagabine 12
Atkins diet 146
  see also ketogenic diet
atomoxetine, use in ADHD 296
atrial fibrillation 230
attention deficit disorders (ADDs) 99, 112, 281, 282, 294–5
management 295–6
atypical anti-psychotic drugs (AAPDs) 298
aura
  dizziness 175
  value in ictal focus localization 30
Australian Registry of Antiepileptic Drugs in Pregnancy 157

B

baclofen, reduction of seizure threshold 215
barbiturates, use in refractory status epilepticus 266–7
battery replacement, vagus nerve stimulation 57
Bcl-2 proteins 260
Beck Depression Inventory-II 284
behaviour problems
  in childhood epilepsy 99, 112
  in intellectual disability 306–7, 308, 309–10, 314
behaviour observation charts 317–18
benign epilepsy with centrotemporal spikes (BECTS) 88
  learning difficulties 98
  treatment 89, 95
benign infantile seizures 64
benign neonatal infantile seizures 64
benign neonatal seizures 64
benzodiazepines 8
  alternative routes of administration 238, 312
  in management of acute seizures 214
  mechanisms of action 141
  use in anxiety disorders 288, 293
  use in catamenial epilepsy 164, 165
  use in infants 70, 73
    in SMEI 74, 75
  use in patients with intellectual disability 310
  use in porphyria 237
  use in status epilepticus 264, 269
bilateral temporal lobe epilepsy 42
biotinidase deficiency 68
bipolar disorders 244, 282–3
  management 289–91
blood dyscrasias in AED therapy 8, 179
blood flow, changes in SE 260–1, 262
bone health, effect of AEDs 4, 179
bone marrow transplantation 221–2
brain development, effect of AEDs 167
breastfeeding 161
breath-holding 105
broad spectrum AEDs 15
bupropion 301
'burst suppression' EEG pattern 69
buspirone, use in anxiety disorders 293

C

caffeine, neuroprotection in SE 272
callosotomy 44
cancer patients 224
carbamazepine 4, 6, 15, 217
  advantages and disadvantages 91
  aggravation of seizures 136, 197, 204
  alternative routes of administration 238
  breastfeeding 161
  in combination therapy 14, 17, 110, 142
    with lithium 291
  comparative studies 125–8

dosing schedule 19–20
drug interactions 5, 143, 144, 240, 242–3, 287, 288, 299–300
   with oral contraceptives 154
generic substitution 15
initiation of therapy 16
mechanisms of action 141
metabolism 93
side-effects 179, 221, 231, 236, 239
   effect on bone health 179
teratogenicity 157
use in bipolar disorders 290, 291
use in children 89, 90, 93
use in elderly patients 180–1
use in infants 70
use in liver disease 234
use during pregnancy 159, 160
use in renal disease 232, 233
carbapenems, interaction with valproate 219
cardiovascular disease 220–1, 230–1
carnitine supplementation, valproate therapy 7
caspase inhibitors 271
caspases 260
catamenial epilepsy 163–5
   perimenopausal seizure frequency 166, 167
catecholamines, changes in status epilepticus 261
cavernomas, detection by MRI 31
cell death, as consequence of SE 258–60
Center for Epidemiologic Studies Depression Scale 284
cerebral palsy 307
cerebrospinal fluid, effects of vagus nerve stimulation 52
CGX-1007 (conantokin-G) 145
chemotherapeutic agents
   drug interactions 224
   reduction of seizure threshold 215
childhood epilepsy 85
   abortive therapy 97, 108
   AED treatment 89
      in absence epilepsy 193–7
      choice of drugs 109
      discontinuation of treatment 98
      evidence-based analysis 109
      in generalized epilepsy 95–6
      in partial epilepsy 89, 95
      pharmacokinetics 107
      topiramate, side effects 11
      valproate, hepatotoxicity 7
      zonisamide, side effects 13
   attention deficit hyperactivity disorder 99, 294, 295–6
   behaviour problems 99
   decision to treat 88
   diagnostic tests 107
   evaluation of first seizure 87
   evaluation of newly diagnosed epilepsy 87–8
   history-taking 85–7

learning difficulties 98–9
psychiatric disorders 99
psychosocial needs 113
safety precautions 99–100
status epilepticus, risk of subsequent epilepsy 255–6
treatment-resistant 103, 115
   co-morbidity 111–13
   confirmation of aetiology and epilepsy type 106
   ketogenic diet 108, 110
   medical intractability 114
   monotherapy vs. combination therapy 110–11
   re-assessment of diagnosis 103–6
   rescue therapies 108
   second- and third-line AEDs 108
   seizure aggravation by AEDs 111
   vagus nerve stimulation 54–5
   see also infantile epilepsy; infantile spasms (West syndrome)
chlomipramine 301
chlorpromazine
   drug interactions 300
   effect on seizure threshold 299
chromosome abnormalities
   in epilepsy syndromes 64, 65
   in pyridoxine-dependent epilepsy 67
citalopram 285, 288
   drug interactions 286–7
   effect on seizures 286
classification of seizures 86, 135–6
clearance sites, AEDs 93–5
clobazam 8, 191, 217
   advantages and disadvantages 91
   for childhood absence seizures 197
   use in catamenial epilepsy 164
   use in children 89, 90
   use in patients with intellectual disability 310
   use in SMEI 74
clomiphene citrate, use in catamenial epilepsy 165
clomipramine, drug interactions 286–7
clonazepam 8, 191, 217
   use in anxiety disorders 288, 293
   use in childhood absence seizures 196, 197
   use in infants 70, 73
   use in juvenile myoclonic epilepsy 201
   use in patients with intellectual disability 310
clonidine, use in ADHD 296
clorazepate 8
closed-loop brain stimulation 146
clozapine 298, 301
   effect on seizure threshold 299
clusters of seizures 224–5
CNS stimulants, use in ADHD 295
co-morbidity 130, 229
   psychiatric 281–2

see also anxiety disorders; attention deficit
disorders; bipolar disorders;
depression; psychotic disorders
in treatment-resistant childhood epilepsy 111–13
co-trimoxazole, prophylactic use in infantile
spasms 97
coagulopathy, as side-effect of valproate 219
cognitive behavioural therapy (CBT) 293–4
in ADHD 296
cognitive function 121
effect of AEDs 113, 179, 239
effect of status epilepticus 255
communication problems in intellectual
disability 307
complementary medicine, drug interactions 241
complications of surgery 45
computed tomography (CT)
in elderly patients 178
in investigation of acute seizures 214
in status epilepticus 261
conantokin-G (CGX-1007) 145
contrast agents, reduction of seizure threshold 215
controlled-release AEDs, implantation into seizure
focus 146
conventional anti-psychotic drugs (CAPDs) 298
cooling, value in status epilepticus 270
corpus callosotomy 44
corticotropin-releasing hormone (CRH), role in
infantile spasms 71
cost of AEDs 15
cost-effectiveness of AEDs 127
creatine deficiency disorders 68
cryptogenic epilepsy 28
cryptogenic partial epilepsy, treatment in
children 89
cycling 100
cyclosporine, neurotoxicity 222, 233
CYP enzymes *see* hepatic enzymes

D

danazol, use in catamenial epilepsy 165
daydreaming 105
deep brain stimulation (DBS) 44, 51, 58, 146
use in highly refractory status epilepticus 269
depression 99, 112, 130, 244, 281–2
association with sexual dysfunction 165
atypical manifestations 283
diagnosis 283–4
in elderly patients 239
indications for psychiatric referral 289
interictal 282
major episodes 283
pharmacotherapy 284–5
choice of drug 286
therapeutic expectations 285
see also anti-depressants

physical symptoms 288
relationship to treatment response 129
risk of developing epilepsy 281
use of vagus nerve stimulation 182
depth electrodes 38
desflurane, use in highly refractory status
epilepticus 269
desipramine
drug interactions 286–7
use in ADHD 296
dextroamphetamine, use in ADHD 295
diabetes
avoidance of phenytoin 236
risk from anti-psychotic drugs 298
diagnosis
in elderly patients 175–6
in patients with intellectual disability 307–8
dialysis, AED therapy 220, 233
diazepam 8
rectal 97, 108, 312
paediatric dosing 95
use in status epilepticus 264, 269
differential diagnosis of seizures
arrhythmias 231
in children 104–6
in elderly patients 176
in patients with intellectual disability 308
discontinuation of treatment
in children 98
in older patients 183–4
dizziness, as aura in elderly people 175
Doose syndrome, seizure aggravation by AEDs 111
dosing schedules, AEDs 19–21
double depression 283
Down syndrome 306
doxepin, drug interactions 286–7
Dravet syndrome (severe myoclonic epilepsy in
infancy) 65
pharmacological treatment 74–5
driving 184
with history of childhood epilepsy 98
drug delivery systems 145–6
drug interactions 5, 15, 17, 143–4, 218–19, 222, 240–1,
242–4
with anti-depressants 286–8
with anti-psychotic drugs 299–300
with carbamazepine 6
with chemotherapeutic agents 224
in co-morbidities 112–13, 130
in elderly patients 180
with felbamate 9
with lamotrigine 10
with lithium 291
with oral contraceptives 153–5
with oxcarbazepine 12
with phenytoin 4, 8, 11
with tiagabine 12

with topiramate 11
with valproate 8
with warfarin 230
with zonisamide 13
duloxetine 288
use in anxiety disorders 292
DWI (diffusion-weighted imaging), MRI 216
dyspnoea, as side-effect of vagus nerve
stimulation 56
dysthymic-like disorder of epilepsy (DLDE) 283

E
E01–E05 studies, VNS 54–5, 140
early AED treatment 122
MESS study 123–4
early infantile epileptic encephalopathy (Ohtahara
syndrome) 65, 75–6
early myoclonic encephalopathy (EME) 75–6
eclampsia 224
efflux drug transporters 145
elderly patients 173, 184–5, 238–9
AED treatment 178–82
discontinuation 183–4
gabapentin 10
aetiology of epilepsy 174
diagnosis 175–6
incidence of epilepsy 174
psychosocial concerns 184
risk factors for epilepsy 174–5
status epilepticus 175
surgical treatment 183
vagus nerve stimulation 182
electroconvulsive therapy
in depression 290
in status epilepticus 269
electroencephalography (EEG)
in acute stroke 221
in children 87, 88
in eclampsia 224
effect of anti-psychotic drugs 299
in elderly patients 176–7
monitoring in critically ill patients 219
in pre-surgical evaluation 31–2, 33
in prediction of seizure recurrence 120
in status epilepticus 257, 258, 267–8
prognostic factors 255
employment implications 129
enflurane, risk of seizures 237
epilepsy syndromes 63, 64–5
epileptic encephalopathies 63, 65
epileptiform transients 177
epileptogenic zone (EZ) 28
identification 29
see also pre-surgical evaluation
escitalopram 285, 288
drug interactions 288
estradiol, neuroprotection in SE 272

ethosuximide 8, 15, 191
combination with valproate 110, 142
drug interactions 144
initiation of therapy 16
mechanism of action 141
use in children 89, 195, 197
evidence-based data, in IGEs 191–2
evidence categories 192–3
excitotoxic hypothesis of cell death 259
extra-temporal ictal foci 28

F
facial weakness, as side-effect of vagus nerve
stimulation 55
fear, ictal 292
febrile seizures, ictal focus 30
febrile status epilepticus, risk of subsequent
epilepsy 256
feeding difficulties, association with intellectual
disability 307
felbamate 9, 15, 96, 148
drug interactions 144, 240, 243, 244
with oral contraceptives 154
initiation of therapy 16
mechanism of action 141
side-effects 179
use in elderly patients 181
use in liver disease 234
use in patients with intellectual disability 310
use in renal disease 232
fertility 130, 162–3
first seizures 87
AED treatment 121–2
MESS study 123–4
recurrence risk 120
FIRST trial 122, 123
FK-506, neurotoxicity 221
FLAIR (fluid-attenuated inversion recovery) MRI
sequences 216
in status epilepticus 262
fluoxetine 285
drug interactions 287, 288
effect on seizures 286
fluphenazine 299
fluvoxamine
drug interactions 286–7
effect on seizures 286
folate supplementation during pregnancy 156
folinic acid-responsive seizures 68, 70
follicle-stimulating hormone, LH:FSH ratios 162
forced normalization 297, 301
fosphenytoin 238
in management of acute seizures 214
side-effects 231
use in liver transplant patients 222
use in status epilepticus 264
fracture risk, AED treatment 4, 179, 239

fragile X syndrome 306
functional neuroimaging 36–7
functionalized amino acids 145

G

gabapentin 10, 15, 197, 216, 217
  advantages and disadvantages 91
  aggravation of seizures 205
  in combination therapy 17
  comparative studies 126
  drug interactions 5, 143, 144, 300
  initiation of therapy 16
  mechanism of action 141
  metabolism 93
  neuroprotection in SE 271
  use in anxiety disorders 293
  use in cancer patients 224
  use in children 89, 90, 93
  use in elderly patients 180–1
  use in HIV patients 223
  use in liver disease 219–20, 234, 235
  use in porphyria 237
  use in renal disease 220, 232, 233
  use after stroke 230
gamma-aminobutyric acid (GABA), intracranial
      delivery 44
ganaxolone 145, 165
gastrointestinal side-effects of AEDs 6, 7
GCP 40116 271
generalized-onset tonic–clonic seizures,
      treatment 194, 198–201
generalized anxiety disorder 291
  pharmacotherapy 292–3
generalized epilepsy, AED treatment in children
  choice of drugs 109
  evidence-based analysis 109
generic substitution, AEDs 15
gingival hypertrophy 4
Gingko biloba, drug interactions 241
glucocorticosteroids, in treatment of infantile
      spasms 71–3, 74
glucose transporter defect 68, 106, 108
gonadotropin analogues, use in catamenial
      epilepsy 165
gonadotropin-releasing hormone (GNRH)
      secretion 162
grapefruit juice, drug interactions 13
guanfacine, use in ADHD 296

H

HAART (highly active anti-retroviral therapy) 223
haemodialysis, AED therapy 220, 233
haloperidol 299
heart, vagus innervation 52
heart transplantation 221, 222
hemimegalencephaly 106

hepatic disease 217, 219–20, 233–5
hepatic encephalopathy 219
hepatic enzymes
  effects of drugs 8, 93–5, 143, 144, 234, 235, 240
  enzyme-inducing drugs, interactions 240–1,
      242–3
  enzyme-inhibiting drugs, interactions 244
hepatotoxicity of AEDs 7, 9
  in infants 70
herpes virus encephalitis 30
high-dose monotherapy 110
highly refractory status epilepticus (HRSE) 267–9
history-taking 30
  children 85–7
HIV patients 223–4
holocarboxylase deficiency 68
hormone replacement therapy (HRT) 166–7, 184
hospitalized patients
  aetiologies of seizures 215
  anti-epileptic drug selection 216–18
      cancer patients 224
      in cardiovascular disease 220–1
      in hepatic disease 219–20
      HIV patients 223–4
      in intensive care units 218–19
      in renal disease 220
      transplant patients 221–2
  evaluation of new-onset seizures 213–16
  obstetric patients 224
hyperglycaemia, non-ketotic 236
hypernatraemia 236
hypersensitivity to AEDs, cross reactions 17
hyperthermia in status epilepticus 261
hypoalbuminaemia 219, 234–5
hypoglycaemia 236
hypohidrosis, as side-effect of AEDs 11, 13
hyponatraemia 236–7
  as side-effect of AEDs 6, 12, 179
hypotension, as side effect of AEDs 231
hypothalamic–pituitary–gonadal axis
      disregulation 162
hypothermia, value in status epilepticus 270
hypothyroidism, association with intellectual
      disability 307

I

ictal confusion, diagnosis in elderly patients 175–6
ictal foci 28
      implantation of AED-containing polymers 146
      localization see pre-surgical evaluation
ictal panic 292
ictal SPECT 36
idiopathic epilepsy syndromes 63, 64
idiopathic generalized epilepsies (IGEs) 191–3, 194
      childhood absence epilepsy 193, 195–7
      generalized-onset tonic–clonic seizures 198–201
      juvenile absence epilepsy 198

juvenile myoclonic epilepsy 201–4
  seizure aggravation by AEDs 204–6
idiopathic partial epilepsy, treatment in children 89,
  95
imipramine
  drug interactions 286–7
  use in ADHD 296
  use in panic disorder 293
immunosuppressive drugs 215, 221, 222, 233, 235
implications of diagnosis 129
incidence of epilepsy 119
  age-specific 174
incidence of status epilepticus 253, 254
infantile epilepsy 63, 66
  epilepsy syndromes 64–5
  investigations 67
  ketogenic diet 76–7
  pharmacological treatment 70, 75–6
    in severe myoclonic epilepsy in infancy 74–5
  surgical treatment 77–8
  vitamin supplementation 66–70
infantile masturbation 105
infantile spasms (West syndrome) 65
  ketogenic diet 77
  patient evaluation 96
  pharmacological treatment 14, 71, 73–4, 89, 97,
    109
    ACTH and oral steroids 71–2, 72–3
    vigabatrin 72–3
  vagus nerve stimulation 55
infants, non-epileptogenic paroxysmal disorders 66
infection risk, vagus nerve stimulation 55
infertility 162–3
inhalation anaesthetics, use in highly refractory
  status epilepticus 269
initiation of therapy 16, 19, 21
INR (international normalized ratio), effects of
  AEDs 230
intellectual disabilities 305–6
  AED use 310–12
  aetiology and severity 306
  behaviour observation charts 317–18
  communication problems 307
  diagnosis of epilepsy 307–8
  impact of epilepsy 309
  need for treatment of epilepsy 309
  physical health problems 307
  psychiatric and behavioural problems 306–7,
    309–10
  rescue medication 312–13
  seizure recording charts 319–22
  treatment choice 310
  treatment evaluation 313–14
intensive care units, management of seizures 218–
  19, 237–8
interictal anxiety disorders 291
interictal EEG 31
  in children 87

interictal psychosis 297
International League Against Epilepsy (ILAE)
  categories of evidence 193
  definition of status epilepticus 252
  treatment guidelines 194
    for childhood absence epilepsy 193, 195
    for GTC seizures 198
    for juvenile myoclonic epilepsy 201
intracarotid amytal (Wada) test 34
intracerebral haemorrhage (ICH) 229–30
intracranial drug delivery 44
intracranial electroencephalography (iEEG) 36,
  37–8, 40
  subdural strip and grid electrode placements 39
intrathecal drug administration 145
investigations
  in elderly patients 176–8
  pre-surgical see pre-surgical evaluation
irritative zones 28
isobolograms 142
isoflurane, use in highly refractory status
  epilepticus 269

J

juvenile absence epilepsy, treatment 198–201
juvenile myoclonic epilepsy
  aggravation by AEDs 111
  treatment 9, 12, 95, 98, 194, 201–4
    choice of drugs 109
    evidence-based analysis 109

K

ketamine, use in status epilepticus 268, 271
ketogenic diet 108, 110, 146
  in glucose transporter defect 106
  in SMEI 75
  use in infants 76–7
ketotic hypoglycaemia 108
kidney transplantation 221–2, 233

L

lacosamide 145
lamotrigine 9–10, 15, 191, 217
  advantages and disadvantages 91
  aggravation of seizures 136, 205
  breastfeeding 161
  for childhood absence seizures 195, 196–7
  in combination therapy 17, 110, 142, 143, 240
    with lithium 291
  comparative studies 126–8
  dosing schedule 20, 21
  drug interactions 5, 143, 144, 288
    with oral contraceptives 154, 155
  effect on sexual function 166
  for idiopathic GTC seizures 199
  initiation of therapy 16, 216

for juvenile myoclonic epilepsy 202
mechanism of action 141
metabolism 93
teratogenicity 157
use in bipolar disorders 290, 291
use in cardiac disease 231
use in children 89, 90, 93
use in elderly patients 180–1, 239
use in liver disease 234
use in patients with intellectual disability 310
use in pregnancy 156, 157, 160
use in renal disease 232
use after stroke 230
Lamotrigine Pregnancy Registry
language lateralization assessment 34–5
lead breakage, vagus nerve stimulation 56
learning difficulties, in childhood epilepsy 98–9, 112
Lennox–Gastaut syndrome
AED treatment 9, 10, 96, 109, 310
seizure aggravation by AEDs 111
vagus nerve stimulation 54–5
lesional epilepsy 28
extra-temporal, surgery 43
leucopenia, as side-effect of carbamazepine 6
levetiracetam 12–13, 15, 191, 217
advantages and disadvantages 91
breastfeeding 161
for childhood absence seizures 197
in combination therapy 17
comparative studies 128
dose schedule 20
drug interactions 5, 143, 144
in first-line therapy 216
for idiopathic GTC seizures 200
initiation of therapy 16
in management of acute seizures 214
mechanism of action 141
metabolism 93
neuroprotective effect 220, 271
use in cancer patients 224
use in children 89, 90, 93
in juvenile myoclonic epilepsy 202
use in elderly patients 181
use in HIV patients 223
use in liver disease 219–20, 234
use in liver transplant patients 222, 235
use in porphyria 237
use during pregnancy 157
use in renal disease 220, 232, 233
use in status epilepticus 265–6
lidocaine infusion, use in highly refractory status
epilepticus 268
lifestyle counselling, JME 203
lifestyle implications 129
lithium 290
interaction with AEDs 291
reduction of seizure threshold 215

liver disease 217, 219–20, 233–5
liver transplantation 221, 222, 235
lorazepam 8
in management of acute seizures 214
as rescue therapy 108
use in porphyria 237
use in status epilepticus 264, 269
loxepine, effect on seizure threshold 299
lumbar puncture 216
lung transplantation 221–2
luteinizing hormone (LH), LH:FSH ratios 162

M

magnet stimulation, VNS 54
magnetic resonance imaging (MRI) 31, 214, 216
in childhood epilepsy 88
in elderly patients 178
functional 36–7
in patients with intellectual disability 308
in patients with VNS devices 57
in status epilepticus 261, 262
magnetic resonance spectroscopy 37
magnetoencephalography (MEG) 35–6, 37
major depression 283
malignant partial seizures in infancy 65, 76
manic episodes 282–3
maprotiline 301
medical intractability 114, 136–9, 206
medroxyprogesterone acetate, use in catamenial
epilepsy 164, 165
memory assessment, Wada test 34, 35
menopausal age 163
menopause 166–7, 184
menstrual cycle, catamenial epilepsy 163–5, 166, 167
mental retardation 112
mesial temporal lobe epilepsy 41–2
mesial temporal sclerosis, association with febrile
SE 256
MESS study 123–4
meta-analyses of AED studies 125
metabolic disturbances 236–7
metabolic epileptic encephalopathies 68
metabolism of AEDs
in liver disease 233–5
pharmacokinetic interactions 143–4
phenytoin 4
methylphenidate, use in ADHD 295
mianserin, drug interactions 286–7
midazolam 8
as rescue therapy 95, 108, 312
use in refractory status epilepticus 266, 267
use in status epilepticus 269
migraine 105, 130
use of AEDs 241
mirtazapine 288
effect on seizures 286

misdiagnosis 103–6, 135, 136
  see also differential diagnosis of seizures
mitochondrial function, effect of valproate 70
MK-108 271
molindone 299
monitoring
  during carbamazepine therapy 6
  during felbamate therapy 9
  during phenytoin therapy 3–4
  value of serum levels 18–19
    in elderly patients 182
monotherapy 17
mood, effects of AEDs 17
mood disorders 289–90
  bipolar disorders 282–3
  interictal depressive episodes 282
  major depression 283
  psychotherapy 293–4
  see also depression
mood-stabilizing drugs 289, 290, 291
mortality rates
  epilepsy surgery 44
  refractory epilepsy 27–8
  status epilepticus 253–5, 266
movements, unusual 104–5
multi-disciplinary conferences, pre-surgical 35
multiple seizures 224–5
myoclonic seizures
  aggravation by AEDs 111
  see also juvenile myoclonic epilepsy

N
N-acetyl aspartate (NAA), NAA:choline and
      NAA:creatine ratios 37
narrow spectrum AEDs 15
National General Practice Survey of Epilepsy
      (NGPSE) 129
necrotic cell death 259, 260
nefazodone, drug interactions 286–7
neocortical ictal foci 28
neocortical temporal lobe epilepsy 42
neonatal epilepsy
  folinic acid-responsive seizures 70
  pyridoxamine phosphate oxidase deficiency 68,
      69–70
  pyridoxine-dependent epilepsy 67, 69
nephrolithiasis, as side-effect of AEDs 179, 220
neurocognitive risks, intrauterine AED
      exposure 158
neuroleptics, reduction of seizure threshold 215
neurological disorders depression inventory for
      epilepsy (NDDI-E) 284
NeuroPace Responsive Neurostimulator
      system™ 44
neuropathic pain 130
  use of AEDs 241

neuroprotection, in status epilepticus 270–3
neuropsychological testing, role in pre-surgical
      evaluation 32, 34
neurostimulation 44, 51
  see also deep brain stimulation; vagus nerve
      stimulation
nitrazepam, use in infants 70, 73
NMDA (N-methyl-D-aspartate) receptor activity, role
      in cell death 259
NMDA receptor antagonists 270, 271
non-convulsive seizures
  in critically ill patients 216
  history-taking 86
non-convulsive status epilepticus 175, 252, 269
  incidence 253
non-ketotic hyperglycaemia 236
non-lesional epilepsy 28
  extra-temporal surgery 43
noradrenaline, changes in status epilepticus 261
norfluoxetine, drug interactions 287
North American Antiepileptic Drug Pregnancy
      Registry 156
nortriptyline
  drug interactions 286–7
  use in ADHD 296
NS1209 145
nucleus tractus solitarius (NTS) 52, 140

O
obesity 130
oestrogen, effect on neuronal excitability 163
Ohtahara syndrome 65, 75–6
olanzapine 298, 299, 300
opioid withdrawal, reduction of seizure
      threshold 215
oral contraceptives
  failure rate 153
  interaction with CYP3A4 inducers 154–5
  interaction with hepatic enzyme inducers 154–5,
      240–1
  interaction with lamotrigine 10
  use in catamenial epilepsy 164–5
orgasmic dysfunction, women 165–6
osteoporosis
  association with intellectual disability 307
  as side-effect of AEDs 179, 239
oxcarbazepine 11–12, 15, 217
  advantages and disadvantages 91
  aggravation of seizures 136
  comparative studies 126, 127, 128
  drug interactions 5, 143–4, 240, 243, 244
    with oral contraceptives 154
  initiation of therapy 16
  mechanism of action 141
  metabolism 93
  side-effects 179, 236, 239

use in children 89, 90, 93
use in elderly patients 181
use in liver disease 234
use in porphyria 237
use during pregnancy 160
use in renal disease 232, 233

P

P-glycoprotein 145
pacemaker implantation, vagus nerve
    stimulation 53, 140
paediatric dosing ranges, AEDs 93–5
palliative surgery 44
pancreas transplantation 221–2
pancreatitis, valproate therapy 7–8
panic, ictal 292
panic disorder 291
    pharmacotherapy 292–3
    prevalence 282
parasomnias 105
parkinsonian symptoms, as side-effect of AEDs 179
Parkinson's disease, polytherapy 140–1
paroxetine 285
    drug interactions 286–7
paroxysmal disorders in infancy 66
paroxysmal dystonias 104
partial epilepsy 10, 12, 13, 15
    AED treatment in children 89, 90, 95, 109
patient selection, surgical treatment 29
peak-dose toxicity 19, 20
pentobarbital
    intracranial delivery 44
    use in refractory status epilepticus 266–7
perfenazine 299
perimenopause, seizure frequency 166, 167
periodic epileptiform discharges (PEDs) 257, 258
periprocedural patients 237–8
pharmacodynamic drug interactions 17
    AEDs and anti-depressants 287–8
    AEDs and anti-psychotics 300
pharmacokinetic drug interactions, AEDs 5, 143–4,
    299–300
pharmacokinetics
    in children 107
    in elderly patients 180
phenobarbital 6–7, 217
    advantages and disadvantages 91
    aggravation of seizures 205
    alternative routes of administration 238
    avoidance with propofol 267
    caution in acute stroke 221
    combination with phenytoin 142
    comparative studies 125
    drug interactions 5, 143, 144, 240, 242
        with oral contraceptives 154
    for idiopathic GTC seizures 199

initiation of therapy 16
intrauterine exposure 158
mechanism of action 141
metabolism 93
neuroprotection in SE 271
side-effects 179, 239
use in children 89, 90, 93
use in elderly patients 180, 181
use in infants 70
    in SMEI 74
use in liver disease 234
use during pregnancy 159
use in renal disease 220, 232
use in status epilepticus 264, 266
phenylcylidine 271
phenylethylmalonamide (PEMA) 7
phenytoin 3–4, 217, 230
    advantages and disadvantages 92
    aggravation of seizures 205
    breastfeeding 161
    caution in acute stroke 221
    in combination therapy 17, 142, 143, 240
    comparative studies 125, 128
    drug interactions 5, 143, 144, 230, 240, 242, 287,
        300
        with oral contraceptives 154
        with oxcarbazepine 12
        with topiramate 11
        with valproate 8
    generic substitution 15
    initiation of therapy 16
    mechanism of action 141
    metabolism 94
    in periprocedural patients 237
    reduction of seizure threshold 215
    side-effects 179, 231, 239
        effect on carbohydrate metabolism 236
        sexual dysfunction 165
    use in children 89, 90, 94
    use in elderly patients 180, 181
    use in infants 70
    use in liver disease 234
    use in liver transplant patients 222
    use during pregnancy 159
    use in renal disease 232
    use in status epilepticus 264–5
3-phosphoglycerate deficiency 68
photosensitivity
    in JME 203
    in SMEI 74
physical examination 30
physical symptoms in depression 288
phytonadione supplementation during
        pregnancy 161
polycystic ovary syndrome (PCOS) 162–3
    association with valproate 8
polymers, controlled-release of AEDs 146

polytherapy 17–18, 140, 147–8
  dosing schedules 20, 21
  pharmacokinetic interactions 143–4
  pharmacomechanistic approach 140–1
  synergistic combinations 142–3
  teratogenicity 157
  toxicity avoidance 143
  in treatment-resistant childhood epilepsy 110–11
porphyria 236–7
positron emission tomography (PET) 36
  in status epilepticus 262
post-ictal psychosis 297
  treatment 300
post-ictal state, in elderly patients 176
post-operative patients 237–8
potassium bromide, use in SMEI 75
pre-surgical evaluation 28–9, 40
  electroencephalography 31–2, 33
  functional neuroimaging 36–7
  history and examination 30
  intracarotid amytal (Wada) test 34
  intracranial electroencephalography 37–8
  magnetic resonance imaging 31
  magnetoencephalography 35–6, 37
  multi-disciplinary conference 35
  neuropsychological testing 32, 34
  psychiatric issues 34
  video-electroencephalography monitoring 32
precipitating factors 87, 136, 237
prednisolone, in treatment of infantile spasms 71–2, 72–3
pregabalin 13–14, 15, 216, 217, 218
  advantages and disadvantages 92
  in combination therapy 17
  dose schedule 20
  drug interactions 5, 143, 144
  initiation of therapy 16
  mechanism of action 141
  metabolism 94
  neuroprotection in SE 272
  use in anxiety disorders 293
  use in cancer patients 224
  use in children 89, 90, 94
  use in elderly patients 181
  use in liver disease 219–20, 234, 235
  use in porphyria 237
  use in renal disease 220, 232
pregnancy 156, 167
  AED therapy
    dosing 159–60
    neurocognitive risks to child 158
    teratogenicity 156–8
  effects of seizures 158–9
  epilepsy risk in offspring 161
  new-onset seizures 224
  seizure changes 159
  use of valproate 8
  vitamin K supplementation 161

primary generalized epilepsy with tonic–clonic seizures alone 95
primidone 7
  comparative studies 125
  drug interactions 5, 143, 144
  effect on bone health 179
  initiation of therapy 16
progesterone
  anti-convulsant effect 163
  use in catamenial epilepsy 164, 165
prognosis, newly diagnosed adult epilepsy 129
prophylactic AEDs 221–2
  after stroke or intracerebral haemorrhage 229–30
propofol, use in refractory status epilepticus 266, 267
propofol infusion syndrome 267
protein binding of AEDs 217, 231
  drug interactions 240
  in older patients 238
proton pump inhibitors, drug interactions 240
protriptyline, drug interactions 286–7
provoking factors 85, 86
'pseudo-temporal' lobe epilepsy 42
'pseudoresistance' 135–6
pseudoseizures 105
psychiatric co-morbidities 281–2, 301
  in intellectual disability 306–7
  prevalence in childhood epilepsy 99, 112
  see also anxiety disorders; attention deficit disorders; bipolar disorder; depression; psychotic disorders
psychiatric issues, epilepsy surgery 34
psychiatric referral, indications 289, 293
psychiatric side-effects, AEDs 17
psychogenic non-epileptic seizures 105
psychomotor slowing, as side-effect of topiramate 11
psychosocial concerns
  in childhood epilepsy 113
  in older patients 184
psychostimulant drugs 112, 113
psychotherapy 293–4
  in ADHD 296
psychotic disorders 297
  prevalence 282
  treatment 298–301
psychotic features in depression 289
psychotropic drugs 112, 113
'purple glove' syndrome 265
pyridoxal 5'-phosphate (PLP) 66–7
  use in infantile spasms 73–4
  use in neonatal-onset epileptic encephalopathies 69–70
pyridoxamine phosphate oxidase deficiency 68, 69–70
pyridoxine-dependent epilepsy 67, 68, 69, 106
pyruvate dehydrogenase complex deficiency 108

Q

quetiapine 298, 299, 300

R

RAG (Red/Amber/Green) behaviour observation
    charts 317–18
Rasmussen's encephalitis 106
rational polytherapy 140–4
recreational drug use 136
recurrent laryngeal nerve 52
refractory epilepsy *see* surgical treatment; treatment-
    resistant epilepsy
refractory status epilepticus 266–9
    cooling 270
remission rates, newly diagnosed adult epilepsy 129
renal calculi, as side-effect of zonisamide 13
renal disease 217, 220, 231–3
renal stones, risk from ketogenic diet 77
rescue therapies 225
    in children 97, 108
    in patients with intellectual disability 312–13
restless legs syndrome 241, 244
retigabine 145
Rett syndrome 108, 306
risk factors, in elderly patients 174–5
risperidone 298, 300
Rolandic epilepsy, AED treatment
    choice of drugs 109
    evidence-based analysis 109
rufinamide 145

S

safety precautions, childhood epilepsy 99–100
St John's Wort, drug interactions 241
SANAD (Standard and New Antiepileptic Drugs)
    study 126–8, 131
SCN1A mutations, SMEI 74
screening instruments for depression 283–4
seizure classification
seizure clusters 224–5
seizure frequency, in definition of treatment
    resistance 138
seizure interruption, vagus nerve stimulation 54
seizure recording charts 319–22
seizure recurrence risk 120–1
seizure threshold
    effect of anti-psychotic drugs 298–9
    effect of methylphenidate 295
    reduction by medication 111, 128, 136, 204–6,
        215, 231, 233
selective norepinephrine reuptake inhibitors
    (SNRIs) 284, 285
    effect on seizures 286
    efficacy 288
    use in anxiety disorders 292

selective serotonin re-uptake inhibitors (SSRIs) 239,
    244, 285
    drug interactions 287
    effect on seizures 286
    efficacy 288
    use in anxiety disorders 292
    value in DLDE 283
serine deficiency syndromes 68
serotonin syndrome 288
sertraline 285, 288
    drug interactions 286–7
    effect on seizures 286
serum levels, value in AED therapy 18–19
    in elderly patients 182
severe myoclonic encephalopathy 65
severe myoclonic epilepsy in infancy (SMEI, Dravet
    syndrome) 65
    aggravation by AEDs 111
    pharmacological treatment 74–5
sexual adverse events
    AED and anti-depressant combinations 287
    AED and anti-psychotic drug combinations 300
sexual dysfunction, in women 165–6
side-effects 91–2, 130, 179, 217, 231
    of ACTH and oral steroids 72
    of anti-psychotic drugs 298
    of atomoxetine 296
    of benzodiazepines 8
    of carbamazepine 6, 221
    in children with co-morbidities 113
    of CNS stimulants 295
    cognitive impairment 113
    in combination therapy 17
    in elderly patients 179, 239
    of ethosuximide 8
    of felbamate 9
    of gabapentin 10
    hyponatraemia 236
    of ketogenic diet 76, 77, 110
    of lamotrigine 9, 10
    of levetiracetam 13
    of oxcarbazepine 12
    of phenobarbital 6, 221
    of phenytoin 3, 4, 221
    of pregabalin 14
    of tiagabine 12
    of topiramate 11
    of tricyclic anti-depressants 296
    of vagus nerve stimulation 55–6
    of valproate 7–8, 73
    of vigabatrin 14, 72
    of zonisamide 13
single photon emission computer tomography
    (SPECT) 36
SISCOM 36
skin rashes as side-effect of AEDs 4, 6, 7, 9, 10, 12, 13

sleep apnoea, as side-effect of vagus nerve
        stimulation 56
speech problems, as side-effect of topiramate 11
spina bifida, association with valproate therapy 8
spontaneous remission 121
sports participation 100
status epilepticus 252
    classification 252
    clinical presentation 256–7
    consequences 257–8, 261, 263
        blood flow changes 260–1, 262
        cell death 258–60
    definition 252
    diagnosis 263–4
    in elderly patients 175
    epidemiology 253, 254
    historical context 252–3
    management 214
        cooling 270
        initial treatment 264
        pre-hospital 269
        second-line treatment 264–6
        vagus nerve stimulation 55
    morbidity 255
    mortality 253–5
    neuroprotection 220, 270–3
    non-convulsive 175, 253, 269
    during pregnancy 159
    refractory 266–9
    risk of subsequent epilepsy 255–6
steroids, in treatment of infantile spasms 71–3, 74
Stevens–Johnson syndrome 4, 6, 9, 10, 12, 13
stiripentol, use in SMEI 74–5
stroke 220–1, 229–30
    as cause of status epilepticus 175, 253
stupor, as side-effect of tiagabine 12
subarachnoid haemorrhage 230
subclinical rhythmic electrical discharges of
        adulthood (SREDA) 177
subdural strip and grid electrode placements 38, 39
sudden unexpected death in epilepsy (SUDEP) 28
    incidence in patients with intellectual
            disability 308
suicidal ideation 289
sulthiame 89
superior laryngeal nerve 52
surgical treatment 27–8, 139
    in children 114
    complications 45
    corpus callosotomy 44
    in elderly patients 181, 183
    extra-temporal 43
    goals 28
    in highly refractory status epilepticus 268
    in infants 77–8
    outcome 45
    patient selection 29

risks 44
    temporal lobe 41–3
    see also pre-surgical evaluation
sustained-release preparations, serum levels 18, 19
swallowing difficulties, association with intellectual
        disability 307
Swedish Medical Birth Registry survey 157
swimming 99–100
symptomatic epilepsy 28
symptomatic partial epilepsy, treatment in
        children 89
syncope 105
synergy, AEDs 142–3, 240

T
tacrolimus, neurotoxicity 221, 222, 233
talampanel 145
tariquidar (XR9576) 145
temporal lobe epilepsy (TLE)
    association with febrile SE 256
    interictal discharges 31
temporal lobe surgery 41–2
    outcomes 42–3
'temporal plus' seizures 42
teratogenicity of AEDs 130, 156–8
    valproate 8
testosterone levels, women 165, 166
tetracosactide, use in infantile spasms 72–3
theophylline, reduction of seizure threshold 215
therapeutic ranges 18, 136
    carbamazepine 6
    ethosuximide 8
    felbamate 9
    lamotrigine 9–10
    levetiracetam 13
    oxcarbazepine 11–12
    phenobarbital 6
    phenytoin 3
    topiramate 11
    zonisamide 13
therapeutic windows 19
thiopentone, use in refractory status epilepticus 266,
        267
thioridazine, drug interactions 300
throat, side-effects of vagus nerve stimulation 52,
        55–6
thrombocytopaenia, as side-effect of valproate
        therapy 8
tiagabine 12, 15, 197
    aggravation of seizures 205
    combination with vigabatrin 142
    dose schedule 20
    drug interactions 5
    initiation of therapy 16
    mechanism of action 141
    use in anxiety disorders 293

use in elderly patients 181
use in liver disease 234
use in porphyria 237
use in renal disease 232, 233
tics 104
Todd's paralysis, in elderly patients 176
tolerance to benzodiazepines 8
topiramate 10–11, 15, 191, 217, 218
  advantages and disadvantages 92
  breastfeeding 161
  for childhood absence seizures 197
  combination with lamotrigine 142
  comparative studies 126, 127
  dosing schedule 20, 21
  drug interactions 5, 144, 240, 243, 244
    with oral contraceptives 154
  effect on cognitive function 179
  for idiopathic GTC seizures 199–200
  initiation of therapy 16
  for juvenile myoclonic epilepsy 202–3
  mechanism of action 141
  metabolism 94
  neuroprotective effect 220, 272
  use in cardiac disease 231
  use in children 89, 90, 94
  use in infantile spasms 73
  use in liver disease 234
  use in liver transplant patients 222
  use in patients with intellectual disability 310
  use in porphyria 237
  use in renal disease 220, 232
  use in SMEI 75
  use in status epilepticus 266
toxic epidermal necrolysis 10
toxicity
  avoidance in polytherapy 143
  phenytoin 4
  see also hepatotoxicity; side-effects
transcranial magnetic stimulation 269
transplant patients 221–2, 233, 235
treatment
  future directions 44
  neurostimulation 51
  see also anti-epileptic drugs (AEDs); surgical
    treatment; vagus nerve stimulation
treatment-resistant epilepsy 135, 205
  in children 103, 115
    co-morbidity 111–13
    confirmation of aetiology and epilepsy
      type 106
    diagnostic tests 107
    ketogenic diet 108, 110
    medical intractability 114
    monotherapy vs. combination therapy 110–11
    pharmacokinetic issues 107
    psychosocial issues 113

  re-assessment of diagnosis 103–6
  rescue therapies 10–18
  second- and third-line AEDs 108
  seizure aggravation by AEDs 111
  new treatment strategies 144–6
  practical treatment approach 147–8
  'pseudoresistance' 135–6
  rational polytherapy 140–4
  recognition 136–9
  see also surgical treatment; vagus nerve
    stimulation 139–40
treatment response 129–31
tremor, as side-effect of AEDs 179
tricyclic anti-depressants
  drug interactions 286–7
  use in ADHD 296
trifluoperazine 299
tuberous sclerosis
  ketogenic diet 76
  vagus nerve stimulation 55
  vigabatrin therapy 72, 89, 97

U
Unverricht–Lundborg disease, aggravation by
  AEDs 111

V
vagus nerve, anatomy 52
vagus nerve stimulation (VNS) 51–2, 57–8, 139–40, 206
  acute side-effects 55
  battery replacement 57
  in children 114
  chronic adverse events 55–6
  cost 57
  device and implantation 53
  efficacy 53–5
  in elderly patients 181, 182
  indications for use 57
  long-term management 56
  long-term tolerability 56
  magnetic resonance imaging 57
  mechanism of action 52–3
valproate 7–8, 15, 191, 217
  advantages and disadvantages 92
  alternative routes of administration 238
  association with PCOS 162–3
  breastfeeding 161
  for childhood absence seizures 195–6, 197
  in combination therapy 9, 17, 110, 142, 143, 240
    with lithium 291
  comparative studies 125–6, 127
  dose schedule 20
  drug interactions 5, 143, 144, 219, 244, 287, 300
  for idiopathic GTC seizures 199
  initiation of therapy 16

for juvenile myoclonic epilepsy 201, 204
in management of acute seizures 214
mechanism of action 141
metabolism 94
neurocognitive risks from intrauterine
    exposure 158
neuroprotection in SE 271
side-effects 179, 219, 239
teratogenicity 157, 158, 167
use in anxiety disorders 293
use in bipolar disorders 290, 291
use in cardiac disease 231
use in children 89, 90, 94
use in elderly patients 180, 181
use in HIV patients 224
use in infants 70
    in infantile spasms 73
    in SMEI 74, 75
use in liver disease 234
use during pregnancy 159, 160
use in renal disease 232, 233
use in status epilepticus 265
velocardiofacial syndrome 306
venlafaxine 285, 288
    effect on seizures 286
    use in anxiety disorders 292
ventricular asystole, as side-effect of vagus nerve
    stimulation 55
verbal memory impairment 32, 34
Veteran's Administration Cooperative Studies 125,
    179, 183, 239
Veterans Affairs studies 125
video-electroencephalography monitoring
    infants 66
    in patients with intellectual disability 308
    role in pre-surgical evaluation 32
vigabatrin 14, 15, 148, 197
    advantages and disadvantages 92
    aggravation of seizures 205
    combination with carbamazepine 110, 142
    drug interactions 144, 243
    initiation of therapy 16
    mechanism of action 141
    metabolism 94
    neuroprotection in SE 271
    in treatment of infantile spasms 71, 72–3, 74,
        89, 97
    use in children 90, 94
    use in liver disease 234
    use in porphyria 237
    use in renal disease 232
Vineland Adaptive Behaviour Scale (VABS) 73
visual field defects, as side-effect of vigabatrin 14,
    72
vitamin B6 disorders of metabolism 66–7, 68
    folinic acid-responsive seizures 70

pyridox(am)ine phosphate oxidase
    deficiency 69–70
pyridoxine-dependent epilepsy 67, 69
vitamin supplementation
    in infantile epilepsy 66–70
    during pregnancy 156, 161
voice, side-effects of vagus nerve stimulation 52,
    55–6

W
Wada (intracarotid amytal) test 34
warfarin, interaction with AEDs 230
weakness, as side-effect of tiagabine 12
weaning from AEDs, children 98
weight gain
    association with valproate 162
    risk from AEDs 17, 287
West syndrome (infantile spasms) 65
    ketogenic diet 77
    patient evaluation 96
    pharmacological treatment 14, 71, 73–4, 97
        ACTH and oral steroids 71–2, 72–3
        vigabatrin 72–3
    surgical treatment 77
    vagus nerve stimulation 55
withdrawal from benzodiazepines 8
women, sexual dysfunction 165–6
Women's Health Initiative (WHI) 166

X
XR9576 (tariquidar) 145

Z
zero order kinetics, phenytoin 4
ziprasidone 298, 299, 300
zonisamide 13, 15, 191, 217
    advantages and disadvantages 92
    for childhood absence seizures 197
    drug interactions 5, 143, 243, 244
    for idiopathic GTC seizures 200
    initiation of therapy 16
    for juvenile myoclonic epilepsy 203
    mechanism of action 141
    metabolism 94
    side-effects 179
    use in children 89, 90, 94
    use in EIEE 76
    use in elderly patients 181, 239
    use in infantile spasms 73
    use in liver disease 234
    use in liver transplant patients 222
    use in renal disease 220, 232
    use in SMEI 75

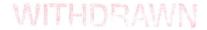